D1823427

Palgrave Studies in Literature, Science and Medicine

Series Editors
Sharon Ruston
Department of English and Creative Writing
Lancaster University
Lancaster, UK

Alice Jenkins
School of Critical Studies
University of Glasgow
Glasgow, UK

Jessica Howell
Department of English
Texas A&M University
College Station, TX, USA

Palgrave Studies in Literature, Science and Medicine is an exciting series that focuses on one of the most vibrant and interdisciplinary areas in literary studies: the intersection of literature, science and medicine. Comprised of academic monographs, essay collections, and Palgrave Pivot books, the series will emphasize a historical approach to its subjects, in conjunction with a range of other theoretical approaches. The series will cover all aspects of this rich and varied field and is open to new and emerging topics as well as established ones.

Editorial board:

Andrew M. Beresford, Professor in the School of Modern Languages and Cultures, Durham University, UK
Steven Connor, Professor of English, University of Cambridge, UK
Lisa Diedrich, Associate Professor in Women's and Gender Studies, Stony Brook University, USA
Kate Hayles, Professor of English, Duke University, USA
Peter Middleton, Professor of English, University of Southampton, UK
Kirsten Shepherd-Barr, Professor of English and Theatre Studies, University of Oxford, UK
Sally Shuttleworth, Professorial Fellow in English, St Anne's College, University of Oxford, UK
Susan Squier, Professor of Women's Studies and English, Pennsylvania State University, USA
Martin Willis, Professor of English, University of Westminster, UK
Karen A. Winstead, Professor of English, The Ohio State University, USA

Nicolas Pierre Boileau

Mental Health Symptoms in Literature since Modernism

palgrave
macmillan

Nicolas Pierre Boileau
Aix-Marseille University
Aix-en-Provence, France

ISSN 2634-6435   ISSN 2634-6443   (electronic)
Palgrave Studies in Literature, Science and Medicine
ISBN 978-3-031-37632-0   ISBN 978-3-031-37630-6   (eBook)
https://doi.org/10.1007/978-3-031-37630-6

© The Editor(s) (if applicable) and The Author(s), under exclusive licence to Springer Nature Switzerland AG 2023
This work is subject to copyright. All rights are solely and exclusively licensed by the Publisher, whether the whole or part of the material is concerned, specifically the rights of translation, reprinting, reuse of illustrations, recitation, broadcasting, reproduction on microfilms or in any other physical way, and transmission or information storage and retrieval, electronic adaptation, computer software, or by similar or dissimilar methodology now known or hereafter developed.
The use of general descriptive names, registered names, trademarks, service marks, etc. in this publication does not imply, even in the absence of a specific statement, that such names are exempt from the relevant protective laws and regulations and therefore free for general use.
The publisher, the authors, and the editors are safe to assume that the advice and information in this book are believed to be true and accurate at the date of publication. Neither the publisher nor the authors or the editors give a warranty, expressed or implied, with respect to the material contained herein or for any errors or omissions that may have been made. The publisher remains neutral with regard to jurisdictional claims in published maps and institutional affiliations.

Cover illustration: Georges DIEGUES / Alamy Stock Photo

This Palgrave Macmillan imprint is published by the registered company Springer Nature Switzerland AG.
The registered company address is: Gewerbestrasse 11, 6330 Cham, Switzerland

Paper in this product is recyclable.

ABSTRACT

'To link madness and writing is to perpetuate one of the greatest commonplaces of our modernity' (Cape 2011: 7). One of the reasons for literature's interest in madness might be found in the symptom of psychic disorder itself, which can be conceived as something else than a 'cyphered message' (Zizek, Enjoy your Symptom! Jacques Lacan in Hollywood and Out, Routledge, London, 1992: 175). According to Lacan, the symptom is also something ineffable, unattainable, which never ceases to remain unwritten (Lacan, Autres écrits. Éditions du seuil, "Champ freudien", 2001: 559). Literature itself has long chronicled the state of those who fail to go through life without troubles and disorders (Mullini, Littérature et Pathologie. L'imaginaire du texte, Paris, 1989). The question I want to raise in this work is *how, thanks to the Modernist forays into the workings of the mind, literature produces, instead of simply reproducing, symptoms,* how the symptoms produced are decoded or made decipherable in a way that medicine leaves out, but also *how the represented illness defies cure and care and resists the attempts currently made to erase symptoms through biomedicine, instead of working from and around them.*

This book will therefore look at various ways of dealing with symptoms of psychological disorders in the literature of the long twentieth century. It is based on the premise that *Mrs Dalloway* set an example in which the author goes beyond the logical explanation of psychological symptoms. *This book's thesis is that the notion of symptoms has never been central to studies of literature and madness, often as a result of a lack of clarity as to what symptoms mean and how they are used in therapy.* Very often, critics and readers have endorsed or resisted diagnostic categorisation; some have followed in the footsteps of dominant medical discourses—currently neurological and biomedical; others have criticised the medical biases and prejudices that diagnoses and methods of treatment reflected; in other words, literary critics have contended with notions of normality, commonality and statistical representations while affirming that subjects were being subjected, reified and stigmatised by psychiatric and 'mental health' discourses. This book shows that literature can, in its questioning of commonly accepted views of this lived experience of psychic symptoms, *help engender new theories* about the functioning of subjective cases.

What happens, indeed, if the symptom is regarded not as that which should be disposed of but as the subjective response to a world that subjects can never fully grasp because of their existence through and in language? The fact that the emergence of 'mental health' care coincided with a global, artistic movement now called Modernism invites us to think about the way in which the history of medical treatment in the twentieth century—ranging from the advent of cognitive psychology and its scientific apparatus to an understanding of the multiple fractures within the fields of psychiatry and psychoanalysis—helps understand new figures of madness in literature, and contributes to producing new symptoms that are not metaphors (Sontag, Illness as Metaphor (1977–78) and Aids and Its Metaphors (1988–89). Doubleday, London, 1978; 1989).

In order to explore these questions, the following novels will be studied: Virginia Woolf's *Mrs* Dalloway (1925), Patrick McGrath's *Asylum* (1996), Pat Barker's *Regeneration* Trilogy (1991–1995), Doris Lessing's *The Fifth* Child (1988), Alan Hollinghurst's *The Line of Beauty* (2004), Rachel Cusk's Trilogy (2014–2018) and Ali Smith's *Seasonal Quartet* (2018–2021). The corpus has been selected for the following reasons: first, the novels chosen are all somehow connected to Woolf and the Modernist era, in ways that I shall explore, so that a history of the evolution of the uses of symptoms can be delineated through a careful analysis of the novels. Secondly, these novels have never been discussed together and some of them have never featured in studies of psychic disorder and symptom analysis. I think it is fruitful to track down symptoms in overt manifestations of psychic disorders (Part I) as well as in discreet ones (Parts II and III), which is arguably the modality of psychic disorders of our contemporary era (Gaspard, Nouveaux symptômes et lien social contemporain, 2010: 357–371). Lastly, most, if not all, of these texts form part of a cycle in their author's writing, either by being overtly part of a trilogy, having a sequel, or by being themselves connected to a certain period of production. It is as if none of these novels stood on their own, as if their authors were fully aware that symptoms are not written out, or off, without consequences. This is the sign that *symptoms persist, because they are not simply a 'cyphered message', but the singular skein of meanings which structure one's being into a functioning entity in the world. The definition of symptoms as a sure sign of an illness that must be cured is what literature disputes,* as can be seen in the representation of psychic disorders in the long twentieth century which will be exemplified in this volume.

References

Capé, Anouck (2011). *Les Frontières du délire: écrivains et fous au temps des avant-gardes.* Paris, Honoré Champion.
Sontag, Susan (1978–1989). *Illness as Metaphor* (1977–78) and *Aids and Its Metaphors* (1988–89). London: Doubleday.

CONTENTS

The Function of Symptoms of 'Mental Health': How Literature Is Situated in the Debate Between Cure and Care

'There are books about' madness in literature 'as much as there are books about most things':[1] sense of place or identity, race, time and space, and other questions that interrogate the alienation of human beings from their reality. Madness and the things people do when they are mad certainly continue to attract much attention, providing 'some of the most powerful images of social disorder and of individual disintegration' (Saunders and McNaughton 2005: 1). It almost appears at times that madness is part and parcel of literature, based on an 'intimate relationship' that 'seems natural' (Capé 2011: 7).[2] This is especially relevant with questions such as the madness of the creative mind (Downie 2005: 49), the social implications of psychiatric treatment (Wall 2018) or more generally the understanding of the madness of literary creation (Felman 1978) and the very quality of language and the linguistic inventions of those regarded as mad (Ferrer 1990; Lecercle 1996). One also immediately sees this theme as having a long history, readily connecting it with medieval studies of melancholia and lunacy or, in an Anglophone context, with the Shakespearean

---

[1] This formulation is inspired by Cusk: 'There are books about motherhood, as much as there are books about most things' (Cusk 2001: 117).

[2] Unless specified in the bibliography, all translations of French texts into English are mine.

© The Author(s), under exclusive license to Springer Nature Switzerland AG 2023
N. P. Boileau, *Mental Health Symptoms in Literature since Modernism*, Palgrave Studies in Literature, Science and Medicine, https://doi.org/10.1007/978-3-031-37630-6_1

explorations of irrationality.[3] In recent years, the collective work by Charley Baker et al. (2010) has mapped out the state of such a topic in the twentieth and twenty-first centuries. They have renewed the interest in the question of madness in the contemporary era by carefully analysing the categories of medical treatment and the evolution of their fictionalisation. They have contributed to reflecting the shift from the equivocal term 'madness' to the more medical expression: 'mental health'. This book pays tribute to existing works on literature and madness but proposes to look at a more specific point: the question of symptoms in 'mental health'. The book will not seek to establish what would inevitably be a long list of symptoms—such as what can be found in the *Diagnostic Statistical Manual of Mental Disorders* (DSM-5)—or to chronicle the evolution of symptomatology as shown in fiction in the long twentieth century (the phrase 'long twentieth century' is intended to indicate that I will be looking at works produced between 1925 and the 2020s). I would like to resist such temptation for a taxonomical approach and side with Bonikowski when he says that we should not play 'a game of symptom or diagnosis spotting' (Bonikowski 2013: 6).

What this book will explore instead is the discrepancy between the way doctors deal with symptoms—for now, suffice it to say that from a medical point of view symptoms are the signs of an illness which patients want to control if not get rid of, and which biomedical science endeavours to erase—and the way literature uses and produces symptoms, especially linguistic ones, to invent characters and account for the experience of symptoms and their significance at the subjective level. The question I want to raise in this work is *how, thanks to the Modernist forays into the workings of the mind and the body, literature produces, instead of simply reproducing, symptoms,* how the symptoms produced are decoded or made decipherable in a way that medicine does not (outside strict causality), but also *how the represented disorder defies cure and care and resists the attempts currently made to erase symptoms through biomedicine, instead of working from and around them. The definition of symptoms as a sure sign of an illness that must be cured is what literature disputes,* as can be seen in the representation of psychic disorders in the long twentieth century which will be exemplified in this volume.

---

[3] The theme has long been commented upon by critics. See for example the issue 'Shakespeare et la folie'. *Revue philosophique de la France et de l'étranger.* (123) 1937, 128. See in particular H. Suhamy's concern that such a common theme be reduced to a simple equation of madness to freedom (Suhamy 1989: 9).

The Literary Diagnosis of Symptoms

In the field of 'mental health', some argue that symptoms are not to be erased but to be nourished as the essential, most singular part of an individual: the enigmatic meaning of the symptom(s) does not preclude a crucial function in the subjects' handling of their lives. Seen from this perspective, the definition of the symptom is related to Lacan's elaborating in the later years of his teaching: the symptom, spelt *sinthome*, is, according to Lacan after decades of clinical practice, no longer that which needs deciphering, or 'a cyphered message' (Zizek 1992: 175), through which, in orthodox Freudian theory, 'the subject gets back... the truth about his desire, the truth that he was not able to confront' (Zizek 1992: 175). The symptom can be defined beyond its analogy to a physical symptom, that is, as a sign to be interpreted in relation to some organic dysfunction and causing pain the doctor seeks to assuage. In contemporary Lacanian psychoanalytic theory, the symptom is a subjective solution that enables subjects to knot together different aspects of their life into a whole that holds; a scaffolding (to paraphrase Woolf in *Moments of Being*); the very essence of their subjective response to the world, the very cause of their discomfort with their being, inherently unsatisfactory, and that which can be manipulated or at least manoeuvred from in therapy and through writing (Lacan 2005). In his essay on Hollywood cinema, provocatively titled *Enjoy Your Symptom!*, Zizek explains that the symptom is 'a particular signifying formation which confers on the subject its ontological consistency, enabling it to structure its basic, constitutive relationship to *enjoyment* (jouissance)' (Zizek 1992: 177). While agreeing with this, I would prefer to use 'singular' or 'subjective' rather than 'particular' because I see the symptom as a formation of the subject. All the same, this definition shows that literature is not only a place where symptoms are interpreted, analysed and given meaning but also one where symptoms are produced.

This book will look at British, mostly English, literature of the twentieth century, and is based on two hypotheses: first, that the mad person characterised by delirium, lack of coherence in speech and thought, and an enigmatic response to the world, like Septimus Smith in *Mrs Dalloway*, more or less disappeared over the course of the twentieth century as a literary trope, a development that mirrors the effects of biomedical psychiatry;[4] secondly, that there has been *little consideration of the impact*

---

[4] The use of specific neuroleptics has enabled most medicated patients to have fewer symptoms of incoherent delirium.

of 'mental health' symptoms and diagnoses in and *on literary representations of madness* and psychic disorders. The evolution of symptomatology towards contemporary 'discreet disease categories', to use a phrase by Micale, has more or less been treated as an insignificant oddity bearing no relation to the question of madness. I will try to determine how, in the works of Virginia Woolf, Patrick McGrath, Pat Barker, Doris Lessing, Alan Hollinghurst, Rachel Cusk, and Ali Smith, these discreet symptoms both enable us to confirm the functions symptoms play in the subjective response to life and invite us to redefine the medical binary of health/illness. With the expression 'discreet disease categories', Micale suggests that the nosography in 'mental health' treatment gradually discarded the notion of symptom clusters with the improvement of biomedicine and now observes other formations which resist the effect of biomedical treatment (Micale 1993: 503).

This *introduction looks at how one can situate the place of literary explorations of the symptoms between, on the one hand, a medical understanding of symptoms as having an organic cause and, on the other hand, a sociological or cultural apprehension of the symptom as a consequence of norms and a crippling effect of society. Literature, I argue, unravels the function of symptoms at the subjective level: their function or place in the character's life.* Symptoms can be seen as potential for creative storytelling (Woolf 1926), in which case medicine's cure is not sought and its authority on the value of symptoms is disputed. There have been many novels, autobiographies and studies of a Foucauldian nature seeking to disparage psychiatric institutions and treatment: we may think of Jennifer Dawson's *The Ha-Ha* (1961), Sylvia Plath's *The Bell Jar* (1963), Janet Frame's *Faces in the Water* (1961) and *An Autobiography* (1987), Susanna Kaysen's *Girl, Interrupted* (1983) and so on.[5] Using novels that are overtly based on 'mental health' therapy and novels that are only discreetly so, I propose that we follow instead the evolution of the psychoanalytic framework. The theory of Freudian repression emerged at a time when psychological disorder was better left unsaid and cure meant the erasure of the symptom, leading many artists and critics to adhere to the logic of inhibition in which the symptom was thought to contain the key to the subject's illness. Nowadays, the symptom is regarded as the persistence of an ungraspable content which is not governed by the logic of inhibition and offers a different perspective on treatment (Lacan 2005; Miller 1999). In order to achieve this,

[5] This is analysed in 'Power and Institutions in Fiction' (Baker et al. 2010: 61–98).

I will look at mostly secondary characters who show, at times discreet, symptoms of psychological disorder in Virginia Woolf's *Mrs Dalloway* (1925), Pat Barker's *Regeneration* Trilogy (1991–1995), Patrick McGrath's *Asylum* (1995), Doris Lessing's *The Fifth Child* (1988), Alan Hollinghurst's *The Line of Beauty* (2004), Rachel Cusk's *Outline* Trilogy (2014–2018) and Ali Smith's *Seasonal Quartet* (2018–2021). These novels are all connected with Virginia Woolf's writings, *Mrs Dalloway* in particular, and the Modernist aesthetics to which they are likened. Woolf's *Mrs Dalloway* resonates with all these novels either in their themes (First World War and post-traumatic stress disorder, or PTSD) or in the presence of secondary characters whose madness or disorders affect the story and the structure of the works, or their voices: what manifests in these novels is the absence of the characters' voices, their mutism or their silencing following the pattern of Septimus; the Modernist or neo-Modernist aspects of these works are constantly re-affirmed because of the novelists' primary concern with subjectivity, an exploration of the unsaid and its effect on the subject's apprehension of life. I argue that their connection lies in the analysis of the characters' solutions for making do without the capacity to articulate their experience—these novels explore the symptom of psychic disorder as a means to explore the limits of literature and the failure of language that is central to *Mrs Dalloway*. The idea for this book is based on the premise that *Mrs Dalloway* sets an example in which the author goes beyond the logical explanation of psychological symptoms. I intend to show that Septimus's symptoms exceed the logic of shell shock and constitute his singularity. Septimus is not reducible to an example of a pre-existing pattern or paradigm.

Secondly, these novels have never been discussed together and some of them have never featured in studies of psychic disorder and symptom analysis. I think it is fruitful to track down symptoms in overt manifestations of psychic disorders (Part I) as well as in discreet ones (Parts II and III), which is arguably the modality of psychic disorders of our contemporary era (Gaspard 2010: 357–371). Lastly, most, if not all, of these texts form part of a cycle in their author's writing, insofar as they either are part of a trilogy, have a sequel, or are themselves connected to a certain period of production. It is as if none of these novels stood on their own, as if their authors were fully aware that symptoms are not written out, or off, without consequences. This is the sign that *symptoms persist because they are not simply a 'cyphered message', but the singular skein of meanings which structure one's being into a functioning entity in the world.*

'ON BEING ILL': ON THE LITERARY APPREHENSION OF ILLNESS

Woolf enables us to identify the fundamental characteristics of a paradox that runs through the twentieth century and that informs our relation to illness, disease and well-being: the more we know about treatment and symptomatology, the less we know about what remains unknown. In her essay 'On Being Ill'[6] (1930), Virginia Woolf wonders why illness does not feature as one of the major themes of fictional works, alongside love, betrayal and friendship since, given that it affects both body and mind, it should be one of the primary concerns of human life.[7] She notes that, oddly enough, illness does not hold this place and she goes on to assert that critics have failed to see its potential for storytelling (Woolf 1926: 10), despite the fact that 'illness often takes on the disguise of love, and plays the same odd tricks' (Woolf 1926: 11). Woolf's essay is a reflection not on pathology but, as always, on fiction writing. It seems to open gateways to a revolution in themes and patterns, tropes and ways of telling central to Modernist concerns. The Modernist context of the 1920s very much revolved around defining new ways of writing and new themes that downplayed the influence of certain questions in order to enhance the novelty of the authors' own vision (Boileau and Estrade 2021).

More specifically, the mid-1920s saw the emergence of a dialogue in publication between Woolf and E.M. Forster centred upon the redefinition of what fiction should be about and the object that it should centre upon. 'On Being Ill' can be construed as Woolf's response to E.M. Forster's series of lectures which were published in 1927 under the title *Aspects of the Novel*. I see Woolf's essay as a partial response to her 'critical friend['s]' *Ars Poetica*.[8] She therefore takes illness as the starting point of her own

---

[6] V. Woolf, 'On Being Ill' (1930), *The Moment and Other Essays*, London, Harvest Book, 1948, 9–23. This text was first published in 1926 under the title 'Illness as Unexploited Mine' in *The Forum* and has attracted relatively less attention than other versions of the essay. See Coates 2012: 1n1.

[7] For a discussion of the relevance of this theme in Woolf's Modernist aesthetics, see Moran (1996): 1–5; 25–39.

[8] 'Morgan is the only one, either side, that matters' (V. Woolf, *Letters*, 4; 54); H. Trivedi, 'E. M. Forster and Virginia Woolf: The Critical Friends' in Das, G. K. and Beer, J., eds., *E. M. Forster: A Human Exploration*, London: The Macmillan Press, 1979. Hoffman, M. J. and Terr Har, A. '"Whose Books Once Influenced Mine": The Relationship between E. M. Forster's *Howards End* and Virginia Woolf's *The Waves*', *20th Century Literature*, vol.45, n°1, 1999, 46–64.

theory: it is to be remembered that the 1920s was a decade of great creativity for Woolf, with the publication of *Jacob's Room* (1922), *Mrs Dalloway* (1925), *To the Lighthouse* (1927) and *Orlando* (1929) as well as many critical essays which are as much about other people's writings as metatextual manifestoes concerning her own writing projects. *The Common Reader* (1925), gathering texts written prior to 1924, sets the tone of essays like 'On Being Ill'.

Both authors influenced each other greatly in their definitions of what writing fiction meant.[9] In his 1927 lectures, Forster declared that love is one of the five 'main facts in human life', thus adopting a taxonomical approach similar to Woolf's, and concluded with a similar diagnosis that these literary concerns invariably fail to take into account what really matters. Forster sardonically argues that the place love is given in literature is disproportionate to the space it occupies in real life, thereby also suggesting that literature needs to open up to other questions, especially those that remain unseen and unrecorded, a category into which illness would certainly fall. The connection between love and illness, and more broadly these two essays, perhaps is not obvious, but what Forster explains helps articulate a connection between them. Forster argues that he can understand why love is different from birth, food, sleep, and death because it is an instrument of connection with others: 'it is the emotional communion, this desire to give and to get, this mixture of generosity and expectation, that distinguishes love from the other experiences on our list' (Forster 1927: 51).

Woolf also reflects upon the great themes of literature and finds them wearisome, just as Forster finds romantic stories hackneyed; and like him, she seeks ways in which readers might relate to the life represented, which is how she justifies the need to include illness in fiction. In 'On being Ill', she advocates illness as potential epic material and elevates something dreaded to the status of something that must be voiced and analysed, taken into account and regarded as a basis for strong human connections.[10] What Woolf underlines about illness is structurally akin to what

---

[9] See, for example, Catherine Lanone's analysis of the tensions between both writers (Lanone 2007: 111–124).

[10] In more recent years, Coates has argued that this connection was also a maternal connection, the text being both conceived as a response to Julia Stephen's manual of caring and a means of emphasising the role of the 'invalid' (word taken from Marcus 1997 qtd in Coates 2012: 3) over the nurse, which Woolf saw as a way of getting freed from her 'Victorian legacy' to become an artist' (Coates 2012: 2–3).

Forster articulates concerning love: both raise a question of connection, with others but also with the literary tradition, and of commonality, illness being as common an experience, and possibly as structuring in one's life, as love (Coates 2012: 10). Woolf is interested in tracking down what history has left behind or left out of its grand narratives and while the domestic novel had noticeably dominated the literature produced by women until the Modernist era (Saudo-Welby 2019), always promoting a heterosexual vision of love that Forster might have had personal reasons to contend with, illness and the affects it causes suddenly seemed conspicuously absent.

As is often the case with Woolf's engaged writings, she almost convinces us that she is right, even when she seems to deny—or disregard—the existence of this theme prior to the Modernist era, especially in Victorian times. Pett asserts that this is a common mistake made by interpreters of the essay, who tend to take it at face value (Pett 2019: 28). Given the improvement of medicine and science throughout the nineteenth century, it is highly doubtful literature would have remained impervious to such cultural concerns (Bynum 1994: 117; Baker et al. 2010: 131). Not to forget, of course, the representations of doctors on stage, in particular the long-lasting imprint of Molière's characters. In true essayistic fashion (Gualtieri 2000), Woolf rewrites history with a purpose, by giving us a quick overview of the works produced through time, only to conclude that illness has indeed been neglected, or at least that it has been overlooked by both writers and critics: 'literature *does its best to* maintain that its concern is with the mind' (Woolf 1926: 9, emphases mine). S. Pett's text is the most comprehensive, detailed and forceful analysis of this major aspect of Woolf's essay to date (Pett 2019: 31 *et passim*).

Should illness be categorised as an ineffable experience, disconnected from the brain and the mind? On the contrary, Woolf argues, physical impairments, what medicine would call symptoms, have a story of their own, or at least a story to tell. By declaring that illness is not used in fiction, she is not commenting on the frequency of the theme or the fact that characters may be ill. What she questions is how literature makes sense of illness and how it conveys illness as only a mental experience, disconnected from the bodily representation. Emphasising the very Christian, and Cartesian, division between body and mind, a division today challenged by cognitive psychology and neurosciences with their emphasis on the activity of the brain or Lacanian psychoanalysis with its notion of the 'speakingbeing' (*parlêtre*),[11] Woolf 'does her best' to stress the negligible presence of disease, illness or ailment in fiction, because she wants to convince us of something else, the erasure of the body despite its enigmatic presence for the subject: 'But of all this daily drama of the body there is no record' (Woolf 1926: 10).[12] For Woolf, the body is a site of representation and fiction, and not just a juxtaposition of organs; it is something that should be spoken (about), and not just observed by the clinician and physician. In particular, Woolf's 'On Being Ill' focuses on small ailments, like colds, flus and fevers, which may easily go unspoken because they fail to convey any sense of drama. Taking 'On Being Ill' as programmatic, rightful observation and food for thought, Part I of this book will analyse the way in which Woolf's own fictional explorations of this subject might have paved the way for a number of writings about illness, or rather how they invite us to look more closely at the fictional apprehension of symptoms. In particular, Part II of the book will explore symptoms connected with psychic representations of the body in the fiction of Alan Hollinghurst and Doris Lessing, which enable critics to address the body and the way it is handled in contemporary works as an ambiguous over-presence concealing a profound misrecognition.

LITERATURE'S SYMPTOMS ARE NOT SURE CLINICAL SIGNS OF ILLNESS

In the field of psychiatry and the history of 'mental health' treatment, the biomedical development of medicine has now become the central, undisputed authority on symptomatology (Laurent 2016; Oyebode 2009). The criticism from social sciences towards psychiatric treatment and mental care has failed to undermine the medical authority on the question of treatment. Few studies so far have looked at the current debate between psychiatry, psychoanalysis and other 'mental health' theories (outside social and historical considerations that I shall return to) in order to engage with literature and how the mad person is now represented both under and against the influence of such theories. My contention is that the

---

[11] This was the main theme of the last conference of the World Association of Psychoanalysis in Rio de Janeiro, http://www.congressoamp2016.com/uploads/e83dfa7a4a4085a825 4f2024e4277f1e2e129c63.pdf

[12] Disability studies have recently initiated a move towards making illness and chronic diseases more visible and central to the analysis of literature. See, for example, De Bont 2021.

twentieth century's major innovations—the Modernist aesthetics and its avatars (Latham 2016)—can be related to the function of language in the Lacanian conception of the subject (Marret 2017: 89). Subjects have to negotiate the inaccessibility of the real due to a lack in language that creates an inassimilable rest. This lack and rest are at the heart of the contemporary understanding of 'generalised foreclosure' (Miller 1998; Maleval 2019). If everyone can be said to be delirious or mad (Lacan 1979: 278), the modalities of neurotic and psychotic responses or symptoms remain different. This new approach implies 'that [therapists] stop approaching psychoses as pathologies' (Marret 2017: 89). The distinction between sane and insane is repeatedly made obsolete because psychosis is regarded as a distinctive response to the 'real' and not as a pathological one. The literary shift towards non-linear narratives and irrational storytelling has been noted in other fields as stylistic fragmentation (Baker et al. 2010), or the collapse of master narratives (Lyotard 1984) but in the corpus chosen, I want to show the presence of 'discreet' symptoms of a radical absence of meaning in apparently mad characters as well as in others, less typical of psychiatric nosography. Since Modernism, I argue, literature has reflected and produced new symptoms related to 'mental health', which teach us about the development of our subjective response to the world, the need to listen to voices and silence, the aporia of traditional, organised and linear representations and the growing awareness that 'mental health' and madness, or neurosis and psychosis, are not peripheral to normality, but indeed central to humanity.

This argument is made within the context of medical humanities as developed by Saunders and McNaughton, and many others since (e.g. see Pett 2019: 26), and more particularly the necessary inter-disciplinary approach to medicine—a science which can only be practised in language:

The doctor always speaks as if they themselves were firmly set in their boots, the boots of love, desire, willingness and so on and so forth. At the end of the day, it is a very off position, and we are likely to have known for quite a while now that it is a dangerous position. It is the position which makes you assume counter-transference, thanks to which you don't understand anything about the ill person you are dealing with. (Lacan 2013: 343)

Woolf wrote *Mrs Dalloway* in 1925 and 'On Being Ill' in 1926, in the wake of the nineteenth century that saw medical knowledge attain a degree of sophistication hitherto unwitnessed (Marret 2010): 'Modern medicine was the product of 19th-century society' (Bynum 1994: xi). She was also a contemporary of new illnesses that posed a challenge to medical science, especially neurological diseases and post-traumatic stress disorder. The late nineteenth and early twentieth centuries were a time of discovery: the nosography of illnesses did not change as much as the awareness that there was so much more to find the cause of, and the remedy to. The internationalisation of scientific practices and the power given to scientists in medical treatment transformed medical practitioners into a profession set apart and ready to tell its own story (Bynum 1994, 142–175).

At a more personal level, Woolf wrote her essay after she had gone through severe bouts of depression herself and had been sent to nursing homes. Leonard Woolf's autobiography, as well as Hermione Lee's biography of Woolf, among others, chronicles the different treatments she received at that time, which may account for her desire to see illness and health as more determining factors in literature than they tended to be.[13] Indeed, Lee notes that 'On Being Ill' was considered by its publisher to be too intimate and personal, prompting us to look at it like a piece of autobiography (see further information about this in Chap. 2 of the book). In any case, it is clear that when Woolf wrote 'On Being Ill', she intended to appropriate the story of illness in ways that had not been tried before. For while medical practice has gradually become biomedical, making it a domain foreign to most, the symptom, especially in terms of its effects on the subjective life of the patient, is in itself not the property of medicine, but of the patient. It is the patient that comes with a request—a *demande* in French Lacanian terminology—to fix a problem. This is even truer of mental or psychological symptoms as they are not always attributed to a physical cause. Thus, symptoms produce meaning and stories but may not be meaningful *per se*.

Woolf did not have medical knowledge, even though as patient she had a long experience of mental care. Thus, in her essay, the words 'illness' and 'disease' are used interchangeably, which explains why she does not stress the underlying dichotomy of connotations between both terms. If she did, she might observe that one word stresses the presence of something evil, difficult or malevolent within, as the etymology of the word 'ill' suggests, while the other word stresses the feeling of discomfort regardless of its possible cause or origin; she might also observe that illness is a positive/positivist term that describes a state of being while 'disease' suggests a negative

---

[13] Interestingly, in France, at about the same time, many writers of the avant-garde had attended medical school and were far more knowledgeable in medical theory than Woolf, but their work similarly criticises treatment and care (Capé 2011, 23–64).

approach which presupposes the existence of a state of ease that is disturbed—in other words, she equates 'being ill' with an affection of the body in its physicality that can be recognised and categorised. What she is arguing for is the presence of something as yet unseen by most, and the acknowledgement of a lack she wishes to work from. She thereby endorses the common idea that the body is ob-scene,[14] un-seen, un-charted and she seeks to unveil the different ways in which it could be put forward by first claiming that a greater place should be granted to illness in fiction.

However, she already subverts the language of science and medicine in doing so. For example, in her essay, 'fever' and 'melancholia' are presented as equally affecting the body, despite the fact that the nosography would place these terms in slightly different categories: fever is a symptom, melancholia a disease; fever is the sign of something else and must be traced back to a source while melancholia is the result of some complex psychological disorder whose main symptoms are depression, dismay and a refusal to live; while fever may lead to despair, melancholia may be accompanied by fever. These categories have been disputed (DSM-5 n.d.: 4) but remain the paradigm of treatment. Woolf therefore treads on slippery ground from the point of view of accurate medical knowledge, but she nonetheless questions the foundations of literary representation and, as often, forces readers and critics alike to rethink the boundaries and stereotypical forces at play in everyday discourse. More importantly, she suggests that the pathological is not just the realm of medicine and that literature can make sense of symptoms, not only by decoding them but also by understanding the logic of their function. DSM-5 recognises this cultural understanding of symptoms: 'Mental disorders are defined in relation to cultural, social, and familial norms and values. Culture provides interpretive frameworks that shape the experience and expression of the symptoms' (DSM-5 n.d.: 14). There is no understanding of a symptom as a purely objective sign.

'On Being Ill' has been read as informing us about medicine as much as any academic text. Recently, the essay has been read as an attempt at weaving together the individual and the collective experience of pathologic bodies (Couser 1997; Lee 1996). It has been regarded as one of the founding texts of medical humanities, a field that is expanding rapidly:

---

[14] Classical Latin obscēnus, obscaenus has been variously associated, by scholars ancient and modern, with scaevus left-sided, inauspicious (see scaevity n.) and with caenum mud, filth (see cœnose adj.). The derivation from scaena scene n., one of several suggested by the Latin grammarian Varro, probably represents a folk etymology (OED).

Sarah Pett asserts that it is the first essay in medical humanities (Pett 2019: 26) while Claire Barber-Stetson does not hesitate to place it within the field of *disability studies* (Barber-Stetson 2016: 48). Lynne Mijangos sees the essay as connecting gender and illness. Woolf is thus said to speak of women's bodies, their representation or lack thereof in public and artistic discourses, the source of which interpretation can be traced back to the French feminist theory of the 1970s, as exemplified by Irigaray and Kristeva (Mijangos 2016). From this critical standpoint, Woolf's essay is perceived as the first steps that were to pave the way for her feminist essays of the later 1920s and 1930s, in which she identifies the loci of women's misrepresentation at the end of the nineteenth and early twentieth centuries: women's bodies, which were paradoxically the object of considerable medical and psychiatric speculation and photographic work (Didi-Hubermann 1982; Showalter 1985). I choose to see the essay as one of the points of intersection between a reflection upon the failings of literature and a reflection upon the influence of illness on one's subjective experience, a valuable starting point for the analyses of the novels I offer in this book.

Indeed, most of the essay is dedicated not so much to the clinical analysis of symptoms and body ailments as to how the experience of the symptom in the body shapes and interacts with the real in ways that escape symbolisation. In other words, her essay returns to the function of language and literature. After stating that 'illness is the great confessional', Woolf (1926: 13) reflects upon the inherent difficulty, indeed the impossibility, for the experience of disease to be shared: 'We do not know our own souls, let alone the souls of others. Human beings do not go hand in hand the whole stretch of the way. There is a virgin forest in each; a snowfield where even the print of birds' feet is unknown.... In illness the makebelieve ceases' (Woolf 1926: 14). Woolf hereby stresses the presence of something unknown to her and others, something that human 'connection', to use Forster's word taken from the epigraph to *Howards End*, cannot alleviate or fix. She views illness as an open door to this *terra incognita*, which then was inevitably going to be interpreted and read as the Freudian unconscious, despite Woolf's self-confessed distrust of the man and his theory.[15] Her understanding of the symptom is perhaps that it has

---

[15] This is a commonplace of Woolf's studies now and many critics only refer to this as fact that is unchallenged. See https://www.charleston.org.uk/virginia-woolf-meets-sigmund-freud/ or Minow-Pinkney for a detailed account of the relationship between Woolf and Freud.

to be deciphered, but more surely that it is the point at which communication fails and language misses its target. As she finishes the essay with a reflection on the value of poetry, regarded as more efficient than prose because in illness we are attuned to sound and other senses rather than the meaning of words which in health is prevalent (Woolf 1926: 19), it gradually becomes clear that illness is a state of acute sensations that the novelist wants to explore for the possibilities it offers of finding new ways to express what is ineffable. This is how we come full circle to the notion of illness and love being both constructed as beyond symbolisation and discourse, and therefore interesting material to the novelist:

> Woolf's primary agenda, after all, is to distance illness in literature from its history of instrumentalization in order that it might be taken seriously as a lived experience, not to divorce it from all meaning nor to render it inexpressible. Throwing meaning and intention so far into question that all hope of interpretive purchase is lost, the strategies deployed in these poems might come to work at cross-purposes to Woolf's attempt to create 'an original language of her own'. (Pett 2019: 46)

For the physical experience of illness would be nothing for Woolf if it did not raise the question of language. In that respect, literature and medical knowledge have much in common, as pathological states are often discovered only through the articulation into words of some oddity, strangeness, pain or suffering which need deciphering by the person these words are addressed to. According to Woolf, literature needs to express or represent the body's ailments because it is a challenge that literature must rise to, lest the body remains *unspoken*.[16] The English language in particular poses a threat to the expression of illness because it 'has no words for the shiver or the headache' (Woolf 1926: 11):

> The merest schoolgirl, when she falls in love, has Shakespeare or Keats to speak her mind for her; but let a sufferer try to describe a pain in his head to a doctor and language at once runs dry…Yet it is not only a new language that we need, more primitive, more sensual, more obscene, but a new hierarchy of the passions; love must be deposed in favour of a temperature of 104; jealousy give place to the pangs of sciatica; sleeplessness play the part of villain, and the hero become a white liquid with a sweet taste. (Woolf 1926: 11)

---

[16] The point is not to take this for granted and to accept her view. Many critics and writers have spoken about illness before, but what is interesting is to follow her in her attempt at delineating that which remains unsaid.

Here again, Woolf's understanding of a 'medical condition' breaks down the connection between illnesses and symptoms, as if she was much more interested in bringing to the fore the body and the subjective experience of it than the medical perspective of what normal and pathological mean.

The desire to bridge the gap between the omnipresence of love and the relative absence of diseases was to be the focus of relentless efforts on the part of Woolf herself. This is apparent as early as in *Mrs Dalloway*, published one year before 'On Being Ill': the diagnoses of Septimus's illness by the two doctors, Dr Holmes and Sir Bradshaw, are proved useless, while his medical condition affects the story and the structure of the text. Beyond the autobiographical inspiration behind the two doctors' portraits (Lee 1996), what is decisive in *Mrs Dalloway* is the impact of the medical discourse on the subject and the responsibility the doctors bear in Septimus's suicide—that is, paradoxically, in making his body disappear offstage, become obscene where it was omnipresent. This is why this book will first look at the way in which misdiagnoses and the relationship between therapist and patient may help consolidate the lack of connection or articulation inherent to illness, especially for mental symptoms. It will try to unravel the many layers of interpretation by showing how literature 'does its best' to grapple with the skein of meanings that symptoms provoke. Woolf seems to use mental symptoms to suggest that language itself needs to be analysed as the engine of, if not the obstacle to, or as the ambivalent means of expression of, these bodily conditions which influence and shape the subjective response to the world and the place of the subject in the world. Woolf gradually moves from a criticism of the representation of health to the question of the ethics of sympathy and the subject's agency.

PSYCHOANALYSIS VERSUS PSYCHIATRY: EVER-GROWING TENSIONS OVER THE NOTION OF HEALTH

The field of 'mental health' and the question of who gets to define what symptoms are and mean are currently a theoretical and institutional battlefield. In 1980, *DSM III—Diagnostic and Statistical Manual of Mental Disorders*—produced by the American Association of Psychiatry, changed the traditional categories of psychiatry that had been used since Pinel and gained international recognition. This American textbook of nosography was intended to put an end to half a century of theoretical conflicts between psychiatry, psychology and psychoanalysis, the latter being particularly targeted (Shorter 1997). DSM implements the methodology of medicine and promotes cognitive psychology and its approach based on the analysis of behavioural and social problems. Its current fifth edition shows that it partly failed to offer not only a case study but also an efficient way of dealing with 'mental health', unless we think symptoms evolve in under a generation of patients. American cultural influence worldwide, together with a strong campaign of communication, may explain why *DSM*s (in their various versions) have now become the reference in terms of psychotherapy in the western world.

Another example of the changes brought about by *DSM* is the fact that the two great clinical categories of the nineteenth century, neurosis and psychosis, still crucial in psychoanalytic practice (Frosh 1991), were discarded, while the notion of 'disorder' suggests the persistence of a division between normal and pathological, or healthy and ill, that Lacanian psychoanalysis refuses. Differential clinic based on behavioural symptomatology proliferated instead, causing each symptom to become the disorder itself. From this perspective, therapy is based on the erasure of the symptom, regardless of the function the symptoms may have for the subject. Nosography is exponentially developing into smaller and smaller categories, the aim being to observe, test, rank and so forth. 'Mental health' is the site of battles that no other scientific discourse seems to have witnessed and that are linked to politics. Discussing the notion of the pathological, Canguilhem notes that psychiatry is a self-reflexive science, and laments that medicine has not shown a similar interest in defining the terms of its practice: 'It is interesting to note that contemporary psychiatrists, in their own field, have rectified and clarified the concepts of *normal* and *pathological*, whereas physicians and physiologists seem to have remained impervious to such teaching if applied to their own practice' (Canguilhem 1966: 91). This battle between two theoretical frameworks manifests for example in the various laws seeking to organise and regulate the practice of 'mental health' therapies (Maleval 2012: 7).[17]

---

[17] In France, there was outrage in 2021 when a bill was brought to Parliament, aimed at banning the use of the talking cure in state-funded mental health institutions. The protest gave rise to an online petition: https://www.change.org/p/tous-les-citoyens-arrêtons-l--arrêté and a forum uniting the main societies of psychologists, psychoanalysts and therapists: https://events.causefreudienne.org/homepage/104-brochure-arretons-l-arrete.html

With the rise of biomedicine, medical imagery, neurology and *DSM*-based therapies, psychoanalysis came to be derided as unscientific (because it was resistant to the methodology of treatment, the tests used by the sciences which pass them and statistical evaluations) and ejected from what is regarded as valid therapy (Rabeyron et al. 2020, 1–41). Psychoanalysis 'is passé', laments Showalter, but 'Freud's message never got through to millions of people' (Showalter 1997: 9). Instead of accepting that psychoanalysis deals with the formation of psychic disorders, 'many people still reject psychological explanations for symptoms: they believe psychosomatic disorders are illegitimate and search for physical evidence that firmly places cause and curse outside the self' (Showalter 1997: 4). Showalter also suggests that the drug market could only benefit from such conceptions of 'mental health'. From the point of view of public health, shorter, drug-induced therapies mean more profits for the pharmaceutical industry and a seemingly efficient handling of the problem for the states.

The 1990s' confidence in a brain-based, drug-treated approach to psychiatric disorders (the well-known Prozac era), and the superiority granted to psychiatric treatment based on the new 'psychiatric Bible' (Micale and Lerner 2001: 1), *DSM*, in turn, led many literary critics to disparage other explorations of madness and to reduce other theories such as psychoanalysis to Freud, its founder, whose ideas can easily be presented as outdated (Burston 2020: 20). Burston calls them 'Freud bashers' (Burston 2020: 31) and agrees with these critics' analyses, as much as he easily opposes the accessibility of American psychoanalysis to the obscurity and vagueness of French psychoanalysis (Burston 2020: 30; 40). For Thiher, who works at the intersection between literature, medical thought and philosophy, 'neurology's great service to date has been to reduce the number of clinical entities we consider to be madness... neurology does this by describing syndromes that, once recognized as a neurological disease of dysfunction, are no longer considered to be part of madness' (Thiher 1999: 11). Thiher therefore thinks madness is a misdiagnosis that will be erased once a physical origin has been established for various illnesses as yet undiscovered: the explosion of symptoms and nosography that has seen a surge in the number of pages of *DSM* is regarded as progress.

And yet, this downplays the fact that psychiatry itself is not just science: it is also a discourse on mental illness that seeks to dominate, in order to wield power over other discourses or to make sure that their therapies and treatments are marketable and profitable. This is a point of view developed by Edward Shorter who sees psychiatry not solely as the development of a scientific method but also as a battle for recognition within the medical sphere: time and again, he uses the vocabulary of battle and power to evoke the building of psychiatry as a medical force. For instance, he describes the way in which people with no medical training could not be granted access to psychoanalytical training during the 'halcyon days' of American psychoanalysis (Burston 2020: 25); or when he evokes the change from hospital-based practice to private practices as a way of gaining symbolic status (Shorter 1997: 113). Unlike Shorter, I think that the 'winners' of this authority race should not be regarded as the only legitimate opinion on the question of symptom analysis.

DSM-5 asserts its function as a 'practical and adjustable guide' (DSM-5 n.d.: iii) and its intention to 'maintain its rank as authoritative guide for diagnosis and classification of mental disorders' (DSM-5 n.d.: 3). Despite its 'paradigm shift' away from the identification of sole biological markers, based on the recognition that some diagnoses were not perfectly reliable (DSM-5 n.d.: 3), some still consider that its authoritative position runs the 'risk of false "epidemics" with harmful excessive treatments' (Frances 2009: 391). Some dispute the idea that *DSM* brought anything new to the field of psychiatry and argue that its multiple versions have only served the purpose of establishing American psychiatry as the provider of a new nosography and symptomatology in a system that is highly competitive: fewer than 20% of mental illness staff are psychiatrists in the United States (Kirk and Hutchins, 28–29; 33). *DSM* has been accused of minimising psychic diseases and wanting to restrict them to biological causes (Maleval 2012). Maleval argues that in spite of high-calibre education in Ivy League universities, *DSM*-oriented practitioners in the United States caused three contemporary pandemics: multiple personalities, false memories and alien abductions. For him, this is caused by 'authoritarian psychotherapy': 'an interventionist type of therapy in which the therapist places themselves in the position of master: from this position of authority, they present themselves as having knowledge about the subject's well-being, a subject who is invited to conform to the therapist's prescription and adjust to the reality that said therapist conceives' (Maleval 2012: 8n2). The high standard of an education based on scientific evidence gives confidence in the practitioner. It is by challenging this discourse of the master, to use Lacan's phraseology (Lacan 1991: 31), that patients produce other symptoms or feed into their symptoms, which can also be seen as a subjective construction against the invasion of something unnameable and unattainable that Lacan calls 'real'. This is why intersubjective effects cannot be reduced to treatment and hormones. Doctors have a way of influencing patients and reflecting social norms and behaviours as well as what resists the organisation of such behaviours (Maleval 2012). To sum up the debate, there are those that will only value theories of mental illness that speak from the medical field, based on pharmaceutical approaches which they see as scientific and therefore the only ones worthy of trust, while other critics are disinclined to accept the medical diagnosis and prefer to see in it the expression of cultural misfitting. Lacanian psychoanalysis recognises the importance of psychiatric clinical expertise while considering that the medical approach leaves aside the question of how the subject experiences the symptoms and what function(s) these symptoms may have, a subjective level central to the novels studied here.

SUBJECTIVE RESPONSES TO SYMPTOMS

In the current dominant approach, madness is no longer a symbol or the other of rationality, as it might be traced through the history of literature from Shakespeare onwards, but an illness that science—namely pharmaceutical science—will take care of. Yet, some critics resist this tendency by trying to locate where madness 'actively defies... formal diagnostic classification' (Bonikowski 2013: 3). The place of subjectivity is the most interesting bone of contention between the different theories and methods in 'mental health' for literary critics and cultural analysts. Analysing the role of the scientists in the Golden Age of progress in the nineteenth century, Sophie Marret explains: 'When they seek to justify their acts by the benefit humankind will get from them, scientists remain blind to the engagement of their own desire and its effects in said acts' (Marret 2010: 33). Diagnoses today tend to reduce the agency of subjective responsibility through the biomedical approach that favours the explanation of syndromes and disorders through brain activity, hormones and other bodily, organic and physical responses to/by which the subject is said to be subjected (Laurent 2016): 'Nowadays, psychiatrists are no longer interested in "madness"', which is why 'they are driven to reifying their patients... You can see them talk about scales, biology, statistics, protocols... not about the subject' (Maleval 2019: 7).

While fierce debates still exist between various forms of 'mental health' care, the question of subjectivity in scientific methods has been left to human sciences: Bourdieu, in the speech he gave when he received the 2000 Huxley Memorial Award, explains how science feigns to objectify reality to the extent that it forgets to think about its own place in relation to the object studied, while human sciences sometimes think of their own subjectivity as autobiographical data instead of taking into account their subjective place in the world as an objective element of their analysis (Bourdieu 1986). Besides, most legal debates focus on 'qualifications', on who is given the right to treat, cure and help patients, without considering the effects of that cure (Gori and Del Volgo 2005: 17). Quite a number of historians argue that the terms 'medical' and 'therapeutic' have lately become synonymous: yet the medical is only one way of curing and caring, based on science, while the therapeutic is based on other, competing or supplementary factors. 'Everyday cases prove that the truth of the patient is not inscribed in the same place in the psyche as the accurate words that the doctor pronounces from a statistical point of view' (Gori & Del Volgo, 216). This is exemplified in the fact that whenever medicine has no cure or cannot alleviate some pain, the public debate focuses on magical practices: scientific accuracy seems to have overpowered care and knowledge of oneself (Gori & Del Volgo, 41). Ultimately the political question of the diagnosis of 'mental illness' and its symptoms is of paramount importance to decide who should be in charge of the patients, how the curing staff should be trained, and what solutions can work (Gori & Del Volgo, 280). This has inevitably been represented in contemporary literature and can be traced in certain forms of representation of cure and care, as will be seen in Hollinghurst's *The Line of Beauty* and Lessing's *The Fifth Child*.

On the one hand, the twentieth century saw the emergence, success and decline of the psychoanalytical discourse, which is a discourse about desire, thus about loss, and about love, that is, a very particular way of assessing and understanding social links and bonds; on the other hand, this discourse has gradually been superseded by the discourse of science which is an endless series of appropriation of laws and which neglects that which cannot be accounted for by its method. From the point of view of truth, science is imperfect because, even if in everyday language truth and accuracy are often equated, science is accurate but not necessarily truthful. Science constantly evolves and expands; its job is to always improve that which is known, that is to always admit to being untrue, or rather only relatively true (Soler 2002). On the other hand, despite its resistance to the categories of science and the methodology of science, psychoanalysis is truthful to many people and scholars. Psychoanalysis therefore remains true and very much dynamic (Seligman 2019), despite claims to the contrary.

What this argues for is the persistence of the relevance of psychoanalysis in the approach to 'mental health', inasmuch as the Lacanian treatment of symptom diverges from other approaches. Madness often is an enigma that raises the questions of good and evil, rationality and irrationality, reality and the real. Jean-Jacques Lecercle explains why it is the founding principle of literature in terms that show exactly why symptoms of linguistic disorders cannot simply be rectified:

> Language is not the instrument of an inscription to the world, or the revelation of some transcendence, in other words it is not the instrument of an appropriation of reality, but a 'whisper', endlessly repeated. The common experience of madness and literature is an experience of that which keeps trotting out; it is not a transcription of an extra-linguistic experience, judged against truth, but a reflexive experience, intra-linguistic, in which language itself is the object of experience. This way of being in language is called delirium if one observes it from the point of view of sanity, and will be called writing, or poetic language, if one observes it from the point of view of literature. (Lecercle 2004: 296)

Lecercle's concept here is akin to Lacan's: both speak of literary language as an invention which, like delirium in psychosis, enables the subject to hold together, if not knot together, the various aspects of experience, the imaginary, the real and the symbolic, three realms caused by the hole left by language in the subject's appropriation of their own experience. Furthermore, they both suggest that literature is not the place where psychiatric and psychoanalytic nosography is replaced, but rather the place that paves the way for clinicians: Lacan repeatedly said that artists do without prior knowledge what he theorises and teaches thanks to them (Lacan 2001: 192–93).

The aim of Lacanian psychoanalysis is not the erasure of symptoms, but the provision of assistance to subjects in how to deal with their symptoms because the latter are the subject's response to *jouissance* (which can be defined as that which meaninglessly remains outside of articulation and symbolisation for a subject, and which agitates them in spite of themselves). Symptoms are the mark of one's individuality and subjectivity as Lacan argued in one of his last seminars in 1975, focused on James Joyce (Lacan 2005: 65). In this seminar, Lacan shows the function of writing for Joyce: writing seeks to keep the hole of experience at bay, to inscribe the inherent lack of the real where it threatened to overwhelm the subject's experience (Lacan 2005: 73). According to Lacan's theory, as the letter is connected with the unconscious, there is perhaps no other art as likely as literature to reveal how symptoms work and what their function is with regards to what is often unseen by most other scientific approaches, that is, the subject's real, which results from the particular way in which various aspects of experience are knotted together for each and every one of us: 'writing has always something to do with the way I am trying to conceive of the knot' (Lacan 2005: 68—the knot being the topological representation in which Lacan accounts for the way each subject knots together the Imaginary, the Symbolic and the Real).

The study of literature and madness is a well-trodden path in the history of literary studies. In the 1960s–1970s, the perception of madness changed radically from the notion that it was the place of truth and revelation. A new school of criticism was to regard madness from the point of view of gender, society, culture and racism. Some of course found this debatable:

> Dominating the field for the past decades have been scholars who doubt the very existence of psychiatric illness, believing it to be socially constructed... who make the case that capitalist society was venging itself on the patients for their unwillingness to work, for a bohemian lifestyle, or even for a revolt against male authority. (Shorter 1997: 48)

On the one hand, psychiatry itself, its theory, its implied ideology and basis, came to be analysed as a historical, cultural phenomenon, giving new insights into its theoretical biases. On the other hand, historians and sociologists changed the ways these questions were examined. In particular, Shoshana Felman recalls the influence of the school of Harvard in those days and how she herself was encouraged to pursue some aspects of her research in relation to these questions: 'The fact that madness has currently become a *common* discursive *place* is not the least of the paradoxes. Madness usually occupies a position of *exclusion*; it is the *outside* of a culture' (Felman 1978: 13). Felman notes this paradox: 'To talk about madness is always in fact to deny it. However, one represents madness to oneself or others, to represent madness is always ... to play out the scene of the denial of one's own madness' (Felman 1978: 252). This is especially ironical when one reads—in Shorter, for example—a celebration of English clinical practices, which he unashamedly opposes to the supposed French knack for theory and useless conceptualisation: 'The Achilles' heel, or genius if one prefers, of English psychiatry was that it was all clinical medicine and little science. The English were known as superb observers' (Shorter 1997: 90). Even so, Britain was also the place to oppose the rule of psychiatry, through the now debated but then hailed movement of anti-psychiatry (Wall 2018). Literary critics often reflect upon madness for the artistic and aesthetic value(s) it possesses, but in doing so, they tend to erase madness or treat it as a cultural symbol of exclusion which may well derive from its original categorisation. 'Madness has become a commonplace term to describe any number of idiosyncrasies in contemporary life and society. The main discourse that sets out to define, describe and encapsulate madness is psychiatry and related psych-disciplines such as psychology' (Baker et al. 2010: 39). Historian Bynum, after asserting the social perspective of his history of medical treatment and hospital (Bynum 1994: xi), sees the birth of hospitals thus: 'The sick were herded in [hospitals] together with criminals, beggars, the infirm, orphans, prostitutes, the unemployed and the mad' (Bynum 1994: 25).

THE RUPTURE OF THE MODERNIST ERA

These new insights into the psyche, which emerged from the development of medical practice and clinic, and the advent of the discourse of (Lacanian) psychoanalysis, took place within a cultural movement that nowadays is regarded as one of the major movements in the arts: Modernism.

Modernism is a cultural and artistic movement that emerged at around the same time as Freud's ideas about a new vision of madness became available in England. These ideas were to influence the field of therapy until the 1950s at least in the United States, sometimes leading to what appear nowadays as aberrations—for example, in some commentators' insistent refusal to admit that 'the psychoanalytic concept of sexuality… can never be equated with genitality nor is it the simple expression of a biological drive' (Mitchell and Rose 1985: 2). The connection between Woolf and Freud is now well established: it is known that his essays were discussed within the Bloomsbury group, that Woolf herself contributed to the printing of his texts in the English language via the Hogarth Press, and that even though she claims that she never read the author and would beware of his ideas, she was aware of some of them. The era was marked by great Oedipal/family narratives as seen in many cultural productions of the time: Ibsen, Forster, T.S. Eliot and Mansfield leave out the notion of a plot in favour of the exploration of family issues and frustration, internal thought processes and introspection. Modernism has now become such a common term that defining it is more of a conundrum than a helpful tool of analysis, with many wanting to extend it well beyond its initial time-frame. Not wanting for it to become, like hysteria, 'a wastebasket diagnosis' (Showalter 1997: 16), one could say that it derives from a radical distrust of nineteenth-century positivist reality as seen in the shattering of the notion of a single, omniscient and scientific point of view: this led to the idea that truth could only be half-said (Lacan 2005: 31), be read between the lines or emerge from the confrontation of all these viewpoints. Many critics have shown the links between Woolf's artistic choices and the Modernist era in which they happened: 'For Woolf, the feminist and Modernist aesthetics converge, at least initially, in this attempt to challenge phallocentricism' (Minow-Pinkney 1987: 5).

But some of these studies were written at a time when psychoanalysis was an authoritative point of reference, used by many beyond psychoanalytic circles, with a vocabulary that was then understood, but mistaken for a philosophical reflection that was thought to be disconnected from clinical practice: 'Questioning the integrity of the "I", Lacan reveals that the fragmentation which Lukacs interprets as the pathology of Modernism is a universal fact of the human subject. Misrecognition (*méconnaissance*) constitutes the ego; autonomy of illusion, fiction' (Minow-Pinkney 1987, 13). The influence of psychoanalysis has waned nowadays while Modernism remains a fertile ground for novelistic experimentations. In *The Female Malady*, Showalter seems to have the intuition that the revolution occurring in medical and psychiatric treatment at the turn of the twentieth century is akin to the aesthetic revolution occurring at about the same time, Modernism. It is this very term she uses without explaining fully the potential implications of this way of qualifying psychiatric treatment. She later develops this notion through a fruitful parallel: 'Though the classic case histories of hysterical women are structured like Victorian novels that end with marriage, madness, or death, the case histories of Freud's male patients... read more like open-ended Modernist fictions' (Showalter 1997: 95). Woolf's essay, which I see as emerging as a consequence of the writing of *Mrs Dalloway* the year before, enables me to return to Showalter's intuition and explore it: Woolf's indecision regarding some of her proposals leads me to argue that the Modernist questions about the place of the subject, therapy and the definition of the pathological have far-ranging implications running through the twentieth century and were influenced as much by the evolution of therapy as by the aftermath of the

Modernist aesthetics and ideas. Zizek is another cultural analyst who links 'the Modernist procedure' to 'a 'symptomal reading':

> confronted with the totality, Modernism endeavours to subvert it by detecting the traces of its hidden truth in the details which 'stick out' and belie its 'official' truth, in the margins which point toward what has to be 'repressed' so that the 'official' totality could establish itself—Modernism's elementary axiom is that details always contain some surplus which undermines the universal frame of the 'official' Truth. (Zizek 1992: 138)

Literature has found many ways of representing madness and no comprehensive study or even taxonomy of religious, philosophical and medical representations of mental illness could easily be established. Yet representation of madness is key to understanding or experiencing the universal truth that SpeakingBeings are, as subjects of a language that fails to express their being, excluded from the symbolic order (Miller 2018: 52). Critics have therefore looked at the arts, and literature, to make sense of madness. In his history of asylums, Foucault starts with the description of a new symbol—the ship of fools (Foucault 1972: 21–28)—that allows him to raise questions about the domination of medical science in the realm of mental illness. However, to guide us through the maze of representations, some elements are worth recalling: until the Renaissance, the mad person was a threat to social order and a figure of the devil on Earth, without being regarded as a mental or medical condition. Figuring the devil or the demon, thereby feeding into people's beliefs and superstitions, the mad person could be either someone showing symptoms of great hysteria (convulsions, somatisation, paralysis and paralexia) or someone affected by illnesses as yet undiagnosed (venereal diseases, for example, epilepsy etc.), or yet again simply people whose speech distorted rationality. For all these reasons, the mad were enigmatic and posed a problem to those who would have liked to explain it all, and to religious and political authorities. 'Something is rotten in the state of Denmark', says Marcellus after Hamlet has been visited by a ghost (I, 4, 90), a sure sign that he is bedevilled. In those days, humour theory sought to explain madness as a question of equilibrium. Foucault argues that madness became a concern for medical staff after leprosy was contained at the end of the Middle Ages (Foucault 1972: 21), while others contend that it is caused by the improved diagnosis of certain illnesses that make madness always the other of diagnosis, the non-diagnosis so to speak. Some illnesses, like hysteria, are sometimes presented as 'a chapter of art history' (Didi-Huberman 1982: 20).

The 'modernity' of twentieth-century disorders is sometimes called 'Modernist' even by scholars with radically different approaches. Thiher, Zizek and Showalter do so, as if they had the intuition that *something had changed with Modernism*, in its literary sense, and this is what I want to explore here by looking at various authors who have claimed or been regarded as having a kinship with Woolf and her Modernist aesthetics. It seems to me that Modernism and its avatars are a valid *starting point* for a re-appreciation of what has so far been neglected, that is, the place given to illness, treatment and disorder in fiction, and the function of symptoms outside their possible meaning(s) at the subjective level. Indeed, Modernism, for all the vagueness of this term, corresponds to a time when truth was challenged through the change in narrative strategies. What emerges from Modernism is the quest for truth based on the knowledge that it is unattainable, or only partly attainable, a quest that destabilises traditional modes of representation and causality, when things were thought to be stable, fixed and unchanging.

This radical change in the way reality came to be perceived seems to have had no effect on medical discourse, at least when looked at from a distance, or on its perception by the general public. Medicine, like many other sciences, presents itself as positivist, something which Foucault has stressed time and again through the notion of the 'suzerainty of the gaze' (Foucault 1963: 4). Disorders are perceived through sound and examination, and through the observation of the patient's behaviour. In the world of the twenty-first century, the omnipresence of the word *'disorder' suggests that science's concern is to re-order*, or at least that there's a normal (order-ed) way of thinking which those afflicted with some disorder challenge. Is the science of the mad only righting wrongs? Isn't there something beyond this notion of 'resistance' that is worth exploring?

Within Modernism, Woolf is a valid influence to choose because given the critical literature published on her, and her own interest in her fiction, it is clear that she was indeed interested in mental illnesses as much as physical illnesses. Woolf also is the site of a debate that I delineate earlier between psychiatric-oriented critics and psychoanalyst-critics. She has now become the figurehead of the mad/afflicted author in the twentieth century, sitting undisturbed on her throne as the queen of illness, be it psychological or psychiatric (was she mad? Who should be afraid of Virginia Woolf?) or physiological (she was prone to headaches, anorexia, etc.). She attracted the attention of critics beyond literary circles for that very reason before she was set up as the undisturbed queen of feminism despite her ambiguous position (Showalter 1985; Moi 1985; Black 2004; Favre 2021). In the 1980s, within the sociological discourse of many historians, psychoanalysts and feminists who sought to stress the relation of powers that belittled women, there were books, such as *All that Summer She Was Mad: Virginia Woolf: Female Victim of Male Medicine*, which explored the diagnosis of Woolf as a mad artist and the medical discourse that underlay this claim. Commenting on the handling of symptoms and illness in literary criticism, Stephen Trombley argues that most diagnoses come from 'lay critics, who have no knowledge of medical science' (Trombley 1982: 1). This claim seems to posit the existence of a reliable, accurate 'knowledge of medical science'. 'Madness' would thus be defined as an illness like the flu, arthritis or cancer, according to a number of rules and treatment protocols that went unchallenged. And yet, for all these illnesses, not to mention what is often vaguely described, in common everyday experience, as madness, ongoing research seems to suggest that knowledge is in fact far from being fixed, that science's real—which consists of a certain number of rules and principles—is in fact nothing like the real individuals make do with: medicine is now turning to the exploration of the notion of pain, which was once assumed to be dependent on the nature of illness and which is now seen as placed in a more questionable dynamic or relationship with a specific 'ailment' or symptom. Trombley's statement is rooted in his belief in the superiority of said medical discourse: 'Clearly, the term "mad", as Bell uses it here, can have no medical meaning, no *serious* significance' (Trombley, 4, *emphasis mine*). And yet, as seen earlier, psychiatry and medicine are hardly regarded as reliable, but as seeking to be so: medical historians and scientists need to take into account the difference between science, accuracy, knowledge and truth. From Trombley's perspective, accuracy is the monopoly of science (despite the many failed attempts to which science leads (Bynum, 83–85)), while literature is frivolous and unwarranted. One of the arguments of Trombley's book is thus that having undergone no medical test (which is untrue), Woolf can only be regarded as sane (Trombley 1982: 9). And yet, when expertise is called for, critics turn to neurology (Thiher 1999: 11), as if science was a definite knowledge about the enigma of madness and could fill in the holes left in the patient's non-linear, non-causal narrative of what has happened.

The Limits of Social Interpretations
of Psychological Disorder

As madness shows the reverse of reason, it appears that madness has a social function of showing the limitation of logic and rationality when applied to human relations. It is a major threat because, by showing the reverse of reason, it logically raises the question of whether it isn't reason itself that is the reverse of irrationality. In Erasmus's *Moriae Enconium*, in 1511, the author shows that the opposite of reason is also a place where those that regard the bases of this world find them insufficiently founded: this argument is based on a series of binaries that frame the logic of late-medieval, early-Renaissance thinkers, as is found in the division between the two cities (Saint Augustine), the King's two bodies (Kantorowicz 1957), the Cartesian and Christian division of body and mind, etc. In such strict distribution between two poles, the mad person sits uncomfortably because 'mad patients' or mentally ill patients are rarely so all the time and in every circumstance; they are rarely outside language altogether and their symptoms are not always those of an ideal of madness that may never return to sanity. This ideal of a mad person who might be expelled from language and reason inevitably flourishes into visions of carnival, the analyses of Bakhtin's dialogism, the joker/idiot/fool type in theatre, all these figures of a mad person who is always so and who highlights what we consider to be normal and standard and which, by virtue of their very existence, they question (Boileau 2023).

Many critics, amongst whom quite a number of feminist critics, have analysed madness as a social and cultural phenomenon, interpreting it from a causal perspective (Showalter 1997: 7). For them, madness is not so much an illness or a clinical condition, as the manifestation of women's resistance (and some men's) to established modes of power: Showalter is quite clear that she wants gender and not class (others might argue that a refined vision would combine gender and class) to be the determining factor in the exploration of the stigma of psychiatric treatment and its underlying ideology. The semantic field of resistance is used: women are 'heroic rebels' (Showalter 1985: 4), 'champions of a defiant womanhood' (Showalter 1985: 5) and right from the introduction she states that Freud's and Ibsen's Nora, 'resist the social definitions that confine them to the doll's house of bourgeois femininity' (Showalter 1985: 5). This work pertains to the so-called second wave of feminism that expressed the need to promote female figures into the canon of artists, social commentators and historical figures. This step was crucial in establishing a discipline (gender and women studies) and in hystorising our culture.[18] Gilbert and Gubar, and followers, showed how fictional representations of madness were often the expression of the authors' personal frustration at being objectified and their weapon to resist a patriarchal discourse that equated womanhood with madness, lack of moderation and so forth.

For all its social and ideological merit, this line of argument results in a negation of the possibility of irrationality itself. Very often this interpretation tends to advocate for a change in social hierarchy and perspectives. However, it runs the risk of considering that mental illness itself does not exist, that it is caused by social factors and can therefore be suppressed by a social and cultural change. Furthermore, it restricts the interpretation of madness to a social and causal phenomenon, while literature, clinical practices and hospitals have seen a persistence of symptoms of madness, or, to use a more contemporary expression, psychological disorders. 'The figure of the mad person understood as a modern cultural fantasy shaped by psychiatry as well as literature was a founding principle in the avant-garde's discourses and textual practices' (Capé 2011: 8). As a means of defeating diagnosis altogether, the clinical interpretation by literary critics often recedes into the background, as does any other explanation that risks jeopardising the accepted view that psychiatry is an institution of power. For example, Showalter, following a method redolent of Foucauldian analysis, considers that the years 1854–1870 were the tipping point: doctors became the supreme reference in the treatment of patients suffering from mental illnesses, conflating physiological and psychological disorders (Showalter 1985: 53). She also homes in on the point that psychiatry was influenced by social Darwinism and eugenics (Showalter 1985: 99–164). Her analysis therefore focuses on a cultural history of medicine, rather than on the effects of medical discourse as they can be revealed in the very treatment that is represented in literary works. Ultimately, she apparently suggests that there was no need for any treatment and any disorder was

---

[18] This word was invented by Lacan for the preface to the English version of his *Seminar, book XI*, in 1976. It brings together various words—history, tora, hysterisation. Among other meanings, the word suggests that history and story are neurotic symptoms, while reminding everyone that the hysteric is the emblematic subjective position of neurosis. Some gender theorists have used the term to show that history should be more inclusive of women.

caused by the medical wish to overpower and reify the patients, psychiatric medicine being the instrument of patriarchy and control (this will be discussed in Part 1 of the present book).

However, all the works quoted earlier tend to see the history of this phenomenon in a very similar fashion. Three periods would seem to exist. The nineteenth century is the tipping point and in the wake of the emergence of a modern scientific discourse (Marret 2010; Bynum 1994: xi), psychiatry and the treatment of psychoses grew more sophisticated. The period before this is often seen as dating back to Ancient Greece (Porter) and having persisted through the Middle Ages (Foucault 1972), while all see the First World War as the ultimate turning point that leaves the nineteenth century very much isolated as a milestone in the development of psychiatry as a discipline, and Modern times a new era when the pendulum gradually shifts to biomedicine with no possible return. Psychiatry, unlike any other branch of medicine, has always been at the intersection of the medical and the social, and its place within the field of humanities often goes undisputed. According to Micale, for example, the discovery and treatment of hysteria originated in a very socio-cultural context and its disappearance in treatment was the result of de-Victorianisation (Micale 1993: 499): the context has as much to do with the diagnosis as scientific discovery. The discipline of psychiatry itself is comparatively recent: 'In most conventional histories of the subject, modern psychiatry begins with Pinel' (Shorter 1997: 12). And yet the list of treatments, diagnoses and misdiagnoses leads us to query whether psychiatry is a discipline or whether it is a site of diagnostic power where sub-disciplines of health care have manoeuvred. Today, the hyper-specialisation of medicine could lead one to agree with Jon Stone: 'Where once there had been a single physician for "nervous diseases" now there are two doctors: one of the brain and one of the mind' (Stone et al. 2008: 13). For instance, biomedical approaches tend to neglect 'ample data' showing 'that conversion symptoms remain very common in neurological practice, a clinical reality that is curiously not reflected in research activity, teaching or public awareness' (Stone et al. 2008: 12). This neglect has often been translated into the idea that hysteria has disappeared. Ongoing research in linguistics on communication of diagnosis within medical practice, the relentless debates around *DSM* and the training of medical staff seem to have gone unnoticed by literary critics, while this has greatly affected the way illness is now perceived and represented, or apprehended. The literature of the twentieth and twenty-first centuries saw the disappearance of the great figures of mad men and women, like the so-called disappearance of hysteria that is now disputed (Micale 1993; Showalter 1997). They were replaced by characters with small symptoms and oddities which develop and proliferate, forcing critics to readjust constantly and renew taxonomy. And yet, in recent years, these problems, internal to the sphere of 'mental health' treatment, have somehow been neglected due to lack of interest in symptoms and in the diagnosis of neurosis and psychosis.

This vision of neurosis and psychosis, which some think of in terms of sane and insane, following the binary patterns of healthy and non-healthy or disabled and normal, has been challenged by many, within and beyond the medical world (Canguilhem 1966). Most see the binary poles of healthy and not healthy on a continuum or a spectrum whose definitions largely depend on medical and scientific evidence as well as social, cultural and linguistic factors which combine for any given scientist to interpret a case. On that point, DSM-5 and Lacanian psychoanalysis are currently developing patterns of diagnosis in which spectrum and continuum are more valid references than clear-cut categories (Maleval 2019). In Lacanian psychoanalysis, the preservation of the traditional psychiatric structures of neurosis, psychosis and perversion seeks to escape the binaries of healthy and non-healthy, or normal and abnormal, by having no subject fall into a category of sanity: all subjects function mainly according to one of these diagnostic categories which orient treatment but the subjects are not free to choose—'You cannot choose to go crazy' ('*Ne devient pas fou qui veut*'), Lacan sardonically comments (Lacan 1981: 24). These terms suggest that each subject is alienated by their lack of being, to which they respond in symptomatic ways; they are the subjects of the unconscious. Even more importantly, current diagnoses tend to emphasise a greater fluidity between the various psychic structures. In Lacanian psychoanalysis, nobody is regarded as healthy or sane from a psychological point of view: subjects are, by virtue of their being caught up in the limitations of their language and in the lack created by the signifier, 'SpeakingBeings', that is, inscribed in a dysfunctional relation between their bodies, their linguistic existence and the real (Miller 2018).

As can be seen in this presentation of Woolf's case and essay, there is still a lot to say about the complex relationship between literature and (mental) illness, both fields being characterised in the contemporary era by a never-ending expansion. Indeed, as medicine became a profession, the specificities of symptomatology, treatment and nosography created separate spheres between medical knowledge and general knowledge of illnesses. In this book, I address the reduction of madness to symptoms and observe how this reduction has effects in literary productions, ways of representing madness and the perseverance of certain symptoms that are said elsewhere to have disappeared. In the field of psychiatry and mental treatment, this reduction of ailments to symptoms that can be cured and erased has sometimes given way to the argument that madness does not exist: this is exactly the point made by Szasz when he introduces the topic of madness by saying that his book will prove that madness does not exist (Szasz 1973: 21). Another example is to be found in Gagneret's use of inverted commas when she uses the term 'to signify prudence and circumspection' (Gagneret 2019: 15).

THE BOOK'S PREMISE AND STRUCTURE

If 'to link madness and writing is to perpetuate one of the greatest commonplaces of our modernity' (Capé 2011: 7), it is only insofar as there is, in the symptom of psychic disorder, something ineffable, unattainable, which never ceases to remain unwritten, to paraphrase Lacan (*'ce qui ne cesse pas de ne pas s'écrire'*, Lacan 2001: 559). Literature itself has long chronicled the state of those that fail to go through life without troubles and disorders (Mullini 1989). The question I want to raise in this work is *how literature produces, instead of simply reproducing, symptoms*, how the symptoms produced are decoded or made decipherable in a way that medicine leaves out, and *how this represented illness defies cure and care and resists the attempt currently made to erase symptoms instead of working from and around them.*

This book will therefore look at various ways of treating symptoms of psychological disorders in the literature of the long twentieth century. *This book's thesis is that the notion of symptoms has never been central to studies of literature and madness, often as a result of a lack of clarity as to what symptoms mean and how they are used in therapy.* Very often, critics and readers have endorsed or resisted diagnostic categorisation; they have followed in the footsteps of dominant medical discourses—currently neurological and biomedical or criticised the medical biases and prejudices that diagnoses and methods of treatment reflected; in other words, they have contended with notions of normality, commonality and statistical representations while affirming that subjects were being subjected, reified and stigmatised by psychiatric and 'mental health' discourses. Literary critics in the medical humanities field have accepted the authority of the symptom as a sure sign of illness and a reliable symbol to interpret. However, to use Pett's words, I do not intend, 'in celebrating the principles and practices of the humanities, and particularly those of literary studies', to suggest that 'both literature and literary studies [are] more sophisticated and more capacious in their approach to representing and interpreting illness' than they really are (Pett 2019: 56). I do not intend to pose as a clinician where I analyse literature, but rather to try and determine what it is writers teach clinicians and how they 'always precede' the theoretical framework elaborated to account for the function of symptoms (Lacan 2001: 192–193) I will try and show that literature can, in its questioning of commonly accepted views of this lived experience of psychic symptoms, *help engender new theories* about the functioning of these cases for each, singular case.

What happens indeed if the symptom is regarded not as that which should be disposed of but as the subjective response, if not the solution, to a world that subjects can never fully grasp because of their existence through and in language? The reason for this inability to grasp what their existence means is to be found in the fact that there is no essence of a subject's sense of being (no meaning or definition of who the subject is). Moreover, subjects emerge in language and therefore can only be situated in their relation to the law of language and the symbolic place they come to occupy. Bearing this in mind, what would be the effect of considering that the symptom is that which must be preserved to ensure that subjects understand how humble and frail they are in relation to language and as one of the ways of accessing a world that supersedes language itself? In Lacanian terms, symptoms and *sinthomes* are a singular, like no other, response to that which threatens to overwhelm each and every one of us, namely the humbleness and vulnerability of being agitated by what cannot be symbolised: 'Thus Lacan could call … the literary use of letters a symptom. It is not that there is a sort of literature which is symptomatic, but that literature itself is a partner of jouissance' (Soler in Rabaté 2003: 93). I will refer to contemporary Lacanian critics (Miller, Maleval, Castanet, Leguil and Marret-Maleval) but also to established critics of literature who conceive of 'rhetoric as having a performative function that is not simply co-extensive with its cognitive function' and see literature as producing rather than carrying out 'a constative or descriptive inquiry' (Felman

1978: 25). The fact that the emergence of 'mental health' care coincided with a global, artistic movement now called Modernism, invites us to reflect upon the way in which the history of medical treatment in the twentieth century—ranging from the consideration of the advent of cognitive psychology and its scientific apparatus to an understanding of the multiple fractures within the fields of psychiatry and psychoanalysis—helps understand new figures of madness in literature, and contributes to producing new symptoms that are not metaphors (Sontag 1978).

The first section of this book will therefore look at the symptom as subverting medical and psychiatric treatment. Taking the examples of *Mrs Dalloway* and its Modernist aesthetics (Chap. 2), in which the symptom is silenced and unheard in its function, I will consider more contemporary novels that continue to explore the production of meaning linked to the characters' symptoms, first through Pat Barker's *Regeneration Trilogy*, which owes so much to Woolf (Chap. 3), and secondly through Patrick McGrath's *Asylum*, which will enable me to point to the fundamental role played by interpretation in the life of the symptom, notably in its being located in sexuality and the body (Chap. 4). In the second section, therefore, sexuality and sexual identity[19] will be explored in symptomatic readings of dysfunctional relationships. First, I look at Doris Lessing's *The Fifth Child* (Chap. 5), which relates the way a woman tries to live with her disabled child and how their relationship becomes symptomatic. Secondly, I study Alan Hollinghurst's *The Line of Beauty* (Chap. 6), in which the psychic disorders of the family's daughter are treated as an inconsequential nuisance while cocaine subverts and distorts all relationships in what is largely a gay community exposed to the AIDS epidemic. In the last section, the book will turn to voices, silences and body-free modes of expression in contemporary refashionings of the stream of consciousness technique in Rachel Cusk's *Trilogy* (Chap. 7) and Ali Smith's *Seasonal Quartet* (Chap. 8). This will enable me to conclude by analysing new modes of enjoyment (*jouissance*) and new symptoms which tell a story that matters less than the core of enigmatic behaviour these new symptoms circumscribe.

---

[19] As will be explained in the chapters dedicated to this question, I understand sexual identity not as sexual orientation but as a singular, subjective relation to the question of sex and sexed bodies.

Bibliography

Primary Sources

Cusk, Rachel (2001). *A Life's Work*. London: Faber and Faber, 2008.
Forster, Edward M. (1927). *Aspects of the Novel*. Orlando, Florida: Harvest Book, 1955.
Woolf, Virginia (1926). "On Being Ill" (1930). Woolf 1948, 9–23.

Secondary Sources

DSM-5   https://cdn.website-editor.net/30f11123991548a0af708722d458e 476/files/uploaded/DSM%2520V.pdf
Baker, Charley, Crawford, Paul et al. (2010). *Madness in Post-1945 British and American Fiction*. London: Routledge.
Barber-Stetson, Claire (2016). "*On Being Ill* in the Twenty-First Century," *Woolf Miscellany*, 48–50.
Black, Naomi (2004). *Virginia Woolf as Feminist*. Ithaca, New York: Cornell University Press.
Boileau, Nicolas Pierre & Estrade, Charlotte, eds. (2021). *Modernist Exceptions*, in *Miranda*, 23: https://doi.org/10.4000/miranda.40824
Boileau, Nicolas Pierre (2023). "*Reading* Hamlet *with Lacan, the Joint of Symptoms, Desire and Time*". J. Tambling (ed.). *The Bloomsbury Handbook of Psychoanalysis and Literature*. London: Bloomsbury Academic.
Bonikowski, Wyatt (2013). *Shell-Shock and the Modernist Imagination, The Death-Drive in post-World War I Fiction*. Burlington: Ashgate.
Bourdieu, Pierre (1986). "L'Illusion biographique". in *Actes de la recherche en sciences sociales*, vol. 62–63, juin 1986, 69–72.
Burston, Daniel (2020). *Psychoanalysis, Politics and the Postmodern University*. Basingstoke: Palgrave Macmillan.
Bynum, W.E. (1994). *Science and the Practice of Medicine in the Nineteenth Century*. Cambridge: Cambridge UP, "Cambridge History of Science Series".
Canguilhem, Georges (1966). *Le Normal et le Pathologique*. Paris: Presses Universitaires de France, Quadrige, 2013.
Capé, Anouck (2011). *Les Frontières du délire: écrivains et fous au temps des avant-gardes*. Paris: Honoré Champion.
Coates, Kimberly Engdahl (2012). "Phantoms, Fancy (And) Symptoms: Virginia Woolf and the Art of Being Ill". *Woolf Studies Annual*, vol. 18 (2012), 1–28.
Couser, Thomas G. (1997). *Recovering Bodies: Illness, Disability and Life-Writing*. Madison: University of Wisconsin Press.
De Bont, Leslie (2021). "'I saw at a glance that your case was exceptional, and that you also were Occult': Comedy, magic and exceptional disabilities in Stella Benson's *Living Alone* (1919)". In N. P. Boileau and Ch. Estrade (eds.).

Modernist Exceptions, special issue of *Miranda*, 23: 2021. https://doi.org/10.4000/miranda.42498

Didi-Hubermann, Georges (1982). *Invention de l'Hystérie*. Paris: Éditions Macula, 2012.

Downie, Robin (2005). "Madness in Literature: Device and Understanding." C. Saunders and J. McNaughton (eds.), 49–66.

Favre, Valérie (2021). "Virginia Woolf et ses 'petites soeurs': Relire *A Room of One's Own* au prisme de sa postérité littéraire, critique et féministe dans l'espace Atlantique anglophone des années soixante à nos jours". Unpublished PhD Thesis, University of Lyon 2, 2021.

Felman Shoshana (1978). *Writing and Madness*, Palo Alto: Stanford UP, 2003.

Ferrer, Daniel (1990). *Virginia Woolf and the Madness of Language*. Geoffrey Bennington and Rachel Bowlby (trans.). London: Routledge, 1990.

Foucault, Michel (1963). *Naissance de la Clinique*. Paris: Presses Universitaires de France, "Quadrige grands textes", 2003. For the English version: http://monoskop.org/images/9/92/Foucault_Michel_The_Birth_of_the_Clinic_1976.pdf

Foucault, Michel (1972). *Histoire de la folie à l'âge classique*. Paris: Gallimard, "Tel".

Frances, Allen (2009). "Whither DSM-V?" *British Journal of Psychiatry*. 195:5, 391–392. doi: https://doi.org/10.1192/bjp.bp.109.073932

Frosh, Stephen (1991). "Psychoanalysis, Psychosis, and Postmodernism". *Human Relations*, vol. 44, No 1, 93–104.

Gagneret, Diane (2019). *Explorer la frontière: Folie et genre(s) dans la littérature anglophone contemporaine*. Unpublished PhD thesis defended at ENS Lyon, 22.11.2019, under the supervision of Prof. Vanessa Guignery.

Gaspard, Jean-Luc (2010). "Nouveaux symptômes et lien social contemporain". L. Jodeau-Belle & L. Ottavi (eds.) (2010). 357–371.

Gori, Roland & Del Volgo, Marie-José (2005). *La Santé totalitaire, Essai sur la médicalisation de l'existence*. Paris: Éditions Denoël, "Champs Essais".

Gualtieri, Elena (2000). *Virginia Woolf's Essays: Sketching the Past*. London: Macmillan.

Kantorowicz, Ernest H (1957). *The King's Two Bodies: a Study in Medieval Political Theology*. Princeton: Princeton University Press, 1981.

Latham, Monica (2016). *A Poetics of Postmodernism and Neomodernism*. New York: Routledge.

Lacan, Jacques (1979). "Lacan pour Vincennes!", *Ornicar?*, 17/18, Spring 1979.

Lacan, Jacques (1981). *Le Séminaire*, Livre III, *Les Psychoses* (1955–56). J.-A. Miller (ed.). Paris: Éditions du Seuil.

Lacan, Jaques (2001). *Autres écrits*. Paris: Éditions du seuil, "Champ freudien".

Lacan, Jacques (2013). *Le Séminaire*, Livre VI, *Le Désir et son interprétation* (1958–1959) J.-A. Miller (ed.). Paris: Éditions de la Martinière.

Lacan, Jacques (1991). *Le Séminaire, Livre XVII, Envers de la psychanalyse* (1970). J.-A. Miller (ed.). Paris: Éditions du Seuil.

Lacan, Jacques (2005). *Le Séminaire, Livre XXIII, Le Sinthome* (1975–76). J.-A. Miller (ed.). Paris: Éditions du Seuil.

Lanone, Catherine (2007). "Entre accord et écart: l'expérience de lecture selon Virginia Woolf et E. M. Forster". C. Bernard & C. Lanone (eds.). "Woolf lectrice/Woolf critique", *Études britanniques contemporaines*. Montpellier: Presses Universitaires de la Méditerranée, 111–124.

Laurent, Éric (2016). *L'Envers de la biopolitique. Une écriture pour la jouissance*. Paris: Editions Navarin, "Le Champ freudien".

Lecercle, Jean-Jacques (1996). *La Violence du langage*, Michèle Garlati (trans.). Paris: Presses Universitaires de France.

Lecercle, Jean-Jacques (2004). "Redondance et surclassement: pour une théorie du superflu en littérature". G. Girard (ed.). *Le Superflu chose très nécessaire*. Rennes: Presses Universitaires de Rennes, 17–32.

Lee, Hermione (1996). *Virginia Woolf.* New York: Random House, Vintage, 1999.

Lyotard, Jean-François (1984). *The Postmodern Condition, A Report on Knowledge*. Minneapolis: University of Minnesota Press.

Maleval, Jean-Claude (2012). *Étonnantes mystifications, De la psychothérapie autoritaire*. Paris: Éditions Navarin, "Le champ freudien".

Maleval, Jean-Claude (2019). *Repères pour la psychose ordinaire*. Paris: Navarin Éditeurs, 2019.

Marret, Sophie (2010). *L'Inconscient aux sources du mythe moderne: les grands mythes de la littérature fantastique*. Rennes: Presses Universitaires de Rennes.

Marret, Sophie (2017). "Importance et enjeux de la psychose ordinaire". *L'agraphe*, revue de la section clinique de Rennes 2017–18, Département de psychanalyse de Paris 8, 89–99.

Micale, Mark S. (1993). "On the 'Disappearance' of Hysteria: A Study in the Clinical Deconstruction of a Diagnosis". *Isis*, vol.84, n°3, Sept.1993, 496–526.

Micale, Mark S. & Lerner, Patrick (eds.) (2001). *Traumatic Pasts, History, Psychiatry and Trauma in the Modern Age 1870–1930*. Cambridge: Cambridge University Press.

Mijangos, Lynne (2016). "Listening for the Voices of Women: A Close Reading of Virginia Woolf's 'On Being Ill'". *Woolf Miscellany*, 64–65.

Miller, Jacques-Alain (ed.) (1998). *La psychose ordinaire. La convention d'Antibes*. Paris: Seuil.

Miller, Jacques-Alain (1999). "Les Six Paradigmes de la Jouissance". *La Cause freudienne* No. 43, 7–29.

Miller, Jacques-Alain (2018). *L'os d'une cure*. Paris: Navarin éditeur.

Minow-Pinkney Makiko (1987). *Virginia Woolf and the Problem of the Subject*. New Brunswick: Rutgers University Press.

Mitchell, Juliet & Rose, Jacqueline (1985). *Feminine Sexuality, Jacques Lacan and the école freudienne*. London: Norton.

Moi, Toril (1985). *Sexual/Textual Politics*. New York: Routledge, 2002.

Moran, Patricia (1996). *Word of Mouth, Body Language in Katherine Mansfield & Virginia Woolf.* Charlottesville: University of Virginia Press.

Mullini, Roberta (1989). "'Pardon my folly in writing of folly': Les ouvrages sur la folie de Robert Armin". Max Milner (ed.). *Littérature et Pathologie.* Paris: L'imaginaire du texte, 245–254.

Oyebode, Femi (ed.) (2009). *Misreadings: Literature and Psychiatry.* London: Royal College of Psychiatry Publications.

Pett, Sarah (2019). "Re-Thinking Virginia Woolf's *On Being Ill*". *Literature and Medicine,* volume 37, n°1, Spring 2019, 26–66.

Rabaté, Jean-Michel (ed.) (2003). *The Cambridge Companion to Lacan.* Cambridge: Cambridge University Press.

Rabeyron, T., Evrard, R. and Massicotte, C., (eds.) (2020). "Psychoanalysts and the Sour Apple: Thought-transference in Historical and Contemporary Psychoanalysis". *Contemporary Psychoanalysis,* 56 (4), 1–41.

Saudo-Welby, Nathalie (2019). *Le Courage de déplaire. Le roman féministe à la fin de l'ère victorienne.* Paris: Classiques Garnier.

Saunders, Corinne and McNaughton, Jane (eds.) (2005). *Madness and Creativity in Literature and Culture.* London: Palgrave Macmillan.

Seligman, Stephen (2019). "The New Psychoanalysis". *Dissent,* vol.66, No. 1, Winter, 97–103.

Shorter, Edward (1997). *A History of Psychiatry, From the Era of the Asylum to the Age of Prozac.* New York: John Wiley and Sons, Inc.

Showalter, Elaine (1985). *The Female Malady, Women, Madness and English Culture, 1830–1980.* London: Virago Press (1985).

Showalter, Elaine (1997). *Hystories, Hysterical Epidemics and Modern Culture.* London: Picador, 2013.

Stone, Jon, et al. (2008). "The 'Disappearance' of Hysteria: Historical Mystery or Illusion?". *Journal of Royal Society of Medicine,* 101, 12–18, DOI: https://doi.org/10.1258/jrsm.2007.070129

Soler Colette (2002). *L'Inconscient à ciel ouvert de la psychose.* Toulouse: Presses Universitaires du Mirail.

Sontag, Susan (1978–1989). *Illness as Metaphor* (1977–78) and *Aids and Its Metaphors* (1988–89). London: Doubleday.

Suhamy, Henri (1989). "Éloge de la folie ou folie de l'éloge". *Actes des congrès de la Société française Shakespeare,* 7, 9–16.

Szasz, Thomas S. (1973). *L'Âge de la folie,* Paris: PUF, 1978 [1973].

Thiher, Allen (1999) *Revels in Madness, Insanity in Medicine and Literature.* Ann Arbor: University of Michigan Press, 2004.

Trombley, Stephen (1982). *All that Summer She Was Mad, Virginia Woolf: Female Victim of Male Medicine.* New York: Continuum.

Wall, Oisin (2018). *The British Anti-Psychiatrists, from institutional Psychiatry to Counter-Culture, 1960–1971.* London: Routledge.

Zizek, Slavoj (1992). *Enjoy your Symptom! Jacques Lacan in Hollywood and Out.* London: Routledge.

PART I

Doctors' Misdiagnoses: Symptoms, Meaning and Function

CHAPTER 2

Symptomatic Silence: Situating the Subject in *Mrs Dalloway*

This is a little out of place, but then so am I. Diary, *vol. 4, 139.*

Set in the highly fashionable centre of London—the hub of British political power—the party Clarissa Dalloway is hosting (and for which she is
first seen running errands) welcomes the highest class of people. A scene
in the first part of the novel sees Clarissa combing her hair and reflecting
upon her social duties, admitting to herself her vexation at having been
shunned by Lady Bruton: 'faults, jealousies, vanities, suspicions, like this
of Lady Bruton not asking her to lunch; which, she thought (combing her
hair finally), is utterly base!' (D, 32). She then wonders where her dress is.
Clarissa Dalloway is a master in the art of 'assembling' the high and low,
the social and the essential, bringing people and values together, if only for
a party, twisting the domestic into much more than a second-rate, down-
graded activity disparagingly associated with womanhood. The novel is
thus far more interested in the lady that is hosting the party than in the
supposedly more important decisions that will be made by men—amongst
whom the Prime Minister, who, interestingly enough, is introduced as an
inconsequential guest (D, 140). Although the society described in the
novel is that of the ruling class, the traditional places of power are neglected
and the narrative casually lingers on the 'outcasts' (D, 79), or at least those
that feel as such. The characters' social status is the way in which Woolf

© The Author(s), under exclusive license to Springer Nature
Switzerland AG 2023

N. P. Boileau, *Mental Health Symptoms in Literature since
Modernism*, Palgrave Studies in Literature, Science and Medicine,
https://doi.org/10.1007/978-3-031-37630-6_2

questions the place of subjectivity in the novel: the narrative focuses on how characters remain hidden or are forced into silence, even though the text at first reads as a general exposition of internal speech through the now well-known stream-of-consciousness technique (Cohn 1978).

Clarissa Dalloway's strolls in the park are an opportunity for her to escape the higher class and reconnect with the more simple, mundane life of an 'elderly nurse' knitting (D, 50), the women of Pimlico 'giving suck to their young' (D, 6), or walk near somebody hearing birds sing in Greek: this is how Septimus Warren Smith is first introduced, in 'his shabby over-coat alone, on the seat, hunched up' (D, 20). At first sight, Septimus is only one in many characters that make but a fleeting appearance in the novel (Bowlby 2011). And yet, disregarding all etiquette rules, Septimus Warren Smith makes a sensational entrance in the highly polished world of the Dalloways, through his suicide, which accounts for Dr Bradshaw's fashionably late arrival. The humble story recounted in this grand setting reveals the defeat of two examples of what Lacan calls the master's discourse (Lacan 1991: 31): on the one hand, the social discourse of an Other that is perceived as the guarantee of right and wrong—a voice of authority made tangible in Rezia's constant concern for what people may think of her husband's disorder; on the other hand, the medical discourse, caparisoned in scientific jargon and methods, which is defeated by Septimus's suicide, a rather radical gesture for someone for whom 'there is nothing the matter' (D, 77), as Dr Holmes keeps repeating.

In the novel, which portrays a high class of social achievers as political figures seeking to help the poor and ill, the social discourse is entangled with the political and the medical: Richard Dalloway may have missed the opportunity to go to the Cabinet; he is keen to work on an Asylum Act. A similar act had been passed in 1875, but the novel suggests it is now time to review it.[1] Richard's concern, thus society's predominant discourse, focuses not on mental illness at large but on the case of those who, like Septimus, show disordered behaviour, especially in relation to the War (Bradshaw 2000; Mosse 2000; Showalter 1997). That war soldiers may be represented in the novel as failing men indicates that some counter-discourse is possible, a fictional discourse that undermines or weakens the so-called master narratives identified earlier, namely the social and medical discourses. The epic nature of the war narrative is avoided thanks to the absence of a war hero (Letissier 2019). During and in the immediate

---

[1] See H. Showalter, *The Female Malady*, for a feminist exploration of mental health laws.

aftermath of the War, the state seeks to avoid an epidemic (of a hysterical nature?) that would keep too many men away from military service. In the history of mental health, this moment is regarded as one of the causes of the first breakthroughs of psychoanalysis in the psychiatric institution (Porter 2002: 192), because the hysterical symptoms that war veterans showed destabilised the psychiatric discourse that had reached a theoretical aporia (Shorter 1997: chapter 'From Freud to Prozac'). Shorter laments the forays of psychoanalysis on various occasions, convinced as he is that psychiatry is on the side of science, unlike psychoanalysis, while recognising that science can only 'wande[r] astray in the world of quotidian anxiety and sadness, in the obsessive traits of behaviour and the misfiring personality types that are the lot of humankind' (Shorter 1997: 288). He goes on to assert that PTSD's existence 'is unclear' (Shorter 1997: 290). In any case, the novel's discussed bill informs us about the public nature of the debate that was going on about mental health care and raises the issue of what Septimus suffers from and whether all of his symptoms should be regarded as originating in the same causality, namely the War and society.

In *Mrs Dalloway*, Virginia Woolf challenges two commonplace ideas about madness, which are situated at the intersection of illness and social identity. First, the victim of psychiatric discourse is not a woman, but a man, unlike in most novels of the nineteenth century (Gilbert and Gubar 1984) and he is a soldier to boot. Elaine Showalter indicates that women were always going to be associated with madness for two reasons:[2] women are statistically more numerous in asylum patients; and there is a cultural tradition which represents woman as mad (Showalter 1985: 3–4). Charcot's hysterics certainly helped fix the association of woman and madness, even if critics like Micale have shown that these assumptions need revising, at least partially, especially in terms of class and the alleged 'pathogenic social milieu inhabited by middle-class Victorian women'

---

[2] This presentation is not accurate because the Great War tended to diminish the role that the female hysterics had played under Charcot's supervision. Diagnosis focused on PTSD. However, the influence of patients' exhibitions at the Salpêtrière, the images of treatment together with the pictures showing Charcot amongst the patients have contributed to perpetuating the long tradition that posits women as likely to be hysteric, because of Hippocrates' conception of hysteria as coming from the womb (Didi-Hubermann 1982). It is only with Briquet in the mid-nineteenth century that the diagnosis was no longer attributed solely to women. And yet, despite this realisation, it is women that continued to be institutionalised in greatest numbers (Chesler 1994).

(Micale 1993: 500). Secondly, Woolf challenges a trait of nineteenth-century therapy: the woman of high social standing is not the one that is a matter of interest, but the poor soldier. Madness is not just a bourgeois disorder as *fin-de-siècle* theatre suggested—in the theatre of Ibsen, Chekhov, Wilde, Shaw and O'Neill for example—and as Freudian psycho-analysis was accused of catering to (Burston 2020: 1–24; 90–95).

Septimus is rarely analysed for the logic of his madness but as a symbol (Gilbert and Gubar 1984: 31), or a metaphor of social disorder (Hawthorn 1975: 31–44). This is for example the thesis of one of the most influential books published on the question of madness in the novel: 'the language of their [Woolf's and Freud's] answers was literary. They wrote, not equations but narratives: not with formulae, but metaphor' (Abel 1989: x). This interpretation gives credit to the notion that Septimus is to be understood as a symbol, and in particular, the object of an attack of something else, namely the psychiatric institution:

> Woolf herself suffered patriarchal oppression particularly acutely at the hands of the psychiatric establishment, and *Mrs Dalloway* contains not only a splendidly satirical attack on that profession (as represented by Sir Bradshaw), but also a brilliantly perspicacious representation of a mind which succumbs to 'imaginary chaos' in the character of Septimus Smith. (Moi 1985:140)

The vision of Bradshaw as a satire of medical treatment and of Septimus as a fictionalisation of Woolf's condition is consensual amongst critics. Hermione Lee refers to it (Lee 2005: 42). Graham and Lewis call Septimus a 'victim of modern war and bureaucratized medication' (Graham and Lewis 2013: 103). This is no surprise as such interpretation of Septimus's behaviour belongs in the 'sociopolitical management of deviance' (Gori and Del Volgo 2020: 228) which continues a long tradition of seeing psychiatric treatment as paradoxically inhumane and a tool to wield power (Foucault 1972). Authoritative voices of Woolf's scholarship have continuously referred to Septimus's madness as somehow meaningful: 'Is Septimus Warren Smith mad or does he have a message? That he is mad would seem indisputable; even sympathetic discussions cast him as a war victim, not a prophet' (Froula 2002: 145).

One way in which this critical bias became widely consensual stems from the fact that the novel itself offers a diagnosis: Septimus is said to be in a state of '*shell shock*' (D, 155). The naming of the diagnosis in Woolf's text is evidence of its validity, accounting for some of Septimus's symptoms. As a result, most literary scholars follow in the footsteps of psychiatric nosography so that their analyses focus on the way in which this nosography manifests and is pervasive in the cultural discourse outside medical staff. Most critical works focusing on Septimus do not question the diagnosis itself (Thomas 1987) or only to update it, noting that 'shell shock' is no longer used in therapy and that the syndrome would now fall into the category of PTSD (Eberly and Henke 2007: 6; DeMeester 2007: 80–81). Some, like Bonikowski, choose to avoid the diagnosis in order to focus on something larger—madness—and probably vaguer: 'Septimus is not just "shell-shocked" but insane', the critic writes, before asserting that Septimus is 'psychotic' (Bonikowski 2013: 132; 159). Others have preferred to oppose the diagnosis because the term itself did not do justice to the disorder, preferring to identify Septimus as a paranoiac (Schlack 1979) or schizophrenic (Eberly and Henke 2007). If the treatment offered by Bradshaw leaves critics sceptical (Toth 2016: 62–64), perhaps there has been insufficient work on constructing Septimus outside the cultural and medical perspective of the 1920s. In other words, the diagnosis may matter less than the usage Septimus makes of his symptom(s).

Shell shock is now regarded not only as a psychiatric condition but also as a political tool thanks to which psychiatry was to align with the social necessity of the time, which enjoined doctors to establish the condition, cure it and possibly give guidance regarding material reparation (Micale and Lerner 2001: 1–3; 7). Because of shell shock, mental illness was no longer defined by the symptom but by its cause, and the same causes are expected to produce the same effects. This tends to make us oblivious to the individual logic at play behind the subjective effect of some symptoms. In that instance, the War is likely to induce comprehension and sympathy in the general public since the Great War was in itself a collective trauma and formed a paradigm of violence that left very few untouched. War had obviously destabilised courageous, if not heroic, soldiers, like Septimus who is covered with medals ('he had won crosses', D, 75) and yet incapable of functioning as a masculine social being.[3]

---

[3] For essential reads on the question of shell shock as a convenient term in psychiatric diagnoses to make sense of what was essentially perceived as a masculine shortcoming, and therefore a threat to the patriarchal institution of the army at a time when war was raging, see Showalter (1985: Chap. 7, 167–194); see also Bonikowski (2013: 6–10).

In the following chapter, I thus intend to trace the reasons why the novel deploys such an interest in the social understanding of illness in order to delve into the psychic intricacies of a character marked by his exclusion from society. This will help me identify the specificity of Septimus's symptoms, which are anti-social in essence and prove the dominant discourse of medicine wrong. Thus, it can be argued that Septimus is in fact barred from using his own symptoms towards fitting back into society because the doctors treating him do not question the function of the symptoms he shows, only wishing them gone.

THE SOCIOPOLITICS OF MENTAL DISORDER: THE SYMPTOMS GENERATED BY SOCIETY

In the novel, the sociopolitical status of the characters and their psychological states intersect. Mrs Dalloway's 'worldly' nature for example attracts her friends' criticism: 'Clarissa was at heart a snob—one had to admit it, a snob' (D, 161).[4] Clarissa's life revolves around lunches out and hosting parties for the greatest ranks of society. She is a snob because she lives in a world where the prime minister might be driving past her flower shop in the morning and might find himself in her house in the evening. Above all, she is a snob because she would rather go and welcome people who are regarded as superior (the Bradshaws), even if she doesn't like them, than talk to her old and dear friends (Sally and Peter). In addition to this, although her husband is a Member of Parliament, she is said to believe that she has married 'beneath her' (D, 161). Clarissa epitomises a certain idea of the socialite, somebody who seems at ease in the world of the high and powerful, even if the novel does not focus solely on the well-off. The pathologisation of dismay and depression amongst the upper classes has perceptible social effects in the Dalloways' circle: almost all the characters, bar Richard but perhaps including the Royals, have had to be seen by Bradshaw. The latter is presented as a successful man for himself but also for the Nation: 'Sir William not only prospered himself but made England prosper, secluded her lunatics, forbade childbirth, penalized

---

[4] The question appears *verbatim* in the novel. Woolf was to use the very term for herself in the 1936 essay 'Am I a Snob?' (Woolf 2002: 62–77). The specific value of the term in the essay has been commented on by many, such as Lee (1996): 682–683, Reviron (2004) and Latham (2003).

despair, made it impossible for the unfit to propagate their views until they, too, shared his sense of proportion' (D, 84). This patriotic aspect links the novel to its post-war context and underlines the social and political function of mental health care at the time.

The stress laid on the social implications of those involved in the treatment of the ill may point to the denunciation of a society that engenders mental disorders, following a neo-Victorian trend. It is equally suggestive of the fact that society and culture produce their own symptoms: 'Septimus's experience of his society's disavowed violence is labelled madness' (Froula 2002: 127). One immediately recognises the Freudian process of repression (Freud 1926: 4–6) in the novel's suggestion that illness, of a psychic nature—and perhaps of a physical nature too, but this is not mentioned—is that which cannot be named or spoken about because society rejects it. Christine Froula calls the silence about one's own state of mind 'censored truth' (Froula 2002: 145). Freudian readings of *Mrs Dalloway* are numerous, and they show a vast range of interests from the revelation of unconscious, hidden meanings (Abel 1989) to the death drive (Bonikowski 2013: 159) or the link between mourning and meaning (Froula 2002), and even the invalidity of Freudian theory (Broughton 1987), for example when repression is interpreted as a symptom instead of being a Kleinian mode of reparation (Coates 2012: 14). And yet, what is most striking is the social insistence that less is more when it comes to speaking about one's emotional state: silence about one's psychic disorders and ailments plays a far major role in the novel's exposition of what hinders intersubjective relations than the actual uncovering of unconscious desires; mental illness is therefore marked by the difficulty, if not the impossibility to be voiced (cf. Woolf's 'On Being Ill').

The paradigmatic response to illness in the novel is silence, as if health was a sheer question of social standing and appropriateness: '[Lady Bruton replied.] "... And how are you?"/"Oh perfectly well!" said Clarissa (Lady Bruton detested illness in the wives of politicians)' (D, 152). If Lady Bruton expresses such strong views about illness, it is because she has noticed a trend in politicians' wives. Miss Kilman, for example, is very happy to share her own suffering and hear the story of other people's afflictions (D, 115), but Mrs Dalloway cannot stand her attitude. When Clarissa meets the Whitbreads in the park, Hugh's reported speech reads: 'Other people came to see pictures; go to the opera; take their daughters out; the Whitbreads came "to see doctors"' (D, 5). 'Seeing doctors' is ironically listed as being on the same footing as any other social activity, showing Clarissa's spiteful opinion about such practice. Evelyn Whitbread might be suffering from 'some internal ailment, nothing serious' (D, 5) but Clarissa is sensitive enough to not ask questions, lest it should belittle her friend—and yet the reader is made aware that Evelyn is going to see Sir Bradshaw. Besides, another sign of the social appropriation of the medical discourse in intersubjective interaction is to be found in the English usage of leaving out the medical title (Dr) for a social title (Sir) when doctors have reached a level of reputation and expertise that sets them apart from regular practitioners. If 'nothing serious' is ever found by the doctors in the narrative, it is still better not to say anything about it, which is a modality of Lacan's 'not wanting to know anything about it', a formulation which reflects the neurotic repression and its social process, known as inhibition (Lacan 1975: 9 and 101–105[5]).

Septimus himself, despite his being presented as vulnerable because of his loneliness and demeanour, is forced into silence for half of the novel. He incessantly fails to meet the doctors with whom he would be allowed to speak; the meeting with Sir Bradshaw is deferred almost until the end of the novel. Septimus's violent outbursts when he is interviewed by Holmes or when Holmes is called for, take him out of his neurasthenia and silence. From Holmes's point of view, illness lends itself to decoding, without involving the subjectivity of the patient. This is partly the vision Freud had at the time: 'Symptom could be said to be a clue and substitute of some satisfaction linked to a drive that could not be accomplished, or again the successful process of repression' (Freud 1926: 7). Clarissa's own illness is, in that respect, quite revelatory. What happened to her before this day in June is only referred to in subtle, discreet signs that are hinted at but never fully explored by the narrator. She had headaches (D, 54), we are told that she had to be bedridden for a while because of a physical illness (D, 31), and David Bradshaw thinks that she might have caught the flue that killed 230,000 British people in 1917–1918 or gone through menopause (D, xxxv). However, this illness has had other consequences (or causes) because she and Richard now sleep in separate bedrooms, and she now is in a room that seems to be situated up in the attic (D, 26–27),

[5] The pages quoted refer to Brink's translation in the English version of the seminar.

maybe as a sly, ironic comment on the nineteenth-century literature's place of women.[6] It is also said that Clarissa, when ill, went to see Sir Bradshaw, which calls for a link between Clarissa and Septimus (D, 155). There is no denying that on a certain level, the text seems to explore the barrier of the repressed, which makes illnesses of a psychological nature jeopardise social norms and conventional, accepted behaviour.

Most characters seem to be guilty of 'the simplest egotism, the most open desire to be thought first always' (D, 146), even the ones who seem to be on the side of sanity: Peter Walsh, whom we see roaming the Dalloways' neighbourhood with the unacknowledged desire to join Clarissa for her party, while casting a patronising eye on her and this society he loathes and loves; Sir Bradshaw and Richard Dalloway, who do not stop over the case of Septimus who they see only as one in a million cases that need legislation, and so forth. In other words, Woolf seems to show a structural impossibility to speak about what upsets the characters, a feature not restricted to Septimus only—a fact that Bonikowski sees as inherent to Septimus's suicide (a public act) (Bonikowski 2013: 162) but which I would see as a more general feature of the society Woolf depicts.

Inhibition is a process that doctors themselves are subjected to, even in their practice. It is almost as if they avoided hearing a truth they may not know about. Dr Holmes refuses to see that which he is meant to check when he is called for. He does not examine his patient's body; he chooses to describe Septimus's state as 'funk' (D, 78), a choice of word that insists on Septimus's cowardly panic. It is not a medical term and sounds like a judgement, if not a criticism. It is also a way of not labelling the illness, if illness it be, and falling short of establishing a diagnosis. When Septimus cries 'You brute! You brute!', Dr Holmes decides to interpret it as 'nonsense' (D, 79), once again a paradoxical reaction that lays the emphasis on common sense rather than medical knowledge, on emotion rather than professional distance. Not to mention that Holmes is contradicted by the scene itself which has depicted his own attitude as brutal towards Septimus indeed, so that Holmes is perceived as incompetent. Dr Holmes is happier to evoke common sense than medical evaluation. He represses what

---

[6] Clarissa's attic could be an allusion to that which contains Bertha Mason in *Jane Eyre*, but Woolf has reversed the values traditionally associated with the 'madwoman in the attic': 'Whereas Bertha's attic is a place of tropical heat and sexuality, of latent physical violence, Clarissa's has the chill atmosphere of a mortuary' (Minow-Pinkney 1987: 68).

Septimus has to say and trusts Rezia to know what Septimus suffers from: she is the one he asks questions about Septimus's suffering. Sir Bradshaw shares this method of examination.

And yet, the repressed cannot be the unique, valid explanation, because Woolf's modernist technique does not rest on binaries, between knowing and not knowing, the rational and the irrational, 'this and that' or 'this is madness, this sense', to parody two expressions that initially give rhythm to the text. What Septimus's response to the doctors, his silence and his sudden outbursts, reveal is the fragility of the subject,[7] here destabilised by the oppressive science of the doctors, a science that Toth describes as an 'authoritarian doctrine' whose power is 'rational and mortifying' (Toth 2016: 62). Bradshaw's discriminatory method can be interpreted along the Foucauldian terminology of 'lines of fissure/fracture' (Foucault 1972: 103) between the normal and pathological:

> The friends and relations of his patients felt for him the keenest gratitude for insisting that these prophetic Christs and Christesses, who prophesied the end of the world, or the advent of God, should drink milk in bed, as Sir William ordered; Sir William with his thirty years' experience of these kinds of cases and his infallible instinct, this is madness, this sense; his sense of proportion. (D, 84–5)

The narrative irony seeks to underline that there is no knowledge that does not fail, even the law of science, despite the social value of the doctor's judgement and its social function.

The social understanding of the symptom is therefore prevalent in the text but it does not account for Septimus's symptoms because Septimus is already outside society, an outcast of sorts who has no relation other than with his wife. I now want to trace the logic at play in his subjective position, the very aspect of this experience which medical knowledge is shown to overlook. As historical approaches to psychiatry have argued, psychiatry's initial function was not to help: 'All of these institutions had solely custodial functions. Traditional society had no notion of delivering therapy to patients' (Shorter 1997: 4). Doctors therefore may not want to cure him. What is noticeable is that Septimus does not show any sign of repression, but all his relations make sure he remains silent/-ced. I will

---

[7] In this chapter, as in the rest of the book, 'subjects' is used in the Lacanian sense of being an effect of language and enunciation, a linguistic production.

argue that his silence is not just his being silenced. Septimus's silence could thus be analysed as a symptom revealing the underlying logic of his subjectivity beyond the social question of etiquette.

Septimus's Silence: A Sign of His Symptoms Being Unheard in Their Function

After reviewing some of the most consensual cultural analyses of Septimus, I will argue that the causality such comments focus on does not take into account the subjective logic exposed in the novel. Critics have documented the many autobiographical echoes underlying the representation of madness offered by Woolf and the social discourse thus evoked. What has been less central is the logic of the therapeutic effect engendered by doctors who silence, instead of listening; who know in advance, instead of being illuminated by their patients' articulation of their subjective logic. I will thus look at the function of transference in the novel in order to highlight what is left out of the causal explanation, which concerns the definition or isolation of a core of being that is ungraspable in language.

Cultural analyses see in the opposition between Septimus (and Clarissa) and the doctors evidence of a reappraisal of psychiatry as a dominant discourse that cripples individuals. In his analysis of Woolf's novels, Whitworth looks at the theme of illness with an eye trained in cultural analysis. He therefore insists that the doctors' approach to Septimus's ailment corresponds to that of the 'rest cure', which, he tells us, was common practice at the time and a well-accepted form of therapy founded partly on common sense (Whitworth 2005: 170–172). The following quote is often mentioned by critics as a sure sign of the cultural phenomenon Woolf is said to be the mediator of:

> Health is proportion; so that when a man comes into your room and says he is Christ (a common delusion), and has a message, as they mostly have, and threatens, as they often do, to kill himself, you invoke proportion: order rest in bed; rest in solitude; silence and rest; rest without friends, without books, without messages; six months' rest; until a man who went in weighing seven stone six comes out weighing twelve. (D, 84)

Indeed, this passage shows that the 'rest cure' is Woolf's reference when she depicts the doctor's response to Septimus's illness, but stopping here does not delve into the logic of the novel, nor does it illuminate the logic of Septimus as a character. It shows the cultural impregnation of such a form of therapy. What it does is affirm that the novel reflects a commonly accepted view of medicine and has cultural significance as a result. Whitworth's initial question, 'What has caused Septimus Warren Smith's breakdown?' (Whitworth 2005: 169), suggests that the novel necessarily shows a logical relation between a state of mind and an identifiable cause, preferably one external to the subject. This runs the risk of making us overlook the fact that Septimus shows great anxiety even when the doctors are not present, and his inner reflections can be likened to that of a delirious person. In other words, he is characterised by symptoms that cannot be fully restricted to the effect of the medical institution.[8] The novel, I argue, does show how 'scientific ideas' dominant at the time influenced the writing of Septimus's case, but Septimus is not reducible to a case study, which would be the statistical attitude of medicine as depicted in the novel. Septimus offers a vision that goes beyond the scientific knowledge and touches upon a modernist vision of enigma and truth perceptible in the shattering of meanings that a character such as Septimus produces.

It is hardly necessary to recall the way Woolf herself reflects upon the fictional function of madness in her *Diary*, given how often this passage is quoted: 'In this book I have almost too many ideas. I want to give life and death, sanity and insanity; I want to criticise the social system, & to show it at work, at its most intense' (*Diary* 2: 248). This and other such comments have led many to use Septimus's representation as a persona for Woolf and the way she derides doctors as an attack on those that tried to cure her during her life. The notion of the double also explains why the mirror effect of the interplay between Clarissa and Septimus enables some to look at another example of this doubleness: the novel's characters are said to be mirror images of Woolf herself. It has been noticed for example that Septimus's name may originate in the number 7, which was Woolf's position among her siblings. More significant still, the symptoms of Septimus have been said to recall some of Woolf's. Woolf's diaries, Quentin Bell's biography and Leonard Woolf's autobiography certainly reveal that there are similarities and referential echoes between Woolf's

---

[8] 'The definition of *DSM-III* however shows its usual psychiatric usage, which ties in together the following three notions: the wrongness of judgement, unshakable conviction and the deviance from a cultural norm' (Maleval 1997: 9). Delirium is no longer a category used in psychiatry, but it has remained extremely fruitful in psychoanalysis where analysts refer to Lacan's seminar on *Psychoses* in order to locate the subject's jouissance and to orient therapy (Lacan 1981).

experience of mental illness and Septimus's. Woolf heard birds sing in Greek, like Septimus (Bonikowski 2013: 138–146); Septimus reads Dante in Italy in 1917, which Woolf also did (Bort 2002). Less anecdotal, Septimus commits suicide, something Woolf herself did in 1941, pressed by the bombings of Southern England, after several attempts. For many, this justifies an autobiographical reading of Woolf's works, especially in authoritative voices of academia: 'Contributors to this volume ground their literary interpretations in the premise that Woolf's artistic *oeuvre* was profoundly affected and shaped by the consequences of the trauma she endured' (Eberly and Henke 2007: 5).

Hermione Lee furthers this idea by choosing to see Woolf's doctors as 'practising equanimity' (Lee 1996: 174) and wonders why Woolf follows the progress of the psychiatric treatment of the time by 'accepting apparently without irony the current official attitudes' (Lee 1996: 187). Lee therefore argues that not only Woolf's life explains her fictionalisation of treatment, but that she shows very little distance from such therapy: 'Virginia Woolf, to an extent, incorporated their terminology [of the law-making doctors] into her accounts of her own states of mind' (Lee 1996: 189), which authorises a vision of Septimus as only a case study (DeMeester 2007: 81). Many biographical critics have worked from this assumption, since the publication of *Sounds from the Bell Jar*, seeking to establish a posthumous diagnosis of the author (Gordon et al. 1990: 186–244).[9] And yet, Woolf seems to have had a very different vision of her own symptoms, as shown in some of her autobiographical writings: elsewhere, I have shown that Woolf's own approach to her traumatic experience was based on undermining most theories of the supposed relevance of certain causes and symptoms in order to offer her own (re)construction of the logic at play in her psychic troubles (Boileau 2014).

The reception of Woolf's factual and fictional symptoms nevertheless shows that some discourses are legitimised by critics, the result of a complex relation between the accessibility of the arguments made by mental health discourse to people outside the medical and caring professions, as well as the construction of public opinion as spread through the upper classes' practices and modes of enjoyment. This is in part what the novel's discussion of the function of illness within the highest ranks of British society serves. It is developed in Woolf's critical historiography. In *Beginning Again*, Leonard explains how during Woolf's 1913–1915

---

[9] These pages refer to a chapter entitled 'Shadows on the brain'.

major fit, often associated with the publication of *The Voyage Out*, he had chosen to be advised by Maurice Craig in Harley Street (in the same street as Bradshaw), and to stop confiding in Sir Savage alone, Virginia's G.P., whose sole therapy was to walk, to get some fresh air and avoid overwork (Woolf 1964: 168–169). Leonard's analysis shows how medical discourse operates by seeking to erase bodily symptoms without necessarily delving into the subjective function these symptoms may have. Woolf was diagnosed as 'neurasthenic', meaning that she suffered from a *disproportionate* form of nervosity: for Leonard, the difference between a normal person and his wife is a variation in degree rather than nature (Woolf 1964: 76–77), like some critics (Rigney 1978: 54). Leonard Woolf concludes that the 'rest cure' was inefficient but he does not raise the question of the symptoms themselves, neither the ones preceding nor the ones produced by the treatment. He only focuses on physical symptoms, in particular the anorexic syndrome that worries him greatly because he sees it as the sign of his wife's weakness, while her words and what she says of these symptoms go unrecorded by him. Leonard's nursing role could not but reinforce the critics' temptation to see Septimus as based on an accurate depiction of an illness Woolf had known regularly throughout her life. This is the case with H. Lee and Poole amongst many. In recent years, scholars have often looked at Woolf's fiction in relation to the question of trauma and psychiatric treatment in order to see how clear-sighted Woolf was about the symptoms of PTSD and to engage with how fiction can fit the scientific knowledge derived from victim records[10] (DeMeester 2007: 81; Moran 2007). Others wonder to what extent the inclusion of scientific discourse is indeed based on knowledge Woolf had acquired: 'It is difficult for the reader to determine the extent to which the author was incorporating [scientific ideas] consciously' (Whitworth 2005: 169).

However, in Lacanian psychoanalysis, symptoms are not just there to be decoded—even if this was Lacan's initial approach, largely influenced by Freud (Boileau 2023). Instead, Lacan proposes that the symptom should be regarded as the production of the subject's response to his *jouissance*, that is, that which, because language fails to name the world, is left over, rejected, and remains unsymbolised. According to Lacan, symptoms are produced in the literary text ('Poetic creations engender, rather than

---

[10] 'Trauma studies are commonly agreed to have begun in the US in 1980 when a campaign by Vietnam veterans influenced the American Psychiatric Association to accept the condition of war trauma under the diagnosis of PTSD' (Anderson 2012: 5).

mirror, psychological creations' (Lacan 2013: 296)) as well as through the enactment of the subject's relation to their own *jouissance*. In *The Sinthome*, Lacan studies Joyce and comes up with a new direction for his theory of the symptom, one in which the symptom no longer is that which needs deciphering, but quite paradoxically, that which remains an enigma (Lacan 2005). The *sinthome* or symptom enables the patient to fit into society by knotting together language and *jouissance*: at this point in his reflection, Lacan asserts that the symptom (renamed *sinthome*) is outside discourse (Miller 2004: 23), that it 'does not say anything to anyone', because it is the operator of the ciphering of *jouissance* (Miller 2004: 24 qd in Marret-Maleval) which enables the subject to circumscribe that which threatens to overwhelm them. In this respect, Septimus also exists outside the reference to Woolf's context because he offers a way of showing how the symptom works: the symptom is stripped of its imaginary dimension (its meaning) but still comprehensible as produced by the intersubjective, therapeutic relation.

Septimus offers an example of a subjectivity that cannot be controlled or administered, thereby signifying the unfixed character of the subject of language, but his presence in the text is also a reminder of the vanity of a knowledge that seeks to cure an affliction—here depressive emotions—that is not so much an illness as a human condition.[11] Medicine disregards the question of the patients' and the doctors' own desires and thus remains blind to the subjective logic that produces symptoms. The literary discourse on the other hand reveals that which is rejected from other discourses. Dr Holmes seeks to find something 'the matter', that is something wrong with Septimus's body and organs; for him, representing a tradition of physical symptomatology, an illness is perceivable through positivist observation. Holmes thus remains ignorant of the effects of the unconscious, both his patients' and his own. In particular, he ignores one of the most undisputed theoretical aspects of Freud's theory in the handling of patients: transference. Transference is the unconscious link between the

[11] 'For a long time, schizophrenia seemed to stand for the prevalent form of madness in our culture's imagination but in the beginning of the twentieth century, it began to be deposed and replaced by ... depression' (Ehrenberg 1998). Jacques-Alain Miller's interview for *Charlie Hebdo* on November 21st, 2007, entitled 'If sadness is an illness, then the whole of humanity is sick' (*Si la tristesse est une maladie, alors c'est l'humanité aussi qui est une maladie*) can be checked at the following link: http://forumdespsychiatres.org/index.php?option=com_content&view=article&id=682:jam-charlie-hebdo-21-nov-2007&catid=90:mdicament&Itemid=45.

patient and therapist. This relation is essential to the role played by the doctor (and by extension and in certain contexts teachers, politicians, clergy people, etc.), even if doctors are not always fully aware of it. The manipulation of transference can lead to 'suggestion', namely 'the influence exercised through the processes of transference that the therapist can cause' (Freud 1912). Freud himself recognised that he had been a victim of the dangerous consequences of transference when he agreed that what he had done with Dora, his patient, was faulty. This is why Porter claims that psychoanalysis could never get rid of its reputation of acting via suggestion (Porter 2002: 188). Jean-Claude Maleval argues that these phenomena can cause very negative symptoms even when the symptoms the patients had first come with have given way to an apparent improvement:

> What is the value of a statistical apprehension of the disappearance of symp-
> toms, when one knows that the eviction of a symptom is compatible with
> the persistence of unhappiness? An anorexic successfully conditioned to gain
> weight and who commits suicide a few months after being discharged, dies
> statistically cured. (Maleval 2012: 11)

He continues to explain: 'one of the data the least challenged regarding the evaluation of therapies contradicts T. Nathan's thesis: most studies come together to confirm that the "therapist" is more important than the kind of therapy they resort to' (Maleval 2012: 28). All of this leads us to establish that symptoms may be related to the psychiatric knowledge that, when totalitarian and authoritative, may lead to the production of even more serious suffering. If it is true that Septimus barely ever speaks, I do not see this silence as a symptom of Septimus's repression but rather as the consequence of his encounter with a discourse that belittles his own mode of *jouissance* which is linked to a difficulty to symbolise the world, i.e. to see words as symbolically referring to, instead of being, the reality. In other words, Septimus may show signs of repression, but he does not obey this logic and his case can only be seen as a very specific way of knotting together various aspects of his experience, a singularity perhaps impossible to relate to other subjects.

The novel unfolds how the encounter between patients and doctors fails because of the logic of Septimus's subjective presence. Holmes and Bradshaw are like Bouvard and Pécuchet, satirical versions of the medical professions, which goes to show that Woolf was not fooled by this dis-course: convinced that they hold an unfailing knowledge which has made them successful, the two doctors approach psychological treatment like physical cure, considering the symptom as a trustworthy and easy-to-grasp gateway to the illness. In the same way, they think of common sense as a form of reason:

> He could see the first moment they came into the room (the Warren Smiths they were called); he was certain directly he saw the man; it was a case of extreme gravity. It was a case of complete breakdown—complete physical and nervous breakdown, with every symptom in an advanced stage, he ascertained in two or three minutes (writing answers to questions, murmured discreetly, on a pink card). (D, 81)

The pantomime of softness and empathy is counterbalanced by the sarcasm of the narration that hides the answers and questions as if to signify that the interview indeed is useless and fails to connect patient and doctor. It is noteworthy that sight (seeing) is immediately translated into a viable and authoritative diagnosis, underlined by the narrative voice, the absence of modality and the phrase 'it was,' suggesting that the doctor answers his own questions. The subject paradoxically disappears in the observation, a very Foucauldian theme:

> The Clinic is not a means of uncovering some truth that would be yet to discover; it is a certain way of using a truth that is already known and to present it in such a way that it systematically seems to appear. [...]
>
> The act of looking does not cover a field, it falls onto a point, which has the privilege of being the central and decisive point; the gaze indefinitely changes, the look goes straight to the point: it chooses and the line it draws in one quick glance produces in an instant the distribution of the essential thing. (Foucault 1963: 59; 123)

Bradshaw diagnoses Septimus because he already knows what a patient like him is supposed to suffer from: Bradshaw's clinical practice is not based on singularity but frequency, not on what the patients' words point to, but on his own knowledge. 'Reflecting on its situation, (medicine) identifies the origin of its positivity with a return—over and above all theory—to the modest but effecting level of the perceived' (Foucault 1963: xii). Foucault shows that medicine thinks of itself as a modest science, one based on common perception. Yet, for all their (common) sense, Bradshaw and Holmes are unaware of this, and their prognosis is not supported by a narratorial diagnosis. Septimus first of all is introduced as someone who needs to be probed and who is inaccessible, even to his wife; it will become clear in his final act that Septimus could not be cured by science because science obliterates the singular mode of *jouissance* which agitates subjects and because science needs facts established by statistical frequency.

Following the Lacanian argument that Hamlet is not a procrastinator but only procrastinates in a certain context (Lacan 2013; Boileau 2023), I want to argue that Septimus is not silent but silence is an effect of his logic. Septimus only remains silent in a very specific context, when faced with questions. The first time he appears, although it is not clear what words he utters, we are told that he cannot stop speaking: 'But no; there he was; still sitting alone on the seat, in his shabby overcoat, his legs crossed, staring, talking aloud' (D, 21). As pointed out later in the novel, talking is by no means a way of communicating and here, Septimus is indeed the negative image of Clarissa, whose talk is always a social means of interaction, no matter how small, inconsequential, the talk might be. By contrast, Septimus's talk is real in the Lacanian sense, that is, inescapable and incommunicable, unrelated to meaning or comprehension. Hence, the fact that it cannot bear to be ended: Rezia's attempts at intervening can only be met with anger from Septimus because she overlooks the function talking has: 'interrupted again! She was always interrupting' (D, 21). Septimus's symptom is here only comprehensible within the context of her question: 'What are you saying?', which is directed at the level of meaning instead of targeting the real presence of the talk, irrespective of its signification 'matter', since language is the site of *jouissance* (Miller 1999). We could say that Rezia does not take into account the enjoyment of the signifying process, and remains deaf to the very act Septimus engages in.

Moreover, Rezia, like Holmes and Bradshaw, misreads Septimus because she interprets what Septimus says or his behaviour along the lines of a subjective division. This is how she thinks she can account for his lack of consistency. This imagined subjective division is akin to the notion of repression and stems from the idea that human beings fail to be transparent to themselves: 'And it was cowardly for a man to say he would kill himself, but Septimus had fought; he was brave; he was not Septimus now' (D, 20). Mixing gender and social identities with the nineteenth-century tradition of exploring division as a split in personality, Rezia sees Septimus as the site of conflicting qualities in relation to masculinity. Bradshaw's idea of a man is also that of a fighter, a soldier, somebody who experiences no fear and doesn't dread the consequences of his action:

'You served with great distinction in the War?'
The patient repeated the word 'war' interrogatively.
He was attaching meanings to words of a symbolical kind. A serious symptom to be noted on the card. (D, 81)

Here Bradshaw, who is associated with science and knowledge, wants to reinforce the ideal self of Septimus with another example of an unflinching discourse, that of war. This affects Septimus's position as subject, since he is not given a say, which effectively turns him into an object of language, forced to accept the suggestion inferred by the rhetorical question. Bradshaw's interpretation of the repetition Septimus provides, in indirect speech, silences that which has been said: Septimus's repeating the word 'war' does not preclude a symbolic meaning, but there is nothing in the speech act itself to suggest it. If anything, the word 'war' could be thought to lead to a metonymic relation with Septimus's current obsession with the death of his friend Evans, since this is what was on his mind before he entered Bradshaw's practice. Another possible interpretation is that the word is repeated because it fails to mean something, and the absence of associations tends to confirm that it cannot be metaphorised, that is, symbolically connected to bravery, danger, bombings, army and so forth.

Besides, Bradshaw is unaware that by mentioning the war, he touches upon what leaves Septimus perplexed and, paradoxically, what makes him talk aloud to himself and others, all the time. The unfailing discourse about War and the ideal of the soldier have precipitated his lack of emotion, which is at the origin of his feeling of anxiety. The resurfacing of that discourse, detached from his experience of war, may account for his disappearance in the realm of language. Septimus's first delirious experience takes place in the park where he is sitting with Rezia, waiting for 'the time' of their appointment with Sir Bradshaw. It is part of Dr Holmes's recommendation that Septimus should not read but should rather enjoy the simple pleasure of a walk (D, 78), so as to retrieve control and 'a sense of proportion' (in the words of Bradshaw, D, 84–85). In social terms, Holmes's 'pushing Shakespeare aside' can also be regarded as an attempt at controlling the lower classes, by confining Septimus to the humble and simple. Foucault insists on the notion that madness is the excess of a science that is based on error and misconception, that is disproportionate, words that echo Bradshaw's own distrust of educated people and literature (Foucault 1972: 39–41). Woolf's subtle irony is also detectable in her giving the doctor and the poet the same first name. It is a similar class relation that is foregrounded when the couple meet Sir Bradshaw, whose social standing is reinforced by the absence of academic title, the motor car, the fees, and the spite he feels against cultivated people. The two doctors' medical knowledge and stance blind them to the content of Septimus's delirium—which is never listened to, nor given any space during the appointments. It is as if what constitutes Septimus's own response to language and reality was uninvited in the doctors' records. In the words of Dr Holmes, it is better to cut him short and force him to focus on something else, as if with a child: '"Look, look, Septimus!" she cried. For Dr Holmes had told her to make her husband (who had nothing whatever seriously the matter with him but was a little out of sorts) take an interest in things outside himself' (D, 18). In that respect, Septimus shares the plight of those who feel 'dejected' like the frumps on doorsteps that Clarissa would prefer to remain oblivious to. This is the result of his being confronted with a discourse that grants him no place. Indeed, Lacan shows how the subject needs to negotiate a place in relation to the discourse of the Other that threatens to belittle him/her and in some cases may reduce him/her to the position of waste (Lacan 2011): 'it might be possible… it might be possible that the world itself is without meaning' (D, 75). The radical absence of meaning suggests that language, for him, is not used for its meaningfulness.

What Septimus's introspective soliloquy—which psychiatry would then have called delirium—reveals however, beyond the meaningful logic of its association of ideas, is the structural place given to science for him—an organising principle in his world. 'Heaven was divinely merciful, infinitely benignant. It spared him, pardoned his weakness. But what was the scientific explanation (for one must be scientific above all things)? Why could he see through bodies, see into the future, when dogs will become men?' (D, 58) Here is made clear how Septimus is belittled by the discourse of the Other ('spare', 'benignant', 'weakness'), a discourse that highlights his defect and lack (another common point with Clarissa, who always feels scolded by Peter) and places him in the paradoxical position of the one who knows more (he sees what others do not) and of the one that is looked down upon. The delusional aspect of his vision, and the fact that his suggestions defy the laws of physics are not questioned but asserted; his reflection is thus taken for granted and he seeks proof of what he already knows, like the (mad) doctors he is faced with. This is what enables me to define his reflection as delirious (Maleval 1997). What his attention is focused on is the logical explanation behind his elaborations, in order to establish that it is not 'nonsense', but something that has a relevant, structural place for him: 'the great revelation took place' (D, 79).

Septimus eventually experiences an epiphanic moment in which the truthful nature of his words dominates their imaginary meaning. The reference to science, which is the very discourse Rezia trusts to save him, can be the sign of a temptation for the rational, but it can also be an ironic comment on an ideal he barely trusts himself. This pervading irony which affects both the way the doctors are presented, the practice of clinical analysis and the tone of Septimus's delirium can be likened to what Jacques-Alain Miller explains when he deals with the difference between irony and humour:

> Irony and humour both make us laugh but their structure differs.
>
> Humour is the comic side of the ego [...]. Humour has something to do with the Other.
>
> Irony on the other hand does not have anything to do with the Other, but belongs in the subject and goes against the Other. What does irony say? It says that the Other does not exist, that social ties are essentially a sham, and that there is no discourse that is not just sheer semblance. (Miller 1993: 7)

This indicates that Septimus's response to other people getting in the way of his own babbling is ironical in the sense that it targets the Other (the scientific discourse, the language of authority) as sham, shaming and ultimately inapt to offer a guarantee of truth. The character's perception is constructed on the basic opposition between the irrational nature of his hallucinations and the scientific method, if not discourse, that seeks to put it at rest, revealing in this rift the irony Miller mentions between creativity and obedience: 'It was merely a question of rest, said Sir William; of rest, rest, rest; a long rest in bed.... "One of *my* homes, Mr Warren Smit", he said, "where we will teach you to rest".' (D, 82–83). Science is presented as a normative enterprise with educational aims. It is a law that Rezia wants to believe in, or some order that would give form to their reality.

In that respect, by making sure Septimus's voice and words remain silenced throughout the novel, Woolf is able to intimate the notion that Septimus's symptom lies in this complex relation between the word he cannot avoid and the failure of language to convey knowledge. Septimus barely ever utters a single word in the narrative, because of this complex skein resulting from his relation to language. And when he does speak, it is reduced to the smallest units, the word 'war', 'Evans', when it is intelligible at all *by the Other* (D, 21). It is thus not innocent that Septimus should find the word 'I' most problematic. It makes him stammer and interrupt his conversation with Bradshaw, despite the benevolence that the latter seeks to perform: '"Yes?" Sir William encouraged him. (But it was growing late.)/Love, trees, there is no crime—what was his message?' (D, 83). Bradshaw is so much after meaning, disturbed by the fragmented nature of the speech, that he fails to see that Septimus is stuck with the word 'I-I-I-I' (D, 83), repeated four times and literally the last word he is able to pronounce before he takes the dramatic step of killing himself.

Septimus is not the only example in the novel of a delirious person whose language is only listened to as some riddle that needs decoding, instead of being seen as a mode of *jouissance* that needs circumscribing. The beggar sitting outside the tube station is another example of language being used beyond its communicative function, and the situation of the episode in the narrative encourages readers to see them as linked—the beggar is heard singing just before Septimus finally gets to see Sir Bradshaw:

> Since she was so unhappy, for weeks and weeks now, Rezia had given mean-ings to things that happened, almost felt sometimes that she must stop peo-ple in the street …And this old woman singing in the street 'if someone should see, what matter they?' made her suddenly quite sure that everything was going to be right. They were going to Sir William Bradshaw; she thought his name sounded nice; he would cure Septimus at once. (D, 70–71)

The occurrence in the beggar's song of the word 'matter' in a some-what enigmatic, cryptic song, connects Septimus and the 'old woman' in a metonymic fashion that is perhaps less optimistic for the reader than it is for Rezia. The metonymic nature of the character's word usage recalls the word 'war' in Septimus's conversation with Bradshaw and the word 'mat-ter' in Rezia's conversation with Dr Holmes. For indeed this is the very word that Rezia keeps using, borrowing it from Dr Holmes, for whom 'there is nothing the matter' with Septimus. This 'matter' in all its mean-ings induces a reduction of the subject to its 'real' existence, barred from access because of the function of language. By multiplying its meanings, the narrative somehow exhausts the possibilities it had to make sense. The question posed by the beggar in her song echoes the radical negation of Holmes and associates the matter to waste, dejection, pointing to a posi-tion of total submissiveness and passivity that could explain Septimus's final act. The parallel between Septimus and the beggar is structurally and symbolically inscribed in the narrative and further develops the association of Septimus with that which can be disposed of—the outcasts of society. The being is all the more associated to waste as the beggar is sitting outside a tube station, belonging to the liminal space between the elevated and the subterranean. However, the logic of the beggar is very different and with both, Woolf explores two modalities of a relation to language that is not based on communicating meaning.

A QUEER SOLDIER: THE FEMINISATION OF SEPTIMUS OR THE INSTABILITY OF IDENTIFICATION

Since the nineteenth century, women have been over-represented in diagnoses of psychiatric disorders and often more numerous in asylums: 'In the early 1990s, Herman and L. Brown addressed the disparity in clinical and psychological trauma studies between attention on trauma affecting men and those affecting women' (Anderson 2012: 6). But modernism was also the time when this declined a little, even if Woolf's definition of madness was influenced by phallocratic, patriarchal perspectives in which the irrational was thought to be a sign of feminine weakness or lack. 'The lens of gender provides a perspective on reading madness that reveals fundamental understandings of masculinity and femininity in modernist fiction' (Anderson 2012: 57). One of the first steps of Woolfian feminist criticism consisted in re-instating female characters for a greater balance with their male counterparts. This social understanding of madness naturally led to analyses of the novel that celebrated mental health as a metaphor of men-women relations, in order to challenge accepted views of the distribution of powers. One sign of this is that the Bible of feminist criticism in the 1980s, Gilbert and Gubar's *The Madwoman in the Attic*, mentions Woolf several times despite the fact that the book focuses on nineteenth-century fiction: this seems to suggest that Woolf was only writing in continuation of her Victorian sisters. Gilbert and Gubar quote this passage from *A Room of One's Own*, which is indeed essential to understand the necessity for a de-gendering of mental illness but also in terms of the cultural impact of diagnoses:

> any woman born with a great gift in the sixteenth century would certainly have gone crazed, shot herself, or ended her days in some lonely cottage

outside the village, half witch, half wizard, feared and mocked at. For it needs little skill in psychology to be sure that a highly gifted girl who had tried to use her gift for poetry would have been so thwarted and hindered by other people, so tortured and pulled asunder by her own contrary instincts that she must have lost her health and sanity to a certainty.... To have lived a free life in London in the sixteenth century would have meant for a woman who was poet and playwright a nervous stress and dilemma which might well have killed her. (Woolf 1929: 57)

Madness is the result of gender stereotypes and gendered conditions: frustration, social pressure and freedom are perceived as a potential danger for women—everything points to gender relations that are unfair. Mental health itself is negated and reduced to the social roots, which is an essential argument to invite to political engagement. Gilbert and Gubar's stance is that women are not mad, but they show symptoms that manifest their opposition to social order through ailments experienced in their bodies: 'Many critics have concluded that the diagnosis of madness in women was, largely, a power struggle' (Chesler 1994: xxiii).

In their influential book, Gilbert and Gubar posit that the mad woman is first and foremost a spokeswoman for the author, if not a double, and this is based on the exploration of *Jane Eyre* (Gilbert and Gubar 1984: 88): 'The madwoman in literature by women is not merely, as she might be in male literature, an antagonist or foil to the heroine. Rather, she is usually in some sense the author's double, an image of her own anxiety and rage' (Gilbert and Gubar 1984: 88). The argument revolves around the idea that asylums and cultures both distribute women into two roles, angel and monster, roles which Woolf herself refers to in 'Professions for Women' (Gilbert and Gubar 1984: 17). What is surprising is that Septimus is unquestionably included in the list of characters on which this analysis is based, despite the obvious fact that he is undoubtedly a male character: 'Woolf projects herself into both ladylike Mrs Dalloway and crazed Septimus Warren Smith' (Gilbert and Gubar 1984: 78). If Mrs Dalloway is defined by her womanhood, nothing comes to describe Septimus in this quote. In the 1970s' analyses of the novel, Septimus's 'homosexual feelings' were readily associated with his vulnerability during the war, as if sexual orientation and courage were shown as connected in the text: 'Certainly, we are told that he develops 'manliness' in the war. But against this...' (Hawthorn 1975: 49–50). Throughout the novel, the adjective 'queer'[12] recurs to define Septimus, underlining a failure, a form of effeminate nature—Septimus's masculine identity is as oddly befitting as the overcoat he is wearing on a glorious day in June. Gilbert and Gubar refer to this in passing when they talk about an upcoming book that they never got round to publishing, *The Lunatic in the Park* (Gilbert and Gubar 1984: xxxii).

It so happens that the sexuated identity of Septimus, much like his suicide, is presented as an unresolved enigma in the novel. He is indeed married, but it is said that he does not want to father a child, and rapidly it is suggested that his marriage to an Italian lady has not been consummated (D, 76).[13] While Holmes encourages Septimus to stand up to 'English husbands' by refusing suicidal ideas and owing his duty to his wife (D, 78), the narrative voice places the scene about Septimus's marriage under the ironic influence of *Anthony and Cleopatra*, which Septimus wishes to read and which neither Holmes nor Bradshaw looks on with a favourable eye: literature shows that which escapes their knowledge and which could cause further distress; it is also that which Septimus looks up to with desire without ever managing to read it. As Shakespeare's play focuses on a failed marriage, the symbolism of this book must be taken into account, not only in its metaphorical power, but also, more openly, as a sign that Septimus himself wants to know more about carnal aspects: 'Love between man and woman was repulsive to Shakespeare. The business of copulation was filth to him before the end. But, Rezia said, she must have children' (D, 75). Irony pervades again with the beginning of the play referring to a kind of love that contradicts Sir Bradshaw's principles: 'This dotage of our general's/o'erflows the measure' (I, 1, 1–2).

Septimus's identity and his identification to the masculine could have made him one of the great patriarchal men of his time. His early life is

---

[12] Woolf's use of the term is ambiguous, referring both to the notion of 'eccentric' and the more colloquial way of suggesting 'homosexuality'. It cannot be interpreted from the point of view of twenty-first-century critics without some contextualising. I do not offer a 'queer' reading of Septimus here but I wish to show that the presence of this term suggests a problematic position in relation to heteronormative structures that must be made explicit and that contribute to the function silence may have for him.

[13] On explorations of this absence of sexuality, see Nancy Topping Bazin in *Virginia Woolf and the Androgynous Vision* and Rigney's causal reading of sexuality as 'due to repressed homosexual tendencies' (Rigney 1978: 51).

summarised in a list of masculine achievements: 'there in the trenches the change which Mr Brewer desired when he advised football was produced instantly; he developed manliness; he was promoted; he drew the attention, indeed the affection of his officer, Evans by name' (D, 73). What made him 'queer' (D, 22), strange, mad, was the encounter with an ineffable experience which he could not escape and which created a hole revealing an enigma that leaves him perpetually unanchored in language and amongst others[14]. When he witnesses the death of his friend, Septimus does not feel anything: 'It might be possible, Septimus thought, looking at England from the train window, as they left Newhaven; it might be possible that the world itself is without meaning' (D, 75). Woolf makes Septimus a sacrificial victim whose suicide makes his life inescapably enigmatic. Septimus understands life as a question of occupying a logical place rather than a meaningful one in his relation with the Other, and his is that of a waste that can be disposed of.

However, Septimus's obsession is with Evans, the fellow he allowed to die in front of him. The death of the latter left him emotionless, in a state where language failed to allow him access to experience. Elaborating a theory throughout the novel, Septimus is shown as having uncovered 'the truth' with the return of that traumatic experience which has failed to be repressed: 'That man, his friend who was killed, Evans, had come, he said. He was singing behind the screen' (D, 119). In this scene, Septimus is seen by Rezia. This point of view reveals an opposition between a positivist approach to life, and the recognition that there is something other than tangible reality, something truthful that constantly escapes. On the one hand, the medical eye, for whom 'there was nothing. They were alone in the room. It was a dream, she would tell him' (D, 120). On the other hand, Septimus's solitude and absence of 'communication' of his real experience. The doctors in the novel are doubtlessly equipped with a knowledge that is legitimised by society and unchallenged, which therefore is represented as unfailing. This is the very reason why their

---

[14] Lacan calls *troumatisme* the effect of the absence of a signifier to represent the subject, in a pun with the word trauma. The wound that the word trauma refers to etymologically is re-interpreted by Lacan as the effect of the lack inherent in language, by which humans have to make do with the impossibility for some meaning to be fixed in the only tool they have to express it (Lacan 1974, lesson 19 February 1974).

knowledge leaves no room for Septimus,[15] who thus is reduced to 'nothing':[16] the image this time is that of drowning and later will be the paranoid expression of a subject that is deprived of their agency and has to respond to the injunction 'must' (D, 125). Science is thus stripped of its rationality to become an embodied instrument of power whose accuracy is irrelevant.

If at first, Clarissa is '*straight* as a dart, a little too rigid perhaps' (D, 65, my emphasis), it is perhaps to emphasise Septimus's attitude which, by contrast, is 'slouched', physically sporting the signs of his marginality and unfitness, a body that escapes the moral principles of being right and proper, a body that is out of place: 'Looking back she saw him sitting in his shabby overcoat alone, on the seat, hunched up, staring' (D, 20); the shabby overcoat is noted several times in the narrative, so that it metonymically evokes his 'queer' attitude and being. When Septimus eventually commits suicide, Holmes's reaction 'the coward!' (D, 127) leaves no doubt as to the humbling, demasculinising if not castrating, effect of medical discourse on the patient. The permanence of the phrase 'they must do as the doctors said' (D, 128), quite ironic after Septimus is dead, together with the last section of the novel that opens with 'one of the triumphs of civilisation' (D, 128), shows how the master's discourse, by placing the signifier in command, conceals the subject or fails to give it a place (Lacan 1991): Bradshaw and Holmes have not failed in their diagnosis, they have failed because by seeking meaning and interpretation, they answered unasked questions and were victims of their social (under)standing. The novel, which was intended to portray sanity and insanity, ends up showing something more significant than the question of 'madness'. The word is incidentally used unquestionably about Elizabeth (D, 110), even if she displays very few signs of it. It reveals how the subject, a body that speaks, is forced into symptomatic behaviour by the medical discourse which, far

---

[15] Following in the footsteps of Hegel, Lacan has analysed this mechanism of anxiety as a response to the absence of lack in the Other; in other words, an Other that is constituted as unfailing is an Other that potentially can intrude upon the subject and this causes a paranoid response (Lacan 2004: 57; 64–68).

[16] This reading of 'matter' does not invalidate Moran's analysis of materialism, the female body and sexuality in her discussion of the relation between Mansfield's 'Bliss' and Woolf's novel. Moran focuses on Clarissa's lesbian resonance and the materiality of women's bodies and she concludes, via a different route that pays tribute to French feminism and the semiotic, with the same idea that the novel explores the anxiety of seeing the embodiment of an other discourse (Moran 1996: 85).

from being a reliable science, is like the social discourse, something the subject interacts with, and responds to: it is the situation that produces symptoms the subject then suffers from. What the doctors fail to acknowledge is the effect of their knowledge on the subject they try to treat: 'to torture is to know how the other can be modified ... it thus often happens that the same type of professionals are to be found in practices of torture and of therapy: doctors, psychiatrists and psychologists' (Tobie et al. 1998: 237). Septimus, just before he acts out, thinks: 'So he was in their power!' (D, 124) which signals his becoming anxious that he has lost his own subjective agency. This somehow makes him a queer hero rather than an ideal war veteran.

The Hole of Knowledge

To return therefore to the complex skein of Clarissa's social life of frivolities, which seems to be set in contrast with Septimus's queer place in society, I now want to raise the question of the persistence of Septimus's symptoms, even after he dies—in the sense that his speech keeps imposing on characters, who are bound to try and decipher it. If Clarissa is first described as knowing 'nothing; no language, no history; she scarcely read a book now, except memoirs in bed' (D, 7), in the following page she reads off *Cymbeline* by Shakespeare, perhaps not the most renowned of his plays, and looks at different books to give Evelyn. The tortuous artistic references in the novel invite us not to take at face value the absence of knowledge that Clarissa affirms but to analyse it at a structural level: it is not so much that she lacks knowledge, but that she doesn't have the encyclopaedic, patriarchal, phallic knowledge that is common in her milieu and which surfaces in conversation. Richard's understanding of Shakespeare is based on moral grounds and his interpretation founded on the relation between the work and the laws he believes in: 'Richard got on his hind legs and said that no decent man ought to read Shakespeare's sonnets because it was like listening at keyholes (besides, the relationship was not one that he approved)' (D, 64). It is possible to think that, like his friend Lady Bruton, 'without reading Shakespeare', he would still be able to quote him (D, 153), together with the other Academicians, portrait painters, etc. who provide food for conversation during Clarissa's party. On the contrary, Clarissa absorbs dribs and drabs of culture, like the conversation about cabbages that she has with Peter, and the random people she walks past in the streets of London. The quote from *Cymbeline* recurs throughout the novel so as to give shape to her life, and she seems to adjust its meaning as she progresses (Minow-Pinkney 1987: 67–68). When Clarissa meets Sally, they exchange books and Clarissa refers to *Othello*, proving once again that elements of highbrow culture are for her not a means of possession, but something that must circulate, something that will adjust to, and frame her experience of reality. For indeed this reality is governed by the phallic power of those in the know, and when Peter blames Clarissa for her shocked reaction to Sally's having had a baby out of wedlock: 'In those days a girl brought up as she was knew nothing' (D, 50), he means that she knew nothing about sex, not nothing about life. Peter thinks 'she trusts to her charm too much.... She overdoes it' (D, 48). The idea of overdoing is here used in relation to the role that gives her a place in this society, which is best satirised by Peter when he thinks of the Whitbreads' pomp (D, 62–63) and compares it with Richard Dalloway's thickness (D, 63–64). However, beyond the many examples that abound in the novel, it is interesting to notice the constant dialectics between the inflation of social standards and the suspicion of emptiness that this very pompousness points to. 'Lord, Lord, the snobbery of the English!... How they loved dressing up in gold lace and doing homage!' (D, 146) Clarissa seems to develop a self that needs aggrandising because otherwise it is reduced to nothing. Is this a symptom? It might well be indeed. Clarissa's symptomatic relation with the other is a singular response to a context in which other women have opted for other solutions.

Clarissa's pompous, social life is always interpreted in relation to the question of life, and even more precisely to reality—or rather what she describes as 'real':

> What she would say was that she hated frumps, fogies, failures, like himself presumably; thought people had no right to slouch about with their hands in their pockets; must do something, be something; and these great swells, these Duchesses, these hoary old Countesses one met in her drawing-room, unspeakably remote as he felt them to be from anything that mattered a straw, stood for something real to her. (D, 65)

This passage interweaves Clarissa's and Peter's voices and plays with the signifier—frumps, fogies, failures—to make us understand that Clarissa rejects the old and untrimmed, the socially unfit, unless 'failures' is Peter's own addition and the way he feels around her and her friends. Social class, and its dialectics of centre and margin, is still the structuring principle.

What is underlined indeed is that Clarissa's social attitude is in fact the symptom of her difficulty to incorporate the real, as if this world of 'partying, and lunching…' was experienced as sham but the real experience remained inaccessible.

This is why Clarissa's feelings about social events are more ambivalent than Peter thinks: 'Every time she gave a party she had this feeling of being something not herself, and that everyone was unreal in one way; much more real in another' (D, 145). This shows that the social is another expression for a deeper, more Proustian opposition between the real and reality, between what is inescapable and what belongs to the imaginary. The recurrence of the term 'real' links Clarissa to Septimus, because it is the suicide of the latter that is the most 'real' event of the novel. The party precisely is the context in which the suicide is announced:

> There was nobody. The party's splendour fell to the floor, so strange it was to come in alone in her finery.
> What business had the Bradshaws to talk of death at her party? A young man had killed himself. And they talked of it at her party—the Bradshaws talked of death. (D, 156)

This is where I situate the junction between Septimus's story and Clarissa's, one that has been less commented upon and which is based in language. Septimus's suicide happens towards the end of the novel and will not be symbolised, in the sense that it fails to be recounted and be inscribed within language. The suicide is not part of a discourse which would account for it, make sense of it, or simply situate it. Bradshaw's only concession to this patient's singularity is the fact that he arrives late at his friend's party—and even that can be turned into a social mishap. The narration mentions that Richard and William chitchat but interestingly the 'matter' of their conversation is far vaguer than in the novel's other conversations. The choice of Clarissa's point of view at this moment is particularly efficient in conveying the remaining opacity of Septimus's suicide. Instead, the reader is informed that Bradshaw is keen to see the bill he is working on be passed in order to institutionalise the mad, heedless as he is of the fact that this was what he failed to do with Septimus. Stylistically, the expression 'fell to the floor' in the aforementioned quote cannot but echo the way Septimus commits suicide, an idea symbolically recurring here in the aftermath of the event.

According to Frosh, the 'modernist impulse to make something good out of chaos' was attuned to 'a vision of creativity as reparation' promoted by psychoanalysis in Britain (Frosh 2003: 117). However, when elaborating on this idea, Frosh comes to the notion that the modernist aesthetic was not only an attempt to stitch up the tears in the fabric of reality, but also to account for or produce something 'active, present, pushing for expression, motivating, causal' (Frosh 2003: 118). In *Mrs Dalloway*, Woolf paves the way for a literature of the war that will seek to fix or repair the existence of those that have come back from the front by juxtaposing the polished world of frivolities with the grave reality of Britain's outcasts. She also tries to circumscribe, to localise and situate, the uncontrollable, unbridled life of impulses and drives which Septimus becomes the spokesperson for, paradoxically in being silenced and in presenting himself as silent. This silence or mutism is shared with Clarissa, who in her own way refuses to speak while indulging in the art of small talk, and this is where Woolf's modernist aesthetics becomes her political engagement. As Squier argues, 'There is a social consequence to Clarissa's tendency to merge with her surroundings. Rather than feeling individual importance as the well-groomed wife of a socially prominent member of Parliament, she accepts kinship with all city-dwellers based on their common love of "life; London; this moment of joy"' (Squier 1985: 96). If the Bloomsbury set [saw in Freudian psychoanalysis] 'a cultural tool... provoking reconsiderations of language, gender, and memory, and of course of the relationships between external "reality" and what has come to be called... the "internal world"' (Frosh 2003: 127), I have argued that Woolf also thinks beyond this division and envisages the foreclosure of subjective split, giving voice to symptoms that can be related to a subjective structure or logic but not simply discovered, and thereby avoiding the pitfalls of 'act[ing] as the one who tames the irrational speech, making it rational, explaining it and taking over' (Frosh 2003: 119). On the contrary, Woolf tries to invent a reform of mental health care which gives voice to irrationality—if only the reform was not the doing of Richard and Bradshaw.

BIBLIOGRAPHY

PRIMARY SOURCES

Woolf, Leonard (1964). *Beginning Again, The Autobiography of the years 1911–1918*. London: The Hogarth Press.
Woolf, Virginia (1929). *A Room of One's Own*. London: Penguin Books, "Great Ideas", 2004.
Woolf, Virginia (2002). *Moments of Being, Autobiographical Writings*. Jeanne Schulkind (ed.), intro. by Hermione Lee, London: Pimlico Edition.

SECONDARY SOURCES

Abel, Elizabeth (1989). *Virginia Woolf and the Fictions of Psychoanalysis*. Chicago: The University of Chicago Press, "Women in Culture and Society".

Anderson, Sarah Wood (2012). *Readings of Trauma, Madness and the Body*. New York: Palgrave Macmillan.

Boileau, Nicolas Pierre (2014). "Trauma and 'Ordinary Words': Virginia Woolf's Play on Words", in T. Beney et A. Stara (eds.). *The Edges of Trauma*. Cambridge: Cambridge Scholars Publishing, 48–60.

Boileau, Nicolas Pierre (2023). "*Reading* Hamlet *with Lacan, the Joint of Symptoms, Desire and Time*". J. Tambling (ed.). *The Bloomsbury Handbook of Psychoanalysis and Literature*. London: Bloomsbury Academic, 189–204.

Bonikowski, Wyatt (2013). *Shell-Shock and the Modernist Imagination, The Death-Drive in post-World War I Fiction*. Burlington: Ashgate.

Bort, Françoise (2002). "Virginia Woolf et Dante: L'enfer de *Mrs Dalloway*". in Bernard & Reynier (eds.) (2002), 91–106.

Bowlby, Rachel (2011). "Real Life and its Readers in *Mrs Dalloway*". C. Bernard (ed.). *Woolf as Reader/Woolf as Critic or, The Art of Reading in the Present*. Montpellier: Presses Universitaires de Montpellier, 19–38.

Bradshaw, David (2000). Introduction to V. Woolf (1925). *Mrs Dalloway*. Oxford: Oxford World's Classics, 2009.

Broughton, Panthea Reid (1987). "'Virginia is Anal': Speculations on Virginia Woolf's Writing 'Roger Fry' and Reading Sigmund Freud". *Journal of Modern Literature*, 14: 1, Spring, 151–157.

Burston, Daniel (2020). *Psychoanalysis, Politics and the Postmodern University*. Basingstoke: Palgrave Macmillan.

Chesler, Phyllis (1994). *Preface* to Geller Jeffrey L. & Harris Maxine, eds. (1994). *Women of the Asylum, Voices from behind the Walls, 1840–1945*. New York: Anchor Books.

Coates, Kimberly Engdahl (2012). "Phantoms, Fancy (And) Symptoms: Virginia Woolf and the Art of Being Ill". *Woolf Studies Annual*, vol. 18 (2012), 1–28.

Cohn, Dorrit (1978). *Transparent Minds, Narrative Modes for Presenting Consciousness in Fiction*. Princeton: Princeton UP.

DeMeester, Karen (2007). "Trauma, Post-Traumatic Stress Disorder, and the Obstacles to Postwar Recovery in *Mrs Dalloway*." Eberly & Henke (eds.) (2007), 77–94.

Didi-Hubermann, Georges (1982). *Invention de l'Hystérie*. Paris: Éditions Macula, 2012.

Eberly, David and Henke, Suzette (2007), *Virginia Woolf and Trauma, Embodied Texts*. New York: Pace University Press.

Ehrenberg, Alain (1998). *La Fatigue d'être soi*. Paris: Odile Jacob.

Foucault, Michel (1963). *Naissance de la Clinique*. Paris: Presses Universitaires de France, "Quadrige grands textes", 2003. For the English version: http://monoskop.org/images/9/92/Foucault_Michel_The_Birth_of_the_Clinic_1976.pdf

Foucault, Michel (1972). *Histoire de la folie à l'âge classique*. Paris: Gallimard, "Tel".

Freud, Sigmund (1912). "Sur la Dynamique du transfert". *La Technique psychanalytique*, Paris: Presses Universitaires de France, 2013, 57–68.

Freud, Sigmund (1926), *Inhibition, Symptome et Angoisse*. Trans. J. and R. Doron. Paris: Presses Universitaires de France, 1993.

Froula, Christine (2002). "Mrs. Dalloway's Postwar Elegy: Women, War, and the Art of Mourning." *Modernism/modernity*, Volume 9, Number 1, January 2002, 125–163, https://doi.org/10.1353/mod.2002 [last accessed 21 October 2021]

Frosh, Stephen (2003). "Psychoanalysis in Britain: The Rituals of Destruction". D. Bradshaw (ed.). *A Concise Companion to Modernism*. Malden: Blackwell Publishing, 116–137.

Gilbert, Sandra & Gubar, Susan (1984). *The Madwoman in the Attic: The Woman Writer and the Nineteenth Century Literary Imagination*. New Haven: Yale University Press.

Gordon, C., Pryor R. & Watkins, G. (1990). *Sounds from the Bell Jar, Ten psychotic Authors*. London: Macmillan.

Gori, Roland & Del Volgo, Marie-José (2020), *Exilés de l'intime, Vers un Homme neuroéconomique*. Paris: Les Liens qui libèrent.

Graham, Elyse & Lewis, Pericles (2013). "Private Religion, Public Mourning and Mrs Dalloway." *Modern Philology*, vol. 111, n°1, 2013, 88–106.

Hawthorn Jeremy (1975). *Virginia Woolf's Mrs Dalloway, A study in Alienation*. London: Sussex University Press, "Text and Context".

Lacan, Jacques (1981). *Le Séminaire*, Livre III, *Les Psychoses* (1955–56). J.-A. Miller (ed.). Paris: Éditions du Seuil.

Lacan, Jacques (2004). *Le Séminaire*, Livre X, *L'Angoisse* (1962–63). J.-A. Miller (ed.). Paris: Éditions du Seuil.

Lacan, Jacques (2013). *Le Séminaire*, Livre VI, *Le Désir et son interprétation* (1958–1959) J.-A. Miller (ed.). Paris: Éditions de la Martinière.

Lacan, Jacques (1975). *Le Séminaire, Livre XX, Encore* (1972–73). J.-A. Miller (ed.). Paris: Éditions du Seuil.

Lacan, Jacques (1991). *Le Séminaire, Livre XVII, Envers de la psychanalyse* (1970). J.-A. Miller (ed.). Paris: Éditions du Seuil.

Lacan, Jacques (2005). *Le Séminaire, Livre XXIII, Le Sinthome* (1975–76). J.-A. Miller (ed.). Paris: Éditions du Seuil.

Lacan, Jacques (2011). *Le Séminaire, Livre XIX, ... Ou pire* (1971–72). J.-A. Miller (ed.). Paris: Éditions du Seuil.

Lacan, Jacques (1974). "Les non-dupes-errent", leçon du 19 février, 1974. Unpublished.

Latham, Sean (2003). *Am I a Snob? Modernism and the Novel.* Ithaca: Cornell University Press.

Lee, Hermione (1996). *Virginia Woolf.* New York: Random House, Vintage, 1999.

Lee Hermione (2005). *Virginia Woolf's Nose.* New York: Princeton UP.

Letissier, Georges (2019). "L'œuvre romanesque du romancier Alan Hollinghurst: contre-épopée anglaise et généalogie d'une culture alternative". *Itinéraires*, 2019, 2 & 3. 10.4000/itineraires.7020

Maleval, Jean-Claude (1997). *Logique du délire.* Paris: Masson, "Ouvertures Psy", 2000.

Maleval, Jean-Claude (2012). *Étonnantes mystifications, De la psychothérapie autoritaire.* Paris: Éditions Navarin, "Le champ freudien".

Micale, Mark S. (1993). "On the 'Disappearance' of Hysteria: A Study in the Clinical Deconstruction of a Diagnosis". *Isis*, vol.84, n°3, Sept.1993, 496–526.

Micale, Mark S. & Lerner, Patrick (eds.) (2001). *Traumatic Pasts, History, Psychiatry and Trauma in the Modern Age 1870–1930.* Cambridge: Cambridge University Press.

Miller, Jacques-Alain (1993). "Clinique ironique". *Revue de la Cause Freudienne*, n°23.

Miller, Jacques-Alain (1999). "Les Six Paradigmes de la Jouissance". *La Cause freudienne* No. 43, 7–29.

Miller, Jacques-Alain (2004). "Pièces détachées", *L'Orientation lacanienne*, lesson of 17 November 2004, unpublished.

Minow-Pinkney Makiko (1987). *Virginia Woolf and the Problem of the Subject.* New Brunswick: Rutgers University Press.

Moi, Toril (1985). *Sexual/Textual Politics.* New York: Routledge, 2002.

Moran, Patricia (1996). *Word of Mouth, Body Language in Katherine Mansfield & Virginia Woolf.* Charlottesville: University of Virginia Press.

Moran, Patricia (2007). *Virginia Woolf, Jean Rhys, and the Aesthetics of Trauma.* New York: Palgrave Macmillan.

Mosse, George L. (2000). "Shell-Shock as a Social Disease". *Journal of Contemporary History*, vol.35, n°1, 101–108.

Porter, Roy (2002). *Madness, a Brief History.* Oxford: Oxford University Press.

Reviron, Floriane (2004). "'Am I a Snob?' de Virginia Woolf: autoportrait d'une femme savante en précieuse ridicule." S. Crinquand (ed.), *Par Humour de soi*, Dijon: Presses Universitaires de Dijon, "Kaléidoscopes", 85–94.

Rigney, Barbara Hill (1978). *Madness and Sexual Politics in the Feminist Novel, Studies of Brontë, Woolf, Lessing and Atwood.* Madison, USA: the University of Wisconsin Press.

Schlack Beverly Ann (1979). *Continuing Presences: Virginia Woolf's Use of Literary Allusions.* Pennsylvania University Press.

Shorter, Edward (1997). *A History of Psychiatry, From the Era of the Asylum to the Age of Prozac.* New York: John Wiley and Sons, Inc.

Showalter, Elaine (1985). *The Female Malady, Women, Madness and English Culture, 1830–1980.* London: Virago Press (1985).

Showalter, Elaine (1997). *Hystories, Hysterical Epidemics and Modern Culture.* London: Picador, 2013.

Squier, Susan Merrill (1985). *Virginia Woolf and London, The Sexual Politics of the City.* Chapel Hill: The University of North Carolina Press.

Thomas, Sue (1987). "Virginia Woolf's Septimus Smith and Contemporary Perceptions of Shell Shock." *English Language Notes,* vol. 25, No. 2, 49–57.

Tobié, Nathan, Blanchet Alain, Ionescu, Serban, & Zadje, Nathalie (ed.) (1998), *Psychothérapies,* Paris: Odile Jacob.

Toth, Naomi (2016). *L'Écriture vive, Woolf, Sarraute, une autre phénoménologie de la perception.* Paris: Classiques Garnier, "Perspectives comparatistes".

Whitworth Michael (2005). *Virginia Woolf.* Oxford, Oxford University Press, "Authors in Context".

CHAPTER 3

Meaning and Interpretation: The Failure of the Psychiatric Method in *Asylum* by Patrick McGrath

Woolf's knowledge of psychiatric treatment, which derived from her own experience of being pathologised by various doctors throughout her life, greatly influenced both the subversion of the doctors' discourse in *Mrs Dalloway* and contributed to her exploration of a different approach to symptom decoding. Patrick McGrath's fiction also derives from first-hand knowledge, inherited from being not a patient but the son of a psychiatrist who ran a hospital for years (McGrath 1989): McGrath spent 25 years on the Broadmoor estate where his father, a 'forensic psychiatrist', was superintendent from 1957 onwards (McGrath 2002: 141). He was brought up and lived there before contemplating becoming a writer. This is how he had access to examples of madness that were to become the primary source of his novelistic experimentations. His experience of madness is therefore one of having a father whose profession was to cure the mad, and his living within the precincts of the asylum where he could observe, meet and exchange with patients. As a young man, he started to work in a psychiatric unit in northern Ontario, where he remembers adopting the therapist/analyst stance of 'listening to the weird incomprehensible shifts and jumps in their [the Oakbridge schizophrenic patients'] talks' (McGrath 2002: 141).

McGrath's fiction is replete with psychiatrists, doctors and practitioners, who are intent on analysing reality with the help of a science that is

© The Author(s), under exclusive license to Springer Nature Switzerland AG 2023

N. P. Boileau, *Mental Health Symptoms in Literature since Modernism*, Palgrave Studies in Literature, Science and Medicine, https://doi.org/10.1007/978-3-031-37630-6_3

thought to be reliable and rigorous, but which often leads them to make unfortunate decisions. Patients do not react according to the textbook cases the psychiatrists studied, and scientific knowledge is thus defeated. In that respect, McGrath's characters could evoke the scientists of the nineteenth century and their adamant trust in the validity, value and possible comprehensiveness of rationality and experimentation: 'Knowledge for its own sake is the one God I worship'.[1] The scientists' trust in one mode of knowledge denotes some pathological attachment to an ideological framework which is presented as unfailing, and which could be at the origin of the late nineteenth century's renewed interest in the gothic (Marret 2010). According to Dupont, McGrath's *Asylum* fits into a general trend in the 1950s and 1960s' popular culture, during which analysts and psychiatrists became tropes of modern-day fiction, with a particular emphasis upon turning them into pathological figures, blinded by their own faith in a dogmatic theory and a veiled neurotic structure (Dupont 2013, par.1). The twentieth century saw the emergence of 'psychopathographic texts' (Keitel 1989) which sought to sound the mental state of those declared mad and in the 1950s and 1960s, memoir and fictional texts which accounted for the experience of the asylum. These various trends have been widely documented (Baker et al. 2010; Gagneret 2019; Boileau 2022; to name but a few).

One cannot deny that when six novels—*The Grotesque* (1990), *Dr Haggard's Disease* (1993), *Asylum* (1997), *Martha Peak* (2000), 'Ground Zero' in *Ghost Town* (2005) and *Trauma* (2008)—out of seven published texts portray psychiatrists who are both characters and narrators of the stories, the emphasis is laid on representing the scientist dealing with mental health, more perhaps than on the patients. Ironically, the therapists supposed to cure the mad are often shown to be mad themselves. There are several aspects to McGrath's productions that need to be noted: first, the 1990s was a decade of intense productivity, marked by an obsessive interest in pathological doctors. In that decade, Patrick McGrath's novels were both critical and commercial successes: David Cronenberg's film adaptation of his novel *Spider* in 2002 testifies to the popularity of the novelist. His interest in a renewal or re-interpretation of the gothic tropes and genre may explain why his novels were commercially successful. In the 2000s, there were two PhD theses defended on the question of the gothic in McGrath's fiction (Falco 2007a, 2007b; Dupont 2008) and the novel

---

[1] Collins (1883): 179. For an analysis of this novel, see L. Talairach (2013).

Asylum was shortlisted for the 1996 Guardian Fiction Prize. Since then, the author has grown out of favour and his production has substantially halted—he has published only two books since and many anthologies do not even mention him (Acheson and Ross 2005; Childs 2012). However, he remains an important voice in studies of the representation of insanity in fiction (Baker et al. 2010).

It could be said that McGrath explored the gap between scientific method and what is left out of the scientific method, namely the subject and their relation to language: 'To be outcast is the most common signification whose investment is universal. The feeling of exclusion come from the subject's initial status, which is shown in Lacan's matheme of the barred subject' (Miller 2018: 52). Because subjects are produced by the symbolic/language, they can only experience themselves as excluded, as having no stable, designated place in the chain of signifiers. McGrath's interest in the limitations of science has been fruitfully analysed as a strategy of unreliability within neo-gothic tropes (Dupont 2007, 2008). Dupont, who is one of the leading critics of McGrath's *œuvre*, calls him a 'postmodern neo-gothicist' (Dupont 2010, par.3). However, what has been neglected in most analyses of McGrath's work so far—and there is yet to emerge a solid body of works on the author—is his secondary characters, the patients themselves, and the production of symptoms that their encounter with a dysfunctional therapist causes. This is what the following chapter intends to probe by confronting the symptoms displayed by the so-called mad characters with the failure of the therapist's knowledge. This failure is connected, as I wish to show, to the subject's real, that is the presence of something that cannot be symbolised or given a logical character to, and yet which cannot be avoided. For lack of a better word, we may call this dimension or this rest, which is not ordered by reason and meaning, subjective experience.

McGrath looks at madness with a heightened sense of what he knows to be psychiatric treatment while turning this knowledge into fictional stories about the limits of excessive trust in science. His fiction seems to convey the idea that by seeking to interpret meaninglessness meaningfully, the scientist fails to acknowledge his own responsibility in enacting the scientific method. In other words, what his novels try to achieve is to present us with the aporia of making sense of the senseless. From a historical point of view, his novels can be understood as the result of the undebated supremacy of biomedical medicine: 'With the antidepressant Prozac throughout the 1990s, the interpretation of human distress has often been recast in terms of pharmacology' (Healey 1997; Kramer 1994)' (Baker et al. 2010: 7). The advent of biomedical treatment also seems to have reduced the influence of anti-psychiatry, which is hardly referred to in his *œuvre*. Patrick McGrath therefore figures as both an authority on the world of psychiatric medicine and a critic offering a slightly different view from the dominant one. Where much psychiatric fiction has focused on medicine as an oppressive model, one that in the wake of studies by Foucault, Szasz, Hacking and others, could be regarded as sole or exclusive instruments of power, the 1990s was a time for challenging these norms and visions. McGrath proposes to look at psychiatry as a science with doubts, a science that is powerless and often defeated by its own patients and for whom drug-based treatment can never be a solution in itself. Towards the end of his productive cycle of the 1990s, McGrath writes:

> I sit there pondering while you tell me your thoughts, and with my grunts and sighs, my occasional interruptions, I guide you toward what I believe to be the true core and substance of your problem. It is not a scientific endeavour. No, I feel my way into your experience with an intuition based on little more than a few years of practice, and reading, and focused introspection; in other words, there is *much of art* in what I do. (McGrath 2008: 5, emphasis mine)

This quote from his novel *Trauma* is used by Baker, who comments: 'This passage … seems appropriate to begin our concluding chapter with a quote from a fictional psychiatrist who is willing to confess that the processes of psychiatry involve much art—a view that goes against the increasingly dominant, biomedical models of madness' (Baker et al. 2010: 184). I would like to pick up on this idea that McGrath tries to work towards conflating literature and psychiatry. This, in turn, enables him to reflect upon the symptom as different from a univocal sign or a key to understand a relatable logic.

Asylum is, surprisingly perhaps, presented by McGrath as a novel about romantic love (Falco 2007b). It is surprising because the summary would seem to lead to a different interpretation. The novel opens on Edgar Stark, a patient who is institutionalised after he killed his wife because he suspected she was unfaithful. The sentence reflects both a context in which 'passionate' crimes were not as firmly condemned as they are now, and an understanding of the beheading of the wife in psychological terms: Edgar is thought to be delusional. This patient could be considered the central character in the first chapters since the narrator, who is his psychiatrist, reconstructs his story to understand how he seduced Stella, the deputy superintendent's wife, had sexual intercourse with her and stole her husband's clothes so as to escape from the hospital and to lead the life of a fugitive who, in the rest of the novel, appears as both perversely manipulative and profoundly deranged. While Edgar remains more or less consistent throughout the narrative, Stella is the character that changes the most and who comes to question the readers' expectations: instead of being affected by the disclosure of her unfaithfulness and of fitting back into her role as an honourable member of society, she manages to find Edgar in London, leaves her home to stay with him in hiding and when found, after she moves to the Welsh countryside with husband and son, she allows the neighbour to have extramarital sex with her, observes her son drown to death without calling for help and eventually returns to the hospital as a patient who soon manages to kill herself.

This summary can easily account for why some have been interested in the resurgence of the Gothic in McGrath's fiction, his relishing the sordid, the gloomy and hyper-tense stories. In the novel, what is at stake is not the madness of delirium and sensational manifestations of symptoms, such as could be seen in *Mrs Dalloway* and the character of Septimus, but the more discreet signs of disorders in which the subjects fail to make what happens to them logical or dialectical. In this chapter, I intend to show how in McGrath's novel *Asylum*, psychiatric discourse is only deceivingly targeted, like in *Mrs Dalloway*, while what is really at stake is the uncovering of what science cannot reach and the symptoms that emerge from a *jouissance* that is unknown and impossible to articulate. The subjective lack that is foregrounded in the narration by the absence of the patients' own stories reveals that the author wants to show how the institution of mental care is characterised by the same lack, a deficiency that is visible in the psychiatrist's inability to perceive their own blindness. In turn, the author ponders the logic of narration and thereby invents another mode of storytelling in which silence and unrepresented events have a much greater impact than the story that is told.

The Shortcomings of Psychiatry: The Failure of the Psychiatrist's Narrative

The novel interrogates the validity, efficacy and legitimacy of psychiatric practice. The place granted to Peter Cleave, in addition to his being the narrator of the story, makes him fully responsible for why the treatments of Edgar and Stella fail. Peter is the colleague of Stella's husband. When the latter leaves, he becomes superintendent and when Stella is brought back as a patient, he allows himself to fall in love with her—his interest in her before the proposal had already intimated the notion that he was entertaining more than friendly feelings for the woman. They agree to get married just before she commits suicide. There are many reasons why Peter may fascinate the reader: he is the psychiatrist who diagnoses the other characters and is in charge of looking after them; he is the one who tells the story based on his impressions intermingled with the stories he was told by the main protagonists; his attitude is both deontologically and ethically debatable but he also fails in his role as a narrator, a firm trait of many narrators in McGrath's œuvre (Falco 2007a: 104). In other words, there is a lot to say about the unreliability of his narrative, his misconceptions, his certitude and inability to produce meaning and his own blindness, to the extent that he could be seen as the perfect target of those who think the psychiatric institution is a prison in disguise (Caminero-Santangelo 1998; Baker et al. 2010). McGrath insists that Broadmoor Hospital was a sort of carceral institution, where surveillance reigned supreme, and the most difficult cases were put safely away from mainstream society (McGrath 1989).

Edgar's escape (A, 55) is the first event that defies the logic of science—none of the psychiatrists involved in his treatment could have thought that this would be possible, both because of the highly technological surveillance of the place and because of the diagnosis. His defiance causes the first dent in the psychiatrists' trust in their ability to master the human mind, prompting the beginning of the plot which, in many ways, unfolds like a detective story. The most obvious aim of the text consists in excavating, or piecing together, the missing parts of Stella and Edgar's stories when they are away from the eyes of their therapist. What is symptomatic from an analytical point of view in the novel, and in many texts by McGrath, is the hole in knowledge that every subject creates, digs or forms, a hole that psychiatry is not excepted from and which, in turn, agitates the characters in spite of themselves, as something that relentlessly returns to signify their incompleteness.

Literary critics have thus sought to delve into the narrative strategies that the unreliability of the narrator creates, rarely linking the narration itself to another genre, less literary but with a long tradition: the clinical case study. In a very recent PhD on the representation of psychiatrists in Anglophone fiction, Jacqueline Hopson painstakingly goes through the various ways in which the unreliability of McGrath's narrators must be seen and distrusted. Her approach is taxonomical but also marked by the underlying suggestion that there exists, or should exist, a reliable account. However, the narration never is given to someone else, so that there is no stable story to rely on or compare Peter's with. I think that what matters is not so much the unreliability of the narrative as the meaning that emerges anyhow and whose effects must be analysed. Jocelyn Dupont, on the other hand, shows how the various masks and guises worked upon by McGrath in the novel can make us ponder whether madness is on the side of those identified as insane and treated for such a condition or the analyst himself, who, despite being in charge of therapy, proves to be animated by unconscious drives he cannot analyse. Dupont concludes that Cleave's blindness to his own motive means he is a pervert, a manipulative man with ultimately 'mad' intentions (Dupont 2013: par.10). Without perhaps commenting on the diagnosis of the psychiatrist, it cannot be denied that Cleave leaves many aspects of his story susceptible to doubts or suspicion. Cleave tells us that Edgar is back in the hospital in the last stages of the novel but the narration never gives us a glimpse of him and nobody else but the narrator seems to have seen him. Furthermore, Edgar's therapy does not seem to lead to any improvement. Stella commits suicide just when she consents to get married, which proves to be Cleave's greatest failure: not only is he blinded by all the crimes that occurred in the novel, but his solutions (that the couple be moved to Wales; that Stella should marry him; that Edgar should return to the hospital) are all thwarted. McGrath clearly is interested in the narrative potential of medical failure. Given that medical science operates with the forcefulness of authority while remaining fallible, some mistakes end up being fatal or criminal and the stories these crimes produce inherently inspire new fictional forms (Dupont 2007: 146).

Yet, the forms of the narrative's incompleteness is what is never discussed as such but which seeps through at every stage of the novel, and this is true of all the characters, patients and doctors alike; it is what keeps being forgotten in therapy and in the narrative but which McGrath himself never leaves aside. As a result, McGrath also provides some comment on the historicisation of diagnoses: McGrath keeps stressing the division in Cleave—who would thus be named after his main characteristic of being cleft—made visible in his inability to be in full command of his effects on his patients, being often puzzled by what they end up doing, as if his diagnosis never was a functioning prognosis. McGrath, on the other hand, does not inscribe division in Stella and Edgar. At a time when schizophrenia was still regarded as originating in a splitting of the self and had been described as the emblematic illness originating in a social condition (Laing 1969; Wall 2018), it is no wonder this would have attracted interest in many readers. Lacan, on the other hand, argues that division is to be found in all subjects, either in a neurotic form in which division manifests but the subject is unaware of it, or in its psychotic form, in which division is foreclosed, meaning that it is missing (Lacan 1981): psychosis is defined by the foreclosure of division and I will show that this is a more valid clinical starting point as it helps construct a structural explanation for Stella's lack of affects.

Love, passion, crimes and failures form the imaginary dimension of this novel which, on many levels, could make readers overlook other, perhaps less obvious, questions that are tackled. The overt themes of the novel are all the more riveting as they are told from the point of view of a man who clearly is not up to the standard he claims to have reached. Structurally the scene that is most central—in the sense that it precipitates the action and Stella's downfall—is a ball scene. This scene is an artistic trope of romance *par excellence*, which can be found in most comedies of manners, romantic comedies and period films and series. It is also a trope of asylum literature, that is, texts dealing with the experience of being an in-patient in a mental health institution. The function, ritual and cultural significance of such scenes has been largely documented (Braun 2008: 54–60; Showalter 1985). During this scene, various transgressions happen: Stella, a respectable woman of high standing, dances with Edgar, whose erection she feels against her thigh. She is both shocked and attracted—the sexual unexpectedly rents through the narrative. Up until then, the text was predominantly gloomy, gothic, and focused on Edgar and his past crime. Straightaway, the intrusion of the sexual in Stella's life makes her demeanour waver: it is the so-called traumatic event that starts her subjective dissolution—adultery, maternal dysfunction with her only son, her non-active participation in her son's death, suicide. The novel therefore explores how this event forces Stella to renounce a life that was socially valued but made her feel destitute and how she iteratively manages to remain positioned as an infamous woman. The three male characters, Edgar, Max and Peter, are affected by Stella's subjective wavering, testifying to the underlying madness that seems to potentially threaten all the characters, and which their encounter with Stella triggers off.

For the novel also interrogates the relation to the other, a threatening tie between subjects that is presented as dysfunctional. In Lacanian terminology, the capital O in 'Other' is to be understood as different from the other people of our lives, with whom one entertains relationships of similitude, comparisons, self-definitions and Narcissistic, ambivalent feelings of recognition and feelings of difference: it is the level of mirroring, in which the other is a duplicate but also an image external to the subject (Lacan 1966). The writing with a capital letter, on the other hand, signifies radical otherness, such as what precedes the subject (language, the law, the structure of society) and the place where the subject is founded in relation to language as him/herself other. In the novel, the symbolic place of the characters is reshuffled all the time: the respectable wife becomes an adulterous, insensitive woman; the criminal is the object of the psychiatrist's fantasy or the ideal lover; the psychiatrist behaves like a father figure but also takes on the role of wannabe husband. The relationships Peter entertains with his patients make Stella's and Edgar's symbolic places shift constantly and this can be regarded as structurally relevant to the understanding of how all of McGrath's characters seem to be represented as mad.

The conflict between love, disease and the function of the cure was first explored by McGrath in *Dr Haggard's Disease*, whose title in itself is a perfect example of irony and paradox. When the doctor discusses what can only be interpreted as the beginning of a romantic affair between a woman and himself, the dialogue suggests that for the doctor, affects are pathologised in their very nature:

> 'But passion always dies,' I said.
> 'Spoken like a medical man,' she said, as our plates were removed. 'For you, passion is a disease. It causes suffering, comes to a crisis and dies.' (McGrath 1993: 23)

This subtext returns in the open in *Asylum* where affect is not perceived as an effect of something else, but simply as something that should be annihilated. Hopson also contends that a similar misuse of transference leads to homoerotic innuendoes among Peter and Edgar. She even suggests that Stella is only a means for Peter to find out about Edgar's sexual fantasies:

> His need to control and possess Stella to obtain information about her relationship with Edgar offers a self-justifying excuse to explore Edgar as sexual being. It is up to the reader to decide what grounds, if any, exist for Cleave's incarceration of Stella. She seems to have broken a social and ethical code but do love and adultery constitute madness? (Hopson 2020: 115).

This argument signifies that Cleave's doubts have consequences on the patients' well-being: the many therapeutic effects he is responsible for and the ever-growing number of meaningful associations he causes, make it difficult for the readers to analyse what his status is, if not a strategic tool designed to remodel genre fiction.

What Hopson also underlines is that psychiatry operates despite the fact that madness itself has not been confirmed. In other words, Peter might be in charge of the narrative, he seems to leave the question of his patients' diagnosis undiscussed. All in all, McGrath denies Peter the symbolic power of the psychiatrist: his narrative does not follow the well-trodden path of psychiatric cases—a valuable tool to discuss treatment and present your work to your colleagues—and his patients seem to interest him in spite of himself, without much reference to their value as a case. He deals with them as he would with friends. McGrath's 'obsessive' writing (Dupont 2007: 143) could delude the reader into thinking that the narrative is as mastered as the authoritative figure the narration is attributed to: in *Asylum*, the psychiatrist constantly refers to his knowledge with confidence and never misses an occasion to refer to his respectable career and his position of authority (A, 203, 208). His tone is almost paternalist, if not simply sexist, when he explains that he wants to help Stella 'with [his] guiding hand' (A, 73). By having him affirm his scientific value and by showing him break a certain number of ethical rules, McGrath makes sure that readers realise how Peter is blinded by his own confidence in some knowledge he is unable to name. In *Mrs Dalloway*, the doctors are made fun of because of their lack of understanding of their patients. In *Asylum*, the doctors are certainly not deprived of a medical knowledge that is sophisticated, but they remain impervious to the rigidity of that knowledge when what they have to analyse is not fixed or stable. It is this tension that McGrath brings to the fore.

BLINDED BY KNOWLEDGE: SUBJECTIVE CREATIONS DEFEATING SCIENTIFIC METHOD

Edgar and Stella are never in charge of the narrative and remain largely opaque to the readers. But what is most surprising is that they should remain enigmatic also to the psychiatrist who, throughout the novel, is baffled by what he is led to witness, as if the patients were far more creative than he expected them to be or as if his diagnostic hypotheses were never right. Edgar's crime regarding his ex-wife Ruth happened before the novel opens (Chap. 1), which means that there will be no elucidation of the crime motives, nor will there be one for his escape from the hospital (Chap. 3) and his relationship with Stella. Everything remains vague and unsorted, despite the psychiatrist's constant assertion of his great capacity and his medical prowess. The novel resorts to a stock of devices offered by genre fiction when soon Stella's trial for having failed to rescue her son who drowns himself to death (ch. 11) and her suicide (ch. 12) become central plot motifs, the circumstances of which Peter seems to investigate like a detective. However, some have suggested that this was a mere smokescreen for other questions, such as Edgar's sexual attraction (Hopson 2020: 155). For none of these subplots hold, since the beginning of the novel straightaway reveals that Stella is gone and that she probably was the second victim of Edgar's. Stella is given no opportunity to correct the version of events recounted by Cleave. If most of the novel is based on the suspense of finding out what happened to Stella, like in most detective fiction, her suicide appears as a narrative artifice that puts an end to a story designed to remain enigmatic and vague: a 'story without a proper ending' (McGrath 2015: xi). The psychiatrist comes out as a failing figure, not without irony from the author's point of view, because Cleave constantly asserts his own knowledge: 'In fact administratively speaking the female wing has been my domain for years' (A, 203). This goes to show that Cleave is unaware of his own shortcomings, because he is repeatedly contradicted by the women under his supervision. His proposal to Stella for example replays Mr Collins's failed proposal to Elizabeth Bennet in *Pride and Prejudice*: he gives a long list of rational reasons for the wedding, and does not mention love, but the medical benefit of her being married again.

Peter therefore is central to the novel and speaks from a position of authority while the author is reluctant to place his discourse within a specific trend in psychiatric theories. Although McGrath is happy to use the nosography of psychiatry in most of his novels, he remains very cautious with psychoanalytic theory: in interview, after admitting to reading Lacan and having enjoyed his theory, McGrath prefers to say very little on the subject because he is no specialist of the question (Falco 2007b: 42), an argument that barely holds water when compared with his second-hand knowledge of psychiatry which he does not hesitate to use in his fiction. In *Asylum*, the border between psychiatry and psychoanalysis is undetermined since the action takes place in the 1950s–1960s, at a historical time when both disciplines were most conjoined (Shorter 1997: 305). The novel does not give us much detail about Peter Cleave's therapeutic orientation. Edgar and Stella are both his patients, despite their suffering from very different symptoms and conditions, and if he seems to give them drugs, he still arranges talking sessions with them. There are no signs of other medical tests, and no definite diagnosis, whether psychopathological or neurological.

Patrick McGrath's primary concern is the work on his novel's structure: 'When I started writing fiction, I wrote genre fiction... I was only interested in genre' (Falco 2007b: 18). The context which McGrath sets for his 1990s novels is a return to his childhood memories, in the 1950s and 1960s, when diagnosis was largely structural, meaning ordered and structured by language and law. The date of the action is indirectly given by a reference to the 'Mental Health Act' which is said to have just been passed (A, 2). This early reference places the text within the context of medical care improvements, an evolution towards greater management of mental health, progress and knowledge and more visibility given to these questions in the public opinion. The retrospective narration adds to this logic by giving the impression until the very end that Peter knows more than readers, that he writes from a place of hindsight and that meaning has emerged now that the events are over. When the first signs of his delusion become too obvious, Peter suggests that Stella's reluctance to tell him everything explains why he did not make the correct clinical judgement.

Yet, the text contains many elements that jeopardise the psychiatrist's positive vision of his own work. There are many instances of clinical judgement with no connection with the patient other than the statistical evidence of a truth that Stella is impervious to: 'I did not tell her that as a function of her relationship with Edgar not only had she begun to identify with the patients, she had eroticized them. She had eroticized the patient body' (A, 27). This is based on external observation and not at all on what Stella tells him, because as a matter of fact, she does not say anything about the relationship. With this suggestion, Peter, like Bradshaw in *Mrs Dalloway*, answers an unasked question and he does not seem to question his own method, as if he was unaware of the effect of transference on his patient. Stella and Septimus also resemble one another in their acceptance of the therapist's silencing.

The absence of a clear diagnosis does not stop Peter from listing symptoms while advocating the necessity of the talking cure, the concepts of transference (A, 216) and counter-transference (A, 246). These psychoanalytic concepts first demonstrated by Freud are used both within the story and as a structural element to understand how the psychiatrist tries to talk the patients into confessing their crimes to him and how attraction and love function for the characters. This is something that Dupont analyses:

> Transference and counter-transference become novelistic tools which act upon the reader, who necessarily finds themselves involved at an ethical level, while the one who is supposed to diagnose needs to be diagnosed. When the perverse action is successful, as in the story of *Asylum*, what takes place is some very special discomfort that can undoubtedly be regarded as a modality of contemporary gothic style. (Dupont 2013: par.22)

In his study of the process of transference, J.-P. Lucchelli explains how Lacan reworks this notion between 1964 and 1967: Throughout his teaching, Lacan insists on the fact that transference and repetition are two separate unconscious processes and his elaboration leads him to create the concept of the 'subject-that-is-supposed-to-know' (Lucchelli 2009: 21), in order to designate the position held by the analyst in relation to the *analysand*. Lucchelli explains that Freud first thought of transference as an affect and therefore as an obstacle to therapy. He thought it was the other scene where the subject becomes the hero of his/her own tale, blinding him/her to the unconscious effects of this position. The concept of transference was established by Freud as a result of the treatment of Dora, a case which incidentally is an example in which it failed to function in therapy. It was reinterpreted later as the condition of the cure, because the attachment it produces to the analyst is what enables the patient to repeat primary scenes (Lucchelli 2009: 27–34). For Lacanian psychoanalysis, there is a 'symbolic overdetermination' of the inter-relation between the analyst and the *analysand*, and this overdetermination needs interpreting. Mitchell and Rose explain this in very clear terms: 'What happens in an analysis is that the subject is, strictly speaking, constituted through a discourse, to which the mere presence of the psychoanalyst brings, before any intervention, the dimension of dialogue' (Mitchell and Rose 1985: 62). Lacan's ethical stance repeatedly consisted in pointing out the necessity for analysts to have experienced transference in their own therapy so as to avoid falling into the loophole of (ab)using it when helping patients out. In his 'brief history of madness', Roy Porter, who incidentally quotes Lacan only in passing, repeats this argument: 'The months Freud spent studying under Charcot in Paris in 1885 proved crucial to his development—which is one reason why psychoanalysis has never been able to shake off the charge that its "cures", no less than Charcot's, are largely products of suggestion' (Porter 2002: 188). This suggestive power is what Freud sought to avoid by giving up on hypnosis and it is shown in McGrath's novel as a fatal mistake made by the analyst who is unaware of transference and its effects, or perhaps ignorant of its manipulative potential.

Other psychological concepts referred to in the narrative include identification and eroticisation, but they are not operational diagnoses because they are asserted as general statements, heedless of the subjective logic at play in the specific cases of Stella and Edgar. It seems that the text refutes these ready-made symptoms by showing that Stella's experience remains beyond articulation: what Peter wants to reconnect to is a meaning, a dialectics of cause and consequence, a logical outcome to what is never articulated or never explained by Stella herself. What Peter mistakes for resistance and psychic reluctance to speak could well be an impossibility to make sense and therefore say that which happens. The retrospective narrative does not give us any hindsight other than on Peter's own delusional method. Elsewhere, we see how he reports Jack's words which describes the crime committed by Edgar (in impressive details) and the dangerousness of his case, as if he wanted to scare Stella away, which fails because he still has not raised the question of why Stella was attracted to Edgar, if attraction is the correct word (A, 69).

Hopson says that 'conjecture', rather than 'fact', is at the heart of Peter's report (Hopson 2020: 154) but what I would like to stress is how he unashamedly, and unethically, mingles his own voice with the voices of his patients, to the extent that Stella's interpretations, while rare, are often silenced by the interpretation of the scientific man who remains deaf: 'This was her interpretation. I suggested that instead it might be connected with anger./What anger? Anger with Max… She was not ready to talk about it yet, and I didn't force her. It would come' (A, 28). While the patient's response could invite him towards another interpretation, Peter is so certain that he knows more, even if he denies it, that he does not listen—a worrying sign for a psychiatrist. Psychiatry therefore is presented as failing to echo what is said and to make sense of the incoherence observed. Cleave's name gives us a key: he *cleaves* to a version of events that can be made to sound rational. While Edgar says nothing of his crime (A, 9) or Stella says nothing of why she was attracted to Edgar (A, 9), Cleave systematically offers his own analysis as if the patients could not form logical links as elaborate as his. In particular, Cleave corrects the characters' versions of their reality: he knows that Edgar does not have a son; he knows that Ruth did not have any lovers; he knows that Stella did not know anything about Edgar's plans to leave and so forth. He does not seem to consider that this factual version of events means nothing for those whose sense of reality is elsewhere. His version of truth is limited to facts, which in turn hinders his capacity to listen to what his patients' version reveals in terms of psychopathological structure—for example, the function this distance between facts and truth could have. Cleave seems to be unaware that if Stella speaks to him, it is because he holds a place in language and discourse. Instead, he pictures his role as one of 'friendly' (A, 164) care: 'We would talk, I would come to know her. Understand her affair with Edgar. Find comfort with me. Safety' (A, 228). Dr Cleave often uses these non-medical terms—'care', 'look after', 'friend' (A, 164)—as if his own place in discourse was not fixed, his role fluid. If Stella cannot deal with lack and the fact that she has no place, then such attitude is likely to make her experience even greater anxiety and instability. The author shows this tension between patients and doctor by fragmenting the narrative and breaking Peter's coherence so that his demonstration fails to convince.

The consequence of Peter's method is that everyone is always odd and strange, as if Peter was the standard against which some behaviour should be judged respectable or acceptable. If we return to the ball scene, Peter is incapable of voicing why the habit of dancing in hospitals makes him uncomfortable: 'Our patients dress eccentrically and move awkwardly, handicapped as much by the medication they take as the illnesses that make the medication necessary' (A, 4). He does not note the subjective perspective of such a statement, remaining perplexed as to why the way they dress should appear eccentric to him. Very few readers will be equipped to recognise the behaviourist framework through which such a statement can be voiced but most will be uneasy at the doctor's admission of his negative vision of patients. In addition, Peter is entirely ignorant of his own prejudices when identifying the 'illness' he diagnoses his patients with. This behaviourist slant, which consists in interpreting someone's behaviour according to norms and levels of acceptation of deviance, is often to be noted in the novel: 'Watching him dance with Stella it was hard to believe that he suffered a disorder involving severe disturbance in his relationships with women' (A, 7). This also recalls a tendency of the time in which psychiatric and psychological treatment was based on strong social and moral prejudices and grounded in the conviction that madness was the effect of being socially awkward: behaviourism emerged as a theory to help people back into normal life (King 2018). When Stella becomes afraid that she could be discovered by Max, her husband, she says 'reading me like a book, finding it written in fragments of behaviour, fleeting nuances of expression, certain absences of response of which I would not be aware. Oh, I must be vigilant, from this point on I must be vigilant' (A, 24). Stella knows that a book is judged by its cover indeed and that some psychiatrists will base their diagnosis on behavioural symptoms, which are those she must be 'vigilant' about.

Peter's clinical observation seems to be only external, and his appreciation of recovery is based on the disappearance of these external signs. Peter admits to this approach when towards the end of the novel he explains:

> Upstairs, no sort of behaviour provoked surprise because it was accepted that all were mad. Being unhappy and bitter and relentlessly derisive, as Sarah was, that was mad, just as mad as picking at threads that didn't exist or becoming agitated about a missed appointment and tasks left undone twenty-seven years ago. You ceased to be mad when you began to behave as though you weren't in a madhouse, as though you weren't locked up with no real idea when you were getting out again. (A, 217)

This definition of madness strikes one as superficial. It puts on the same footing obsessive worries (appointments and tasks left undone), absolute affects (what is this derision that is referred to and what is it directed to or towards?) and behaviour without questioning the subjective logic of each specific symptom for the patient. This kind of example makes one think that the psychiatrist believes super-egoistic considerations could prevail or should prevail in Stella, as if he considered that everyone was subjected to inhibition and repression: when he does not simply remind us of her social status, he uses it to imagine the logic behind her action (A, 11). It seems that her behaviour—which consists in being unfaithful to her husband while the servants and her mother-in-law are in the house (A, 14), the fact that she does not look after her son or that she is not upset that she is having sex with the neighbour in what is clearly a debasing relationship that means nothing to her—never alerts Peter to the possibility of another *jouissance*, a boundless and unbridled *jouissance*, against which the Freudian theory of repression would be one type of defence, and not necessarily the most useful one:

The Woman is implicated... in phallic sexuality, but at the same time it is 'elsewhere that she upholds the question of her own *jouissance*' (PP, 121), that is, the question of her status as desiring subject. Lacan designates this *jouissance* supplementary so as to avoid any notion of complement, of woman as complement to man's phallic nature... But it is also a recognition of the 'something more', the 'more than *jouissance*' which Lacan locates in the Freudian concept of repetition—what escapes or is left over from the phallic function, and exceeds it. Woman is therefore placed *beyond*.... That 'beyond' refers at once to her most total mystification as absolute Other ..., and to a *question*, the question of her own *jouissance*, of her greater or lesser access to the residue of the dialectic to which she is constantly subjected. (Mitchell and Rose 1985: 51; see also 52–57 for a more detailed exploration of this)

Peter only envisages oedipal inhibition in which division is a sign of repression and censorship. This hinders his capacity to question Stella's iterative, or repetitive, attraction or emotional attachment to dangerous partners. Stella's excessive behaviour defying all norms is never perceived as having a logic of its own.

On the contrary, because Peter remains oblivious of the unconscious, of the split between the real that is excluded from the subject's experience, and the symbolic that fixes reality, he cannot understand the logic behind the absence of dialectics: 'The psychiatrist sees his patients as following predictable paths of madness and this prevents him from closely observing them with an open mind. This repeatedly undermines his psychiatric expertise' (Hopson 2020: 164). This can be illustrated thus:

Despite the fact that we were friends, or perhaps because of it, Stella was inhibited with me at first by what I assumed to be a sense of shame .... I realized a little later that it wasn't shame that made her reluctant to talk to me but uncertainty about my attitude to Edgar.... I told her that as a psychiatrist I wasn't in the business of moral judgements. She seemed to need this reassurance. (A, 19)

This means that Cleave remains unaware of a psychological process evidenced by Lacan, foreclosure. According to Lacan, in psychotic subjects, lack has not been symbolised, which affects the subjects' relation to language because absence is absent, as it were; or the function of lack lacks, which often manifests in the subject's encountering the impossibility to say, to articulate, or to structure what happens to them and to make what happens to them dialectical. This is called 'foreclosure', the absence of the symbolisation of lack and the overwhelming, iterative presence of this lack (Lacan 1981: 21, distinction between *Verneinung* and *Verwerfung*).

In that respect, M. Falco's remark about McGrath's narrative hesitation is illuminating:

> McGrath explains ... that he changed the narrator while he was writing *Asylum*—initially the narrator had been Stella. The fact of having Peter Cleave tell the story, he continues, created a network of diffracted points of view on Stella's story. Thus, as psychiatrist, Cleave can re-invent Stella's story and the initial narrator's story too. (Falco 2007a: 105)

For Falco, this is evidence of McGrath's complex, postmodern narrative strategy which offers many narratological breakthroughs (Falco 2007a: 95). I, on the other hand, would argue that above all McGrath's decision to change narrators shows that Stella's story could not have been consistent, because McGrath conceives her as marked by an impossibility to symbolise what happens to her, that is, to articulate it in a dialectical or symbolic fashion. As a result, the novel barely ever makes us hear Stella through direct speech and in the second half of the novel, when she is secluded in her Welsh home or when she is back in the hospital as a patient, fulfilling her initial idea that she was 'more eccentric than the general population' (A, 7), she is never heard at all. Her silence is the object of Peter's bewilderment. Falco insists that the multiple layers of narration and discourses come to signify the sham of scientific discourse in relation to the underlying madness of the scientist (Falco 2007a, 283). For all the value of such an analysis, it does not account for the absence that is central to the novel, other than by evoking the pleasure derived from such narratological prowess. It is fair to say that critics have failed to see Stella as an interesting psychiatric case: she is never discussed in the major books on the question of literature and psychiatry, even by feminist critics who could have easily continued a tradition of feminist criticism which analyses the patriarchal institutions of power that lead women to crimes and accusations of madness (Gilbert and Gubar 1984). Dupont, Falco and Hopson have certainly looked at McGrath's œuvre, Baker *et alii* too, but *Asylum* never is the central novel of their analyses and when it is, they tend to look at Peter more than Stella: 'In *Asylum*, it is not the perception of the psychiatric patient that needs decoding but that of the authoritative psychiatrist.... It is also obvious that Edgar not Stella is the patient of psychiatric and probably erotic interest to the psychiatrist' (Hopson 2020: 151 & 184). I take this neglect as a sure sign that Stella is indeed the one whose opacity and silence should interest us, another point of connection with the character of Septimus.

STELLA: THE FAILURE OF LOVE
AND THE OTHER JOUISSANCE

In 'Writing Asylum', the preface to the second edition of the novel, McGrath indicates that Stella is the matter of his novel: 'Now I had a story. It would be about the wife' (McGrath 2015: xi). If she is on every page of the novel, and was first thought to be the storyteller, why should she be neglected by critics? My contention is that she embodies the unspeak-able—not because of moralistic or ethical reasons—of a *jouissance* (here of a sexual nature) which cannot be articulated into language and therefore returns as that which has never been symbolised. In that respect, McGrath's suggestion that the novel is first and foremost a love story ('catastrophic love affair' are the very first words of the novel, A, 1) also points to the unquantifiable feelings experienced, an absence of measure that baffles scientific method: Stella is no guinea pig; she is a singular subject whose encounter with sex has left marks on her body but has also made her liter-ally speechless. She does not become delirious like Septimus; she is charac-terised by subjective emptiness: events are not inscribed, they remain distant from her and this disconnection from the world is reflected in her careless attitude towards her body, her sexuality, thus her life, to the extent that she commits suicide. Stella is incapable of caring for herself (Gori and Del Volgo 2020; Foucault 1972). Stella is first shown like an incurably romantic figure, seeking out her lost lover, but it turns out that she is a prisoner of a loving killer, a violent lover, someone both irascible and irra-tional. Opposing all 'logical' explanations, she admits that this does not matter and that she is not afraid, or at least not afraid of that: 'Then she discovered she didn't care' (A, 91). Cleave himself thinks he cares, but what he wants to do is alter. At one point, Stella admits that there is no care that will cure her: 'She looked at him without fear. It didn't matter now. Nothing mattered' (A, 117). Stella remains unaffected by what hap-pens to her or what she makes happen. It is as if she was not there herself, and Stella can therefore be killed, or dead, as she is fully engaged in the enjoyment of a mode of *jouissance* that cannot be channelled: 'Now he was going to murder her. Oddly, the idea held no horror for her, she was detached from everything around her' (A, 130). 'Oddly' underlines the feeling Peter has when faced with this subject that is impossible to fit in.

For Stella, sexual relationships are how she questions the enigma of her identity. This means that love is a symbolic operation—of exchange and connection with other beings—and this operation reveals that subjects, by virtue of their being lodged in a sexed body, are fundamentally alienated to language. Lacan has argued that language does not symbolise two sexes, that there is an absence of symmetry between the unconscious relation to the signifier: some are defined by the meaningless signifier, while others are only partially so (Lacan 1975). Without going into the detail of this, what can be retained here is the idea that sex is intermeshed with language, unconscious processes and the body. It manifests as an enigma for *all*. *Asylum* shows how Stella tries to knot these sexual dimensions into something that would function but she only makes her failure to articulate this back to the symbolic order apparent.

Stella's madness is first identified by her alleged lack of maternal love. When faced with the policemen that want to know why she didn't cry for help when her son was drowning, the narrative states: 'they couldn't understand it; she has no feelings, they said, she is not human, she's a monster. Or perhaps she's mad./She was mad. How could you explain it, unless she was mad?' (A, 199). And yet, saying she is mad is no explanation, as Peter should know. It could be an excuse to avoid a trial at most, but many patients of psychiatric asylums would not let their child drown or would shout—in other words, her lack of words is no clear symptom of a pathology, in the sense of that which guides us back to an illness with no clear nosography. However, it might be a symptom in the sense of a singular response commanded by a certain subjective position. In any case, after the child's death, to paraphrase Lacan, she is 'defamed' (Lacan 1975: 79). This pun is evoked when Lacan explains that a woman is not born a woman, but rather is said to be a woman, which in French translates as '*on la dit femme*'. This resonates with 'defame'—'*Dit femme* and *diffâme* are homonyms in French', writes R. Fink in his footnote to explain the translation (Lacan 1975).[2] The passage in which Lacan makes this pun is complex and would take us very far from our current concern with McGrath's novel but quoting it here resonates with this scene: Stella's exclusion from language is not unrelated to her feminine position and to the *jouissance*

---

[2] The English translation is to be found in the 1998 translation of the text, Fink 1999, 85, n24.

she encounters. For Lacan, some people, because of a lack of a signifier for sexual difference, are essentially marked by exclusion, and statistically this asymmetry has favoured men over women. Hence, the long history of women's exclusion and representation as the radical other of rationality (Mitchell and Rose 1985: 52–53).

Stella is the only woman of the novel. Of course, there are other female characters: Ruth, the dead wife, Mrs Bain, the servant who loves a good gossip, Brenda, Max's widowed mother and spokesperson for morality, or Mair, Trevor's wife, unsexed, not even remotely interested in what her husband and her neighbour do under her nose. All these other female characters are flat, secondary people in the life of Stella and of the novel. They do not engage in any sexual activity, while Stella is immediately presented as highly sexualised; her body is sexed: 'I know she was considered beautiful... She was rather a fleshy, full-breasted woman, taller than the average and that night she was wearing a single string of pearls that nicely set off the whiteness of her neck and shoulders and bosom' (A, 5). As is often the case, women's sexuality appears as the dark continent of psychiatry: 'all his insight, all his psychiatric expertise, none of it could penetrate her womanly shield' (A, 88). McGrath himself points this out in his preface to the second edition of the novel: 'It was then about ten minutes before feminism properly arrived in the south of England' (McGrath 2015: xii). He therefore uses the trope of woman as an enigma to signify that which cannot be tamed, controlled or classified into standard nosography, that is, *jouissance* and the symptom that emerges from the encounter between this and language: 'It had of course occurred to me that she might do something like this, but I'd rather thought she would listen to me. I didn't rightly gauge' (A, 100).

The novel proceeds through a gradual unveiling of the function of the sexual at stake in Stella's subjectivity by showing the many mistaken senses that are attributed to it first. In an interesting reversal of the orthodoxy of pop-Freudianism which consisted in thinking that everything was a substitute for some sexual wish, desire or trauma, Cleave thinks that Stella's behaviour towards Edgar may only be a smokescreen to conceal her true concern: 'Let me ask you to consider a possibility. That this love of yours was just a blind for something else?' (A, 212) And Peter never stops offering comments on Stella's sexual relationships without realising that what is at stake is not the fantasy of completion that love sometimes is a symbol of, as Lacan explains in a rhetorical question: 'Is Eros a tension towards the One?' (Lacan 1975, trans. Fink: 5). It is rather the tragic insistence of that which can never be written:

Perhaps that's the whole point about infidelity, I suggested, not that one has
sex but that by doing so one puts at risk someone else's happiness? It's not
the blunt fact of the thing, it's all in the effect it would have if known. The
thing itself is insignificant. She agreed with me, in principle. But none of
that was relevant anymore. (A, 32)

In these suggestions, one may recognise an analytic discourse intent on
interpreting everything according to sexual drives. Freud is named (A, 42)
but without any clear sign of allegiance or defiance, and no other psychiatric theorist is evoked, despite the constant reference to Cleave's great
knowledge of the human mind. Max, Stella's husband, also seems to operate via suggestion, as if Stella's silences and the few words she utters had
no consistency. These men hold a position of knowledge and take it for
granted that Stella, like Clarissa in *Mrs Dalloway*, does not know anything:
'"It was Edgar in the water."/He nodded. "I thought it probably was".'
(A, 202). It turns out that Stella is not present in the narration, that she is
effaced, defamed, and I argue that there is a structural conclusion to draw
from her relentless absence of answer, which is never said to be a refusal to
answer, even by the blinded witnesses that she encounters: 'She was in the
police station and she didn't have an answer there either' (A, 198–199).
The sentence is clear: she does not have an answer; it is foreclosed.

The novel clearly pits men against women when it comes to pathologising attitudes. Edgar killed his wife, and the novel does not tell us anything
about the police inquiry. When Stella commits a crime, she is the object of
the greatest scrutiny. It is as if she was blamed for her encounter with *a
jouissance* that cannot be named and which baffles everyone. One of the
most discreet ironies of the novel is Cleave's idea that in order to fix Stella's
destiny, he should propose to her. Cleave, unable to conceive of a jouissance that is founded on a failed encounter with men, offers that which, as
a matter of fact, is symptomatic for Stella (the union with men at a symbolic level). For what is more symbolic indeed than the institution of marriage? The proposal suggests a union that leaves unnamed the failure of
the encounter between men and women that Lacan conceptualises with
the notion of an other jouissance. It is indeed in her relationships with
men that Stella strains herself to suicide—examples abound, starting with
her uncontrollable drinking (A, 88), and her many lies. Cleave does not
seem to see that her smile every time marriage is discussed echoes her
enigmatic laughter when Edgar first leaves the hospital: 'Her reaction
astonished her. That she should want to *laugh*—what did this mean?'

(A, 28) Instead of acknowledging the function of this absence of meaning, Peter is keen to cover it with an explanation of his own which defeats the possibility for him to understand the logic of the case.

Stella's reactions are in no way logical from an imaginary point of view, but they make sense if one distinguishes the symbolic level where sex as intercourse and the sexual as a signifying operation of language can be differentiated. Peter seems to have a very basic approach to these questions, as if sex was a popular magazine's topic to be discussed along the lines of satisfaction or dissatisfaction: "'Was Max really so unsatisfactory?" … "I suppose he must have been or it wouldn't have happened'" (A, 217). For Peter, there is no understanding of the relationship with Edgar beyond the moral notions of unfaithfulness and infidelity. And yet, in itself, this infidelity can only be taken into account from a moral point of view. From a psychological point of view, there is no such moral ground and what matters is where the satisfaction is lodged or could be located for the subject in the act that is performed. Stella's concession is almost like a perfunctory acquiescence. In other words, Peter clings to the law and fails to hear what Stella says. Stella agrees to the suggestion that adultery is bad, but her actions show that she cannot resist the attraction and all the reader is left with is the assurance that Peter's interpretation fails.

Cleave in fact points to what is central to the ball scene that Stella recounts without realising how much this ball scene frames the narrative, giving it structure and substance. McGrath's writing consists in ensuring punches in the narrative are both silenced and structurally blatant:

> The essence of it, she told me, was that while they were dancing she became aware that what was pressing against her groin, through his trousers, was, in fact, his penis, and it was getting hard. She said she kept remembering, first, her incomprehension when she felt it, and then, an instant later, her realization that it was, yes, what she thought it was…. At no point then or later did her composure fail her. She was almost sorry when the music stopped and he turned abruptly and went back to the other side of the room. (A, 16)

This example can be interpreted as the intrusion of a *jouissance* that is real, in the Lacanian sense of it: Edgar's sex literally is improper and misplaced; it pierces through the romantic, imaginary dimension of the ball which is supposed to be a civilised place of social bonding. This experience is marked by incredulity, lack of sense, but also guilty pleasure (she was *almost* sorry) and none of it will ever be inscribed in Stella's story ('At no point then or later did her composure fail her'). It is a moment of suspension of disbelief and a moment in which language and meaning fail. However, Stella is still driven to the man and the experience, as if on an impulse. What remains of the experience is the undeniable and permanent mark on Stella's body ('her groin') of the other's desire for her, which she cannot resist. However, the question is not to see Stella as a woman under the yoke of a patriarchal representation in which women are seen as subjected to men's desire, but to see how the narrative strategy consists in displacing the real penis that she felt against her groin to the symbolic level of the phallus, which raises the *question* of her *jouissance* that she cannot articulate: 'Stella told me that it was while Charlie was clinging like a monkey to the shaft of the spade that she felt the first stirring of interest in the man' (A, 10). The phallic symbols structurally return where the real has overwhelmed the subject and it is this logic that prevails, the logic of symbolised sex rather than the actual organ with which Stella, so to speak, will never have to deal again, even if her actions will try to retrieve that moment in intercourse.

The role played by the intrusion of Edgar's penis during the ball scene can structurally be set against Max's lack of interest in sexual intercourse— a detail enabling the unfaithfulness to take place repeatedly without his noticing—as demonstrated by the fact that the couple he forms with Stella has only had one child, at the end of the 1950s, that is before the advent and easy access to contraceptive methods. Nothing is said of this fact, nor is anything said about Trevor Williams's becoming her sexual partner later on in the novel. What the narrative emphasises is Stella's lack of pleasure and pro-active participation in sexual intercourse, when it happens with Edgar, with Nick (Edgar's friend and partner in crime) and Trevor Williams. As a result, one is led to think that, in order to comprehend it, the function of sex is to be seen at the level of the real—that is at the level of what rents through reality and leaves its meaningless trace—and at the symbolic level of language: 'She first had sex with Trevor Williams in the middle of November. It was not her doing, it hadn't occurred to her to think of him in that way' (A, 168). This is a perfect example of the intermingling of Stella's and Peter's voices, the sentence shows two logics, one of meaninglessness and lack of participation, one of interpretation where there can be no lack. Cleave remains alienated to the cultural and meaningful sense of love and the vision of a sexual life regulated by the law, even when faced with a patient whose own relation to sex invites for another understanding.

Peter constantly insists that Stella's relation to sex is unhealthy, which he notes in her reluctance to talk about it: 'It has not been easy to talk to Stella about the sex. She naturally finds it distasteful to be explicit. But she has described to me in detail how it began' (A, 22). Again, he falls prey to understanding this reluctance as inhibition. This dimension is easily delusional indeed and some critics have also tended to use it against the novel. Hopson stresses the paradox that Cleave struggles with. He blames Stella for refusing to speak to him about sex. Yet he reports scenes of a fairly crude sexual nature that she is supposed to have told him—Hopson describes the details as 'salacious' (Hopson 2020: 178)—or that he has conjectured: 'she knelt on the bed holding the headboard and pushed against his thrusts with her eyes closed and her mind empty' (A, 169). Hopson intimates that this is what makes the novel unrealistic because she thinks the crude details are Peter's doing (Hopson 2020: 178–179). In fact, the critic is here victim of the same illusion as Cleave; these characters do not exist. What the narrative does, however, is play out the failure of the encounter between the psychiatrist and his patient for lack of sufficient understanding of the symbolic dimension of the sexual and its central, structural role in the subject's real experience. Stella's attitude and demeanour were steady until the ball scene. After that, she is overwhelmed by something which her will is not sufficient to stop and which iterates in her life. This is destructive when the subject has no imaginary means or symbolic prop to set up barriers against an excessively open and invasive identification to this iterative real. Stella's incapacity to articulate her thoughts is relentlessly attributed to inhibition, an explanation that covers up what the sexual encounters do and how they are something that cannot be symbolised or didacticised. She does not mind the sordid details of intercourse but sex means an overwhelming reaction of her body that she cannot control and which she is alienated to as a result: 'she was sure he couldn't see her clearly through the kitchen window, but he put his hand on his groin and rubbed it, and she couldn't help smiling' (A, 178). Just like the shaft of the spade, the return of the signifier 'groin' structurally (or linguistically) inscribes the return of the ball scene, which enacts the vision of the organ and Stella's smile, uncontrolled and inappropriate to the scene, signals it.

This is a far cry from Peter's vision of marriage, unfaithfulness and love as the coupling of two souls. Peter sets himself the task of having to decode

Stella's symptom and to interpret it by giving it a meaning—which could be paraphrased as: Max is not good enough; you were fooled by a man who did not love you; I shall marry you to make up for your sense of loneliness. But McGrath's text instead seeks to localise this reiterated *jouissance* by emphasising many aspects of Stella's life which, like sex, find no expression. Stella therefore will be shown to have no other relation than relations of a sexual nature: she does not have any friends; she barely ever connects with her son; she is not involved in life outside the hospital. In fact, from day one, she is a patient for whom the hospital is an asylum indeed, where she finds her body enclosed. Other hints become meaningful when approached from the perspective of this symbolic lack. Stella has to make do with Max's mother but she has no parent herself, or relatives: 'she was the daughter of a diplomat who'd been disgraced in a scandal years before. Both her parents were dead now' (A, 1).[3] Not only are these people dead but she never mentions them, they are gone and have no symbolic inscription. In her life, Stella has no apparent memory of her past or her childhood; her life has no other milestone than her sexual encounter with Edgar or her failure as a mother. The novel painstakingly camouflages Stella's reduction, but it still shows, especially in Peter's constant or incessant mistaken judgements: 'She tried, she said, not to dwell on Charlie, but without much success, I suspect' (A, 104). McGrath's style is revealed here in the parallel of the construction: 'she said' is soon followed by 'I suspect'. This enables McGrath to intermingle both voices but in this particular example, it ironically reveals Peter's professional fiasco. When his patient claims that she is not where she is supposed to be, he insists on re-instating her (Boileau 2022).

It is not impossible that *Asylum* may also be a critical reflection on novelists' habit of appropriating madness in the same way as authoritarian psychiatrists do, to assign the patient to a place where they cannot be. McGrath shows great awareness of the suspicion one may have regarding the ethics of certain psychiatrists: in 'Ground Zero', the narrator who is asked to help a patient who lives a dysfunctional love story with an ex-prostitute traumatised by 9/11 asks her patient to spy on him and his girlfriend so that she can gauge who that other person is (McGrath 2005), a debatable practice which seems to ignore the symbolic aspect of therapy and the fact that therapy should help patients realise the symbolic

---

[3] This sees the return of Stella's reputation being 'defamed', a fact inscribed in the family drama of her past.

scaffolding of their unconscious, which bears but little resemblance with reality. The psychological representation of a subject can never be compared with objective facts. Elsewhere, McGrath also interrogates the notion of 'connection' as imagined from a perspective of meaning. Visited by the son of a patient who recently died and with whom he had been involved romantically, Dr Haggard tries to instil the idea that illness indeed is not to be interpreted solely as meaningful:

> 'But tell me, what do you mean, "connected"? What was her illness connected with?'
> Silence. 'I don't know,' you said at last.
> 'Connected with the atmosphere at home. With the arguments. With my father being so angry all the time. I felt as if she were being punished.'
> I was beginning to understand. 'Illness isn't a form of retribution,' I said gently. 'It's not a sign of moral failure.'
> 'Oh I know.' (McGrath 1993: 15)

This exchange enables us to see that meaning is a deceptional aspect of treatment and even if Dr Haggard is a Doctor of Medicine and not of psychiatry, he has to deal with ailments of the body which tend to be interpreted as something other than just physical facts. In that respect, doctors are like novelists—as Woolf says—because they have to deal with heightened impressions and subjective affects caused by the illness but also detached from the physicality, organicity and nosography of medicine alone. Peter can therefore be regarded as a second-rate detective-novelist: 'The problem was that the further she moved away from the hospital the harder I found it to reconstruct her experience, to shape it into something with a shape and a meaning I could recognize' (A, 112). Peter seeks to fashion Stella like a creator, only because of his lack of awareness of this danger, his oblivious sense of what it means to suggest and to precipitate meaning. He pushes Stella towards enjoying her symptom even more, and therefore to be annihilated by it. Current conceptions of psychopathology informed by neuroscience and biomedicine assume that they can explain symptoms and even feelings through biology (Pommier 2004). In other words, they assume that the human brain functions universally and that the standardisation of practices, behaviour and emotions of individuals is conducive to acceptation and social bonding (Gori and Del Volgo 2020). In so doing, they are reluctant to accept the failing of language which cannot express love (McGrath 1993: 95) or illness (Woolf 1926): Stella is an enigma, to herself and to others, and failing to take that into account in order to transform her into a divided subject inevitably fails because it negates her singularity.

CONCLUSION

'To unravel the narrative puzzle of *Asylum*, it is necessary to recognise the text as offering much information about Cleave's deceptions, and very little reliable information about any other character' (Hopson 2020: 186). I hope to have shown the exact opposite of this assertion. What is supposedly 'very little' is not a sign that there should be more, but the discreet sign of the nothingness which Stella enjoys. The character is marked by an incapacity to dialecticise and make sense of what happens to her. As such, the novel points to the failure of psychiatric nosography not because it suggests the madness of a character that is not, properly speaking, mad, but because it reveals the mistakes made by psychiatry in identifying the singular, perhaps unique, modes of enjoyment that subjects create and which literature, on the other hand, feeds on. This is how McGrath renews the genre of the detective novel and the *roman noir* by resorting to the clinical case study. Eventually, we are presented with a form of madness that is not the negative side of the normal, not madness as pathological, but madness as the impossibility to invent ways of channelling or even keeping *jouissance* at bay. For madness is a condition that affects everyone, if we are to consider that it derives from human beings' entry into language. This is Stella's intuition, perceptive as she may be because of her own experience: '"We're all mad." She remembers the moment distinctly. She was sitting on the bench in the shade of the garden wall, and Edgar was up... "I don't think you're mad"' (A, 16).

With Stella, we also come to understand that Edgar himself cannot say anything about what agitates him and that sexuality, although it is the central element of his misbehaviour, is something that he has not thought through: 'Although he functioned at a high level of intelligence he never showed any insight into why he had killed his wife' (A, 8). The only thing that this points to is that, by virtue of his lack of symbolisation of sex, his relation to the Other is violent and lacking. During an interview with Cleave, Edgar retorts to Peter by saying what is covered up in Cleave's transference strategy, what is unknown to him, with a brutality and bluntness that evoke a lack of linguistic prowess suggestive of a subjective emptiness: 'The question is, what would she want with an old queen like you?'

(A, 236). Transference is love. However, love is enigmatic and cannot be established universally. McGrath therefore creates a psychiatrist in love with his patients to work upon the danger there is in wanting to cure patients like these instead of helping them control what remains meaningless. Like genre novelists who reduce characters to types, psychiatrist novelists run the risk of reducing patients to predetermined cases.

Asylum offers another vision of madness which is not based on grand manifestations such as in the hysterics of Salpêtrière or the sociopaths of Hollywood films, and which is more discreet than the likes of Septimus Warren Smith: Stella is not delirious in speech, but her reality cannot find a common ground with others. In the novel, what is mad is the absence of meaning which goes lacking everywhere, except in the perverse suggestions of the psychiatrist himself. The text's structure leaves no doubt as to the sexual origin of Stella's wandering while the psychiatrist never manages to situate the case within the logic of the absence of sexual relation at the symbolic level. In other words, the psychiatrist does not see the foreclosure which the text exposes and then seeks to fill in with meaning. The other aspect which is defeated is the law of realist fiction and detective fiction, these generic structures which McGrath claims to enjoy. These traditional generic tools—murder, love, the psychiatric ward—are much less convincing than the opacity of the central character, or rather the one character that the narration manages to slowly make central. The text's fragmentation of stories, multiplications of versions, owes much more to the Modernist aesthetic than the generic tropes of *roman noir*. The obsession with the failed relationship and the absence of eroticism in what appears at first as carnal scenes and carnal knowledge also invite us to rethink the sexual in terms of not only what is opposed to language but what is irretrievably related to language, insofar as it is built both by its being articulated in language and by its being ejected from language.

BIBLIOGRAPHY

PRIMARY SOURCES

Collins, Wilkie (1883). *Heart and Science*. Stroud: Alan Sutton, 1994.
McGrath, Patrick (1993). *Dr. Haggard's Disease*. London: Viking.
McGrath, Patrick (2005). *Ghost Town, Tales of Manhattan Then and Now*. London: Bloomsbury, 2006.
McGrath, Patrick (2008). *Trauma*. New York: A. A. Knopf.
Woolf, Virginia (1926). "On Being Ill" (1930). Woolf 1948, 9–23.

SECONDARY SOURCES

Acheson, James & Ross, Sarah E. (eds.) (2005). *The Contemporary British Novel Since 1980*. Edinburgh: Edinburgh University Press.

Baker, Charley, Crawford, Paul et al. (2010). *Madness in Post-1945 British and American Fiction*. London: Routledge.

Boileau, Nicolas Pierre (2022). "Suburbia, or *Para*-urbia: Rachel Cusk's Gendered Readings of Suburban Spaces and the Role of the Writer in *Arlington Park*." M. Bouchet, I. Keller-Privat et al. (eds.) (2022). *Suburbs. New Literary Perspectives*. Rowman and Littlefield.

Braun, Alice (2008). *Janet Frame: Le Féminin et la Marge*. Unpublished PhD thesis defended in Paris Nanterre under the supervision of Prof. Claire Bazin.

Caminero-Santangelo, Marta (1998). *The Madwoman Can't Speak, Or Why Insanity is Not Subversive*. Ithaca: Cornell University Press.

Childs, Peter (2012). *Contemporary Fiction: British Novelists since 1970*. London: Palgrave Macmillan.

Dupont, Jocelyn (2007). "Récit de l'obsession et obsession du récit chez Patrick McGrath." M. Amfreville and C. Fabre (eds.). *Les Formes de l'obsession, vol. II*. Paris: Michel Houdard Éditions, 139–149.

Dupont, Jocelyn (2008). *Intertextualité et autorité dans l'œuvre de Patrick McGrath*. Unpublished PhD thesis under the supervision of Prof. Max Duperray.

Dupont, Jocelyn (2010). "Du pastiche idéal à la parodie du pastiche: Patrick McGrath et la fin de l'angoisse de l'influence." J. Dupont & É. Walezak (eds.). *L'Intertextualité dans le roman contemporain de langue anglaise*. Perpignan: Presses Universitaires de Perpignan, 153–169. Available online: https://books.openedition.org/pupvd/32112

Dupont, Jocelyn (2013). "Les psychiatres fous du Dr McGrath." H. Machinal (ed.). *Le savant fou*. Rennes: Presses universitaires de Rennes. Last checked 12/21 http://books.openedition.org/pur/52928

Falco, Magali (2007a). *La Poétique néo-gothique de Patrick McGrath*. Paris: Éditions Publibook Université.

Falco, Magali (2007b). *A Collection of Interviews with Patrick McGrath*. Paris: Editions Publibook Université.

Fink, Bruce (1999). Translation of J. Lacan's seminar *Encore. On Feminine Sexuality, The Limits of Love and Knowledge*, 1972–73, New York: Norton Editions.

Foucault, Michel (1972). *Histoire de la folie à l'âge classique*. Paris: Gallimard, "Tel".

Gagneret, Diane (2019). *Explorer la frontière: Folie et genre(s) dans la littérature anglophone contemporaine*. Unpublished PhD thesis defended at ENS Lyon, 22.11.2019, under the supervision of Prof. Vanessa Guignery.

Gilbert, Sandra & Gubar, Susan (1984). *The Madwoman in the Attic: The Woman Writer and the Nineteenth Century Literary Imagination*. New Haven: Yale University Press.

Gori, Roland & Del Volgo, Marie-José (2020), *Exilés de l'intime, Vers un Homme neuroéconomique.* Paris: Les Liens qui libèrent.

Hopson, Jacqueline (2020). "Malevolent, Mad or Merely Human: Representations of the 'Psy' Professional in English, American and Irish Fiction." PhD defended in September 2020 at the University of Exeter, unpublished: https://search-proquest-com.lama.univ-amu.fr/docview/2497503683?pq-origsite=summon [last checked on 5 May 2020]

Keitel, Evelyne (1989). *Reading Psychosis: Readers, Texts and Psychoanalysis.* London: Blackwell.

King, Pamela (2018). *L'American Way of Life: Lacan et les débuts de l'ego-psychologie.* Fontenay-le-Comte: Éditions Lussaud.

Lacan, Jacques (1966). "Le Stade du Miroir comme formateur de la fonction du Je telle qu'elle nous est révélée dans l'expérience psychanalytique" (1949). *Écrits* I. Paris: Éditions du Seuil, "Essais Points", 1999, 92–99.

Lacan, Jacques (1981). *Le Séminaire,* Livre III, *Les Psychoses* (1955–56). J.-A. Miller (ed.). Paris: Éditions du Seuil.

Lacan, Jacques (1975). *Le Séminaire, Livre XX, Encore* (1972–73). J.-A. Miller (ed.). Paris: Éditions du Seuil.

Laing, Ronald David (1969). *The Divided Self,* New York, USA: Pantheon.

Lucchelli, Juan-Pablo (2009). *Le Transfert de Freud à Lacan.* Rennes: Presses Universitaires de Rennes.

Marret, Sophie (2010). *L'Inconscient aux sources du mythe moderne: les grands mythes de la littérature fantastique.* Rennes: Presses Universitaires de Rennes.

McGrath, Patrick (1989). "A Childhood in Broadmoor Hospital". *Granta,* Dec. 22, 1989. https://granta.com/a-childhood-in-broadmoor-hospital/

McGrath, Patrick (2002), "Problem of Drawing from Psychiatry for a Fiction Writer." *Psychiatric Bulletin,* 26, 140–143.

McGrath, Patrick (2015). Preface to the second edition of *Asylum.* London: Penguin Books.

Miller, Jacques-Alain (2018). *L'os d'une cure.* Paris: Navarin éditeur.

Mitchell, Juliet & Rose, Jacqueline (1985). *Feminine Sexuality, Jacques Lacan and the* école freudienne. London: Norton.

Pommier, Gérard (2004). *Comment les neurosciences démontrent la psychanalyse.* Paris: Flammarion, "Champs Essais".

Porter, Roy (2002). *Madness, a Brief History.* Oxford: Oxford University Press.

Shorter, Edward (1997). *A History of Psychiatry, From the Era of the Asylum to the Age of Prozac.* New York: John Wiley and Sons, Inc.

Showalter, Elaine (1985). *The Female Malady, Women, Madness and English Culture, 1830–1980.* London: Virago Press (1985).

Talairach, Laurence (2013). "'Knowledge for its own sake, is the one God I worship': Les Savants fous dans *Heart and Science* de Wilkie Collins". H. Machinal (ed.), *Le Savant fou,* Rennes, Presses Universitaires de Rennes, 127–143: https://books.openedition.org/pur/52903

Wall, Oisin (2018). *The British Anti-Psychiatrists, from institutional Psychiatry to Counter-Culture, 1960–1971.* London: Routledge.

CHAPTER 4

From Physical Symptoms to Subjective Creations in Pat Barker's *Regeneration* Trilogy

Pat Barker's *Regeneration* trilogy almost straightaway became a modern classic: successful among the public, it was hailed by critics, the press and academia, and the third volume was awarded the 1995 Booker Prize. The novels partake of a renewed interest in the collective trauma of the First World War and a critical obsession to save literature from the aporetic postmodernist strategies. Catherine Bernard argues that the 1980s' political context is decisive to understand the logic of a return to the fictional potential of the war: 'the 1980s' novelists write with a double certitude: that literature has reached a point of exhaustion and that it is necessary to write after the end, at the junction between the end of fiction and its ultimate power' (Bernard 2018: 26). The trilogy gradually moves away from the factual and historically based story of psychiatrist Rivers's involvement in Sassoon's conscientious objection and return to the front (*Regeneration*), to the fictional character of Billy Prior (*The Eye in the Door* and *The Ghost Road*). Most critical works have revolved around the expression of trauma, the re-interpretation of shell shock and how Barker interrogates the grand narrative concerning the effects of the war upon British civilisation. 'Not surprisingly, essays on the trilogy have focused principally on three themes: history, gender and psychology' (Brannigan 2005: 168). The novel's historical perspective, foregrounded by Barker's 'Notes' at the end of each novel, is often treated in relation to the 'ineffable' nature of the horror of

© The Author(s), under exclusive license to Springer Nature Switzerland AG 2023

N. P. Boileau, *Mental Health Symptoms in Literature since Modernism*, Palgrave Studies in Literature, Science and Medicine, https://doi.org/10.1007/978-3-031-37630-6_4

the war (Brannigan 2005: 4), which justifies that the author resorts to historical truths. Facts constitute a solid basis for her fictional work, a sure sign of her postmodernist inspiration and reliance on 'historiographic metafiction' (Brown 2005: 187). Therefore, many have focused on the tensions between the meaning of the war and the way people can cope: 'Pacifism is not depicted as a solution in the *Regeneration* trilogy, yet a profound conflict between the necessity for participants in a particular form of evil (war) and horror as its consequences remains' (Ross 2005: 137).

The war has arguably been the first point of connection between Pat Barker's and Virginia Woolf's Modernist strategy (Brannigan 2005: 169), especially because it is represented as that which alienates men (Vickroy 2004). There is much in common between *Mrs Dalloway* and *Regeneration*: if Barker's novels are set during the First World War while Woolf's takes place in its immediate aftermath, thematic interpretations of the novels have focused on the First World War consequences; they both try to express the ineffable experience of war; they are both structured around sexual repression. More specifically, Septimus Smith in *Mrs Dalloway* comes to mind because Barker explains that she sees the cause of his break-down as originating in some emotional repression of the war years and had characters like him in mind when she wrote the trilogy (Interview of Pat Barker in Saunders & McNaughton 2005: 230). With regard to trauma and her interest in therapy, which extends beyond the trilogy to such novels as *Border Crossing*, Pat Barker claims: 'My books are about recovery [even more than they are about trauma]' (Saunders and McNaughton 2005: 224), but she also explains that '[Rivers's] belief [is] that traumatic experience should be faced… you should sit down and desperately remember' (Saunders and McNaughton 2005: 228). What is left out of the remembering process? What is it that insists, or returns, and is never exhausted in the desperate repetition of the act of remembrance? Those are questions which I wish to address in the following chapter, some 15 years after the heyday of critical interest in the trilogy, and I will do so by exploring how symptoms are produced in the novel.

The commemorative aspect of the novels may also account for the number of studies interested in the notions of spectrality and 'ghosts', the return of the repressed and traumatic iterations—all of which are suggested by two of the novels' titles: *Regeneration* and *Ghost Road*. In her study of the late twentieth century's British art and literature, Bernard notes a British tendency to strategically use wars in arts because they gather notions of trauma and remembrance and a reflection on the process of re-membering: 'For British writers and artists, the war, close or remote, global or latent, offers a dramaturgy revealing rents in the body politic, rents which often manifest on the body itself because time and again, the body is reflecting matter' (Bernard 2018: 71). Since these seminal analyses, critics have also turned to other narrative strategies: Barker's reevaluation of realism (Bernard 2007), Barker's feminist realism (Walezak 2021), Barker's representation of English landscapes (Paul 2005; Cavalié 2015) and more generally sexuality. The central volume, *The Eye in the Door*, deals with Prior's bisexuality and explores the latent meanings of the first volume, disclosed by Barker herself in interviews. She 'has hinted at Rivers being homosexual', leading many commentators to think 'the book's concern is with mutism and stutters, emotional repression and denial' (Childs 2012: 75). A central concern in one of the case studies on Barker's works is how the sexual[1] affects her characters and how it can be related to the subjective experience of war: 'Barker defamiliarizes some of the effects of war in order to illuminate a neglected facet of war neuroses: sexual anxiety' (Monteith et al. 2005: xii).

There is no denying that in Barker's trilogy both therapists and patients are afflicted with symptoms which tempt readers and critics to analyse their relationship along a preconceived grid of sexual repression and neurotic behaviour—neurotic in the common sense of disorderly. The 'talking cure' is advocated by Barker herself as a matter of fascination (Stevenson 2005: 181), which accounts for the emphasis laid on transference instead of hypnosis in her work (Barrett 2012: 247). What I would like to explore here, and possibly further, is Bonikowski's proposal: 'The soldier's symptoms not only repeatedly disrupt the doctor's attempts to create a clear causal explanation but also present a signifying excess, pointing beyond the war to other areas of experience, such as sexuality' (Bonikowski 2013: 15). This suggests that any interpretation oriented exclusively by the question of the imaginary dimension of causality would neglect the surplus, which is not interpreted, the 'signifying excess' that the text is the repository of. It resonates with what has already been discussed about *Mrs Dalloway* and *Asylum*, in the problematic and symptomatic experiences of

---

[1] The sexual is to be understood here as the skein of experiences and meanings created by the relation between the body as sexed, the process known as gendering—and its social and cultural determining factors—as well as the unconscious experience in which the relation between the sexes cannot be written or articulated (Lacan 1975).

the sexual causing constant subjective reconfigurations. Sexuality, as noted by Bonikowski, may be the site of the exploration of such an excess. It is in fact the place where Prior re-entangles various aspects of his existence into something that holds together, albeit imperfectly. For I wish to uncover as well what Barker's novels do that the author is less aware of, or that she does not put forward. The novels indeed present themselves as well documented and as conveying a message about the History of British psychiatry, and Britain at large. Some critics have been tied to this interpretation, insisting that the works carefully and accurately 'examine the chronology of diagnostics' and are interesting for what they reveal of 'how biographical facts "inform" the fiction' (Baker et al. 2010: 58; 68).

In the following chapter, I will show how the encounter with the therapist, when he interprets his patients' symptoms, enables the patient to create their own solution to the excess of *jouissance* that the war, rather than being a cause of it, is more likely to have simply enhanced or 'opened up'. It is the relationship itself that becomes symptomatic: in his study of love, *Encore*, Lacan explains that the tension towards making one in a relationship is always fiction, because it is based on a denial of the 'impossibility of establishing as such, anywhere in the enunciable, the sole One that interests us, the One of the relation "sexual relationship"' (Lacan 1975, trans. Fink: 7). I suggest that Prior be read in his relationships with others as a way of making this absent relationship take place anyhow, a refusal of and a shelter from the *jouissance* he cannot keep at bay: since 'no relationship gets constituted between the sexes in the case of speaking beings' (Lacan 1975: 63/66), Prior's endless attempts at intercourse and forming particular bonds with people can be regarded as his treatment of the subjective sense of lack he experiences. In particular, I will be interested in untangling the historical facts of the repressive hypothesis (Freudian in particular, and as pinpointed by Foucault) with the production of symptoms created by fiction. I will thus start by looking at medical symptoms before I analyse the Freudian echoes of the text and the subversion offered by the patients to the Freudian hypothesis of repression, before I move on to explore the characters' *sinthomes*, that is, the individual, singular response allowing them to contain what is excessive and produced in spite of themselves, what Lacan calls *jouissance*.

The Limitations of Medical Treatment

The novel opens on Dr Rivers's qualms regarding his patient, Sassoon, whose conscientious objection poses a question of war ethics: Rivers 'want[s]' Sassoon to be ill (R, 8) because an illness is supposed to make his work with him relevant and would save Sassoon from the opprobrious reputation of having left the front on a whim, or for lack of bravery.[2] The factual nature of this also serves to contextualise the fact that shell shock had not been fully theorised yet or become such a pervasive cultural diagnosis as it was to become, before being replaced by the more encompassing acronym 'PTSD' (post-traumatic stress disorder): 'Only in Britain did the shell-shock story generate a rich literary tradition that became absorbed into the national cultural canon' (Micale and Lerner 2001: 22). Therefore, psychiatrists had to be innovative in order to deal with patients that were more puzzling to them than expected. The 'epidemic' (Showalter 1985: 168) nature of the illness of hysterical conversions among soldiers, together with the gender of the patients, 'force[d] a reconsideration of all the basic concepts of English psychiatric practice' (Showalter 1985: 167). Showalter is an essential reference to understand the context of the novels because her work is cited as an inspiration for the book (Barker 1991: 251–252); however, there have been critical revisions of her argument, such as Lerner and Leese, who both show that there was a far wider range of innovations regarding the treatment of shell-shocked patients than what is inferred in Showalter's and Barker's renditions, as well as a much longer tradition of dealing with male hysteria, which was only re-evaluated in the war years and not discovered then (Lerner, 142; Leese, 215 in Micale and Lerner 2001). Notwithstanding the historical debate about the accuracy of the doctor's exceptionality (also noted in Brannigan 2005: 95), Rivers's initial concern lays the emphasis on his own anxiety that he may not be able to treat the psychological disorder of his patients. He would thus be more comfortable having to deal with an organic cause. The social and cultural associations of 'trouble' with illness (R, 8) are exposed in the very beginning, setting the tone of the repressive hypothesis that we have seen at play in *Mrs Dalloway* too: there are things better left unsaid and unseen, and Showalter offers a solid analytical reference in the area.

---

[2] On the relevance and meaning of these for masculinities, see Brown (2005), Showalter (1985) and Stevenson (2005).

In the novel, symptoms are first and foremost shown from a medical, clinical viewpoint—'clinical' in the sense explored by Foucault in his early works where he clearly asserts the disappearance of the patient as subject. Foucault writes:

> paradoxically, the patients are only external items in relation to that which they suffer from... Hence the strange character of the medical gaze...: it addresses what is visible in illness—but does so from an ill person that conceals the visible object by showing it; in other words, the doctor must recognize in order to cognize. (Foucault 1963: 8)

The importance Foucault gives to the gaze in clinical practice is in keeping with what is found in the novels, but I am more interested in the process of selection this gaze produces than in the questions of visibility it raises. In particular, many reactions by Rivers make us suspicious as to his capacity to open up to new forms of disorders, as if his gaze had been trained in recognising symptoms, while other unknown, discreet signs are left unnoticed and fail to be theorised. When troubled by Sassoon's demand that he read his poems, Rivers declares that he wants to 'see' the poems (R, 13), just as he wants to see his patients, as if his gaze could pierce through the nature of the illness without any reference to what the subject who produced them has to say.

Furthermore, the novel does not entirely espouse Rivers's view and shows that the patient defies the doctor's gaze. The patients' physical symptoms often remain enigmatic to the clinician: 'Pale skin, purple shadows under the eyes. Apart from that, no obvious signs of nervous disorder. No twitches, jerks, blinks, no repeated ducking to avoid a long-exploded shell.../So far, he hadn't looked at Rivers' (R, 10). Symptoms manifest here in their absence, in relation to a classification that is Victorian, that is, taxonomical in nature and medical in practice: 'nervous' is not synonymous with psychic but with organic, the psychiatrist wanting to cure the mind through the physical manifestations of symptoms which he sees as the signs pointing to the ailment in the brain, that is, what he, as a practitioner of medicine, must do to handle the case. The clinician sees the absence of what he expects to observe and thus fails to note the presence of what is unseen. Such description evokes the first novel's title, which 'derives from Rivers's interest in the regeneration of nerves after injury' (Childs 2012: 74). However, the description of the case cannot be reduced solely to the application of a nosography that Barker would know about.

In it, one notices that the psychiatrist immediately interprets the symptom as a 'cyphered message': 'no repeated ducking to avoid a long-exploded shell'. It is to be imagined that Rivers would not question the ducking, as it is immediately connected to some imaginary relation of cause and consequence due to the backdrop in which such disorder takes place. As shown by Foucault, this also underlines the fact the patient himself is not the primary concern: Rivers first looks at symptoms before noticing that there has been no eye-contact. He may as well be looking at a corpse. This is certainly ominous in the context of a hospital treating patients with war injuries.

Rivers is therefore tempted by this practice of medicine, but the novel shows the tension there is between his classical training and his more modern interest in the patient he is meant to cure. Diagnoses are often quoted in reported speech, as if they were external to his own method, such as when he meets Prior: 'Diagnosed neurasthenic... deep reflexes abnormal' (R, 50). He questions Prior, asking him what his symptoms are and hearing Prior's voice, miraculously recovered, he notices that it 'had the curious effect of making *him* look different' (R, 49). Rivers identifies the subject in the patient; he thereby notices that which makes a body singular. The patient's gaze and their voice are two of the objects *a* identified by Lacan as foundational to the subject. The voice, which Prior has lost and which is the object of so much scrutiny throughout the novel (Stevenson 2005: 176), is one of the most difficult theoretical points in Lacan's theorising of object relation: 'The core of the difficulty in understanding what the voice is about is to grasp that the voice, unlike other objects *a*, first needs to be lost in order to be found'. This is how Maleval addresses the issue in a way that can easily be related to the novel: before Prior can find his voice, in volume three of the trilogy, he needs to have lost it and recovered it. The voice as object *a* remains a matter of great debate among Lacanians and would deserve a discussion of its own but suffice it to say for now that it is not just the phonetic combination of sound production or speech acts: 'The voice is not sonorous but aphonic... and should not be conflated to a question of intonation' (Maleval 2010: 186; 190). This quote already indicates that Prior's voice is indeed the mark of 'something extracted in the realm of the Other' (Maleval 2010: 188). I understand this as meaning that the voice participates in a symbolic exchange that creates the condition for desire too. These insights into another approach to the symptom are not followed through immediately in *Regeneration*, and Rivers's side-comments do not converge towards establishing new diagnoses. In spite of his best intentions, Rivers is still largely influenced by his culture and expertise, so that when he himself manifests symptoms of 'war neurosis'—sweating, a constant need to urinate, breathlessness, irregular heartbeats (R, 139–140)—he needs to be reminded of the obvious notion that psychic symptoms are no less significant than physical ones: 'as we keep telling the patients, psychosomatic symptoms are REAL. I think you should take some leave' (R, 140). Here, it becomes clear that medical knowledge is conducive to repression, because the word 'psychosomatic' has the effect of directing his medical gaze away: by naming the symptom, he refuses to interrogate it. By seeing the symptom, he is forced into an interpretative method based on statistical representation, without necessarily managing to interrogate the place where the symptom is lodged in the psychic structure of the subject forming them, or the place he, as therapist, holds in the production of said symptom (Lacan 1991: 122–134).

The comprehension of the symptoms of war neurosis as contextual prevails in most of the novels, but more specifically in the first one, and it is in keeping with Showalter's analysis that 'symptoms of mental impairment' first were thought to have to be traced 'to an organic cause' (Showalter 1985: 168). This question of the physical cause of symptoms is addressed first as a question of class. Rivers notes: 'It's almost as if for the… laboring classes illness *has* to be physical. They can't take their condition seriously unless there's a physical symptom. And there are other differences as well. Officers' dreams tend to be more elaborate' (R, 96). This quote foregrounds one of the obstacles to the comprehension of hysterical conversions up until Charcot and Freud. It has often been used in relation to a social understanding of the novel, which is extremely valuable, especially because Barker also explores the question of Britishness. Cavalié considers that this is the premise of Barker's structuring her novel on a binary opposition between Prior and Sassoon, stressing Sassoon's more privileged status (Cavalié 2015: 138–139) and regarding Prior as 'a being who, originating from the margins, comes to disturb the social order' (Cavalié 2015: 138). Given the way in which organic causes have continued to be favoured throughout the twentieth century with the advent of neurobiology and neuroleptics, and seeing how the psychic explanation gradually receded in the background, I think what matters more is Barker's heightened sense that a social explanation is easily formulated, that it runs through the diagnoses and perhaps serves to conceal another approach, while something more universal is expressed by the novel: otherwise,

Rivers himself would not be developing these psychosomatic disorders which clearly escape his control, as if by contamination. The social explanation, which served well in the nineteenth century, needs revising for the author of the end of the twentieth century. Class is one factor of treatment, but the stereotypical vision of illness as necessarily physical pervades society as a whole, and class division, like gender, has more to do with the way therapy is manoeuvred (Chesler 1994; Wall 2018) than with the way individuals imagine what the origins of their symptoms may be.

As Brown argues, the historical figure of Rivers enables Barker to strategically embody the progress made by therapists and psychiatrists in handling symptoms of a psychic order: 'The sheer range of W.H.R. Rivers's expertise and interests makes him an ideal figure to embody a transition from Victorian self-confidence to modernist doubt... and from the totalizing grand narratives of modernity to the "*petits récits*" of post-modernism' (Brown 2005: 188). If we take up on Cavalié's suggestion that Barker uses doubles to structure her narrative, it is tempting to look at the function of Dr Yelland as Rivers's exact negative version: his methods are clearly Victorian, which I mean as authoritative, and based on an approach in which the symptom must be eradicated at all costs, even if that involves extracting a part of the patient's body too. His neglect of the 'talking cure' (R, 233), and his narcissistic assertion of being able to 'cure' patients (R, 233) are set in stark contrast with Rivers's doubts, the time the latter spends listening to his own patients and the meaning he seeks to unveil, causing him nightmares and much speculation—which interestingly enough, he does not treat as pathological or requiring therapy. Dr Yelland, on the other hand, ironically announces to one of his patients, Callan: 'You must speak, but I shall not listen to anything you have to say' (R, 231). When Callan is asked to leave, he is forced to thank the doctor for 'be[ing] cured' (R, 233). His instructions are all oriented by the symptom, as if the latter was not connected to the subject that presents it and as if the symptom had a message of its own that he alone understood.

The ironical expression which Dr Yelland repeats, 'Remember *you must talk before you leave me*' (R, 229; 230), is an injunction that the contemporary reader will readily associate with the talking cure. But it is subverted here because the doctor does not listen: what he wants is a clinical observation to make sure that the patient, after going through a medical act that is intrusive and possibly damaging, is still capable of using a bodily function 'normally'. Unlike Rivers, there is no indication here that Yelland takes into account another apprehension of the voice, as Lacan does in his seminar on Anxiety and which derives from the many hospitalised patients who do hear voices (Maleval 2010). Perhaps it is no wonder that the author gives pride of place to medical jargon in this scene of ECT, 'lumbar spines', 'long pharyngeal electrode' (R, 229), to signify Yelland's inscription in the academic discourse, his medical practice and certitude, and possibly the relish he experiences in handling these bodies from the standpoint of a knowledge he trusts unabashedly. The stylistic echoes show Rivers and Yelland as negative versions of each other, but they also resound with parallel visions of the practices of medicine and the practices of war: the authoritarian voices, the mortifying use of a language which is opaque to most people outside the profession, etc. This has been forcefully analysed by Brannigan (Brannigan 2005: 105–106) in relation to the place of psychoanalysis in the novel as one of the discourses of modernity (which, the critic argues, fails to explain humankind). Others have suggested this contrast was perhaps too reductive: 'Barker's *Regeneration* dramatizes a simple and stark opposition between the vicious physical treatment by electric shock by the neurologist Lewis Yelland and the sympathetic, analytic interpretative method pursued by Rivers... *Regeneration* retrofits the Great War with modern trauma theory' (Luckhurst 2008: 53). Barker finds in this opposition a creative crucible for exposing the turmoil doctors and patients have to cope with now that they are faced with new disorders or symptoms.

The connection with *Mrs Dalloway* and *Asylum* is reinforced in this structural presence of the double. Indeed, the two novels also play with duplicates or mirrored characters: Clarissa and Septimus, Stella and Edgar, and the couples of doctors—Bradshaw and Holmes, Cleave and Max Raphael. However, Barker offers a way out of the pessimistic stories by Woolf and McGrath, because there is at least one patient who becomes more stable and a doctor who revises what he has been told to hold as true. The effects of not questioning medical knowledge are still explored fully.

Secondary characters in particular are subjected to this method of psychiatric treatment in which they disappear from view, while the doctors take pride in their capacity to identify symptom clusters designed to structure the case and 'make a case for' an illness that can be treated or taken care of:

> Dundas suffered from abnormal reactions in the air. Where healthy pilots experienced no sensation at all, Dundas reported feeling his head squashed

into his body, or a loss of movement in his legs. He suffered from nausea.
More seriously ill, he had more than once experienced the preliminary stages
of a faint. (E, 60)

Barker subtly underlines that the doctor does not want to recognise
that the symptom is not as interesting as the way it is presented by the
patient themselves: 'He thought Dundas might be minimising his symptoms. It wasn't a good moment for that particular perception to strike' (E,
62). The experiment carried out by Rivers and Head, recounted in the
second novel (E, 141–143), shows that the body remains the gateway to
the subject for Rivers, in true medical fashion, while the novel seeks something else: Barker stresses that Rivers is in search of a 'vocabulary to
express' Prior's 'divisions', a term that is far from innocent in the context
of Freudian notions of the split nature of subjects and the author's own
reference to Jekyll and Hyde (E, 143; 229). Moreover, it points to the way
in which the doctor tries to inscribe the body into the symbolic, by labelling things that happen to the patients and would otherwise overwhelm
them. All of this serves to show Rivers's own duality regarding his practice
and profession, as well as his gradual lack of complacency towards what his
patient might teach him: 'There was one genuinely disturbing feature of
the case' (E, 143). Accepting the failure of ready-made associations
between the sign and the illness, of the symptom as a message, Rivers
becomes the agent of a reappraisal of the symptomatology and Craiglockhart
hospital an experimental institution.

Through Rivers's handling of treatment, Prior changes status and his
symptoms evolve. This is the result of transference, which Steffens laments
because she wishes Barker had focused instead on the failure of the talking
cure in order to highlight the aporia inherent to the traumatic experience
(Steffens 2014: 39). When he was speechless, or rather voiceless, he
becomes voluble and produces a range of symptoms that does not compare with what he had when he was first admitted for treatment. In the
second novel in particular, there is a significant surge in symptom formations—dreams, sexual encounters, encounter with a lover, the unobserv-
able fugue state and so forth. Prior is subjected to new symptoms that
could evoke an evolution in his response to the world; after a panic attack
in the street, we are told of his feelings and his interpretation of such an
act: 'like being naked, high up on a ledge, somewhere in full light, with
beneath him only jeering voices and millions of eyes' (E, 26). The panic
attack therefore is no longer treated as the symptom, as what needs

deciphering, like his initial voice loss, but the explanation he gives is: the whole scene is recounted in the absence of Rivers, outside the therapeutic session, giving here full voice to the character. Is the comparison a sign of Prior's poetic use of language, akin to the interest laid on poetry writing in the first novel of the trilogy? Or should it be read as an imaginary or dialectic exploration of his feelings? In any case, it is clear from the quote that what is at stake is the object cause of desire, extracted here in eyes and voices, a feeling of exposure that nakedness comes to signify.

From this moment on, it is the gaze that is presented as central to his relation to other people, to his actions in the world, to his social bonds as indicated in the title of the novel which is referred to here—a major displacement from his initial voice problem: 'Prior sat back against the wall. He was finding the eye in the door difficult to cope with' (E, 40). The symptomatic creation is unambiguous when he starts having hallucinations: the images he forms after a 'tepid bath' are real in the Lacanian sense of what cannot be avoided. In these images, he is looked at, observed, and the images are said to have power ('powerful'/'the power of this image') and be inescapable: 'he could do nothing about it.... He found himself resenting … [t]he claim [this image] made on his sympathy' (E, 54).

The most obvious aspect of the symptom in the novels of the *Regeneration* trilogy is its physicality and materiality that leaves the doctors baffled by a diagnosis that is inoperant. This naturally leads us to unveil another meaning of the symptom which is structural to the subject:

> There would be no hypnosis, no artificial creation of dissociated states for experimental purposes, no encouraging Prior to think of the fugue state as an alternative self. Even so. It had to be remembered Prior was no mere bundle of symptoms, but an extremely complex personality with his own views on his condition. And his imagination was already at work, doing everything it could to transform the fugue state into a malignant double. (E, 143)

Such passage, central to the second novel and thus to the whole trilogy, shows that the novel fosters another approach to symptom interpretation, in which the decoding must be related to an overall strategy of defence against *jouissance*. In order to be entirely free to operate from the symptom, rather than against it, the psychiatrist and patients must fight back the discourse on repression which, ironically, represses any attempt at finding another path. The novel itself invites us to criticise the role of psychiatry, presented as that which is impervious to perception, and to turn to the novel for a different clinical gaze: 'You want perception, you go to a novelist, not a psychiatrist' (R, 164).

FREUD, HYSTERIA AND THE END
OF THE REPRESSIVE HYPOTHESIS

The Freudian terminology used at times in the novel cannot but influence our understanding of the psychosomatic symptoms experienced by the characters. It reflects the dominant way in which such symptoms would have been perceived by practitioners, and therefore patients, at the time of the novel's story: 'I see. A negative transference. Is *that* what you think we've got?' (R, 65). It is interesting in that respect that some critics try to make do without the influence of Freudian psychoanalysis (Bernard 2007), even when dealing with therapy (Whitehead 2005), while others use this influence in an almost accusatory fashion: 'Barker's eloquent and influential trilogy... has contributed to a Freudianization of shell shock' (Barrett 2012: 238). And yet, shell shock became dominant also because Freud had helped promote hysteria as a worthy area of study. The subject that is central to Rivers, because of his Freudian influence, is the split subjectivity—one may be tempted to call it 'dual', 'ambivalent', 'divided' or any other term. The reference to Jekyll and Hyde cannot stress enough how common and fruitful the image of psychological division had been throughout the nineteenth century, from the heightened sense of self induced by opium eating in De Quincey's 'impassioned prose', to the many monsters peopling the gothic revival and the *fin-de-siècle* novels such as Wilde's *The Picture of Dorian Gray*. This is in keeping with Freud's notion of the unconscious as that which is barred from access to the conscious self, and which returns through the operation of repression. Repression is a process that erases the thought or feeling or impulse in the same time as it inscribes it at its missing place (Freud 1926: 7)—an evocative process for the question of remembrance which is central to the trilogy (Bernard 2007).

Freudian psychoanalysis is often quoted and underlined as a major influence both to Rivers, the historical man, and Rivers, the fictional character. The major influences of Freud would be the refusal of hypnosis as stated above (Freud 1905a, 1905b: 96), the favouring of talk as a mode of access to the subject's truth and the notion that nervous disorders may have a cause in the family drama developed from the Oedipus complex (Freud 1923: 121–123).[3] Stevenson's seminal essay is an extremely valuable piece to understand the logic at play in the novel, in her intricate and complex way of reading Rivers's transference, Freudian psychoanalysis and the palimpsest text of R. Louis Stevenson (Stevenson 2005). My own development does not invalidate such reading, far from it, but wishes to prolong it into the poststructuralist era. For after all, novels speak to us not only because of their accurate rendition of certain past processes. Pat Barker's novels also continue to speak to us because they produce modes of thinking, as Stevenson remarks about Prior, who 'as his name implies, precedes his doctor in the psychoanalytic process that Rivers will take further as he remembers his past in *The Ghost Road*' (Stevenson 2005: 228). This is in keeping with what Lacan declared about Marguerite Duras in his 'homage': 'it should be kept in mind that as Freud said, in his/her matter, the artist always precedes and [psychoanalysts] must avoid playing the psychologist where the artist clears the way for them' (Lacan 2001: 192–193). I intend to take the novels from a slightly different angle, because instead of reading them as the gradual uncovering of the subject's guiding the psychoanalyst, I will start from the Lacanian perspective that if Rivers is so critical of psychologists (Stevenson 2005: 225), it is because his job is presented as needing to create rather than iterate, to produce rather than fear or repress, the symptoms the patient came to dispose of or complain about. Rivers is never shown to envisage curing his patients in the sense of making them leave stripped of their symptoms.

From a factual perspective, the progressist nature of Rivers is shown in the novel as linked to his adopting the talking cure, a fact connected to the real Rivers too (Childs 2012: 75–76). Rivers uses the psychoanalytic theory even in his address to his patient: 'Manning, he knew, had read a certain amount of Freud' (E, 157–158). This allows him to ask questions with the vocabulary of the emerging theory of psychoanalysis. Freud is treated like an item of culture, his name and some of his ideas on the interpretation of dreams and repression clearly having seeped through into the dominant discourse. Right from the beginning of the novel, the place given to dreams is quite significant: in chapter 4, a dream is recounted, analysed (R, 46) and given 'meaning' to (R, 47). 'Is not the dream, when analyzed, an eye of the door into the psyche?' asks Stevenson after all

---

[3] In a footnote of his chapter 'On Female Sexuality', Freud challenges the idea that Œdipus be applicable to women (Freud 1931: 140).

illuminating analysis of the ambivalence, mirror-effect and emergence of the gaze as an object of transference between Prior and Rivers in *The Eye in the* Door (Stevenson 2005: 224). In other words, dreams are clearly and unquestionably material for analysis, in a very Freudian fashion that no contemporary reader of the 1990s could have missed. However, the *talking* part of the therapy is overlooked in the said analysis of the dream, in favour of the content of what is enunciated/said. Elsewhere, Rivers notes his own dream and analysis of it on the notepad (R, 45), in a fashion redolent of Sir Bradshaw in *Mrs Dalloway* when listening to Septimus, clearly not intending to show it to someone else. Unlike Sir Bradshaw, however, Rivers is making forays into the analysis of dreams because he listens to his patients', records his own, taking notes so that his clinical work may one day lead to some theoretical elaboration. Barker pictures Rivers as a man who seeks to change perspective and be enlightened by his patients, rather than as a man of science who knows it all already.

The dream is analysed for what it tells rather than how it is told and its function in the subject's existence. Again, Freudian influence manifests in the vocabulary used by the author: 'The *manifest content* didn't take long. Except for the cutting of his arm, the dream was an unusually accurate reproduction of events that had actually occurred' (R, 46, italics mine). The enigmatic meaning is what Rivers seeks to unveil because he trusts that there is some meaning and truth lurking behind, ready to be discovered. Rivers does not posit that the dream could be a production of the psyche revelatory of a subjective relation to the unconscious, doomed to remain meaningless. His trust in the undisclosed meaning and the latent signifying presence is the reason of his taking some distance from the orthodox views of some ('doctrinaire supporters'): 'He was more inclined to seek the meaning of the dream in the conflict his dream self had experienced between the duty to continue the experiment and the reluctance to cause further pain' (R, 47). Rivers senses that the repressive hypothesis is not entirely satisfactory, but keeping the dream to himself, in no relation of transference, he is not invited to go beyond the revelation that the dream offers and to situate it in relation to a psychic structure. At this stage in the novels, he fails to allow himself to be guided by the function of the dream outside its immediate, contemporary context. The dream is convincingly accepted as a function, which makes impossible the contemplation of another operation, namely that it be some indecipherable core that would correspond to Bonikowski's 'surplus'.

The same interpretative process dominates Rivers's reluctant decision to read Sassoon's poems: 'Rivers knew so little about poetry that he was almost embarrassed at the thought of having to comment on these. But then he reminded himself they'd been given to him as a therapist, not as a literary critic, and from that point of view they were certainly interesting' (R, 25). Not only does Rivers look at these poems as if they were 'interesting' in themselves, but he does not question the reason for Sassoon's request or demand that they should be read. And yet, this aspect is what is crucial to the understanding of the function these poems have for Sassoon in his transferential relationship with his analyst. Once again, the repressive hypothesis—consisting in imagining that the unconscious is the result of a censorship process and the transformation of libidinal drives into other images which re-iterate the lost event or affect—is visible in Rivers's resort to super-egoistic elements that cover up the potential structuring function these poems have in guiding him towards, if not clearing up the way to, the understanding of Sassoon's case. It is true that the novel itself invokes this: 'In advising his young patients to abandon the attempt at repression and to let themselves *feel* the pity and terror their war experience inevitably evoked, he was excavating the ground he stood on' (R, 48), a passage which can be analysed thus—'this passage remarks upon the dangers of Rivers's psychoanalytic method' (Brannigan 2005: 98). But it can also be regarded as a foray into another approach to the symptom where it is not made meaningful but structural.

The central reason why Freudian psychoanalysis should hold a decisive place in the analysis of the novels is obviously its contemporary relevance and the central question of what all these men seem to suffer from. Throughout the novel, the diagnosis hesitates between the new syndrome of 'shell shock' or the more common term of 'hysteria'.

> A withdrawn, almost drugged look, like extreme shock or the beginning of orgasm. Then abruptly the features convulsed with pain, and Prior, teeth chattering uncontrollably, raised his shaking hand and rocked it against his chest.... It was a common symptom of hysterical disorders, but knowledge of it would only serve to reinforce Prior's belief that the alternative state of consciousness was a monster with whom he could have nothing in common. (E, 262)

Once again, the libidinal origin of unconscious signs is only too clear in the alternatives envisaged by Rivers and points back to a long tradition of seeing hysteria as first a woman's condition, and secondly, even when men were diagnosed with the illness, as related somehow to a dysfunctional substitution of libidinal energy. 'Throughout history, hysteria has served as a form of expression, a body language for people who otherwise might not be able to speak or even admit what they feel' (Showalter 1997: 7). Showalter concludes that it is 'a cultural symptom of anxiety and stress' (Showalter 1997: 9), while Didi-Huberman sees it as an illness in which subjects 'offer themselves to the gaze' and can 'captivate [their] doctor' (Didi-Huberman 1982: 223). Both definitions are relevant to the passage of *The Eye in the Door,* but they are even more forceful if one follows in the footsteps of Lacanian analysis, which is oriented by the subject's *jouissance.* Prior's lack of control and convulsions—the so-called conversion symptoms which remain 'very common in neurological practice' but which are now a 'clinical reality that is curiously not reflected in research activity' (Stone et al. 2008: 12)—are offered to the clinical gaze of Rivers, time and again, as if Prior wanted his doctor to be the witness of his suffering. This indicates that, if we are to follow the notion that he precedes Rivers in his discovery of the illness which is his, he is signalling towards symptoms that have not yet been inscribed in his story and whose subjective relevance needs articulating into a whole. The reference to 'orgasm' is like an ironic comment on an explanation that is perhaps too simple. However, the most determining aspect here is the use of the word 'monster', which evokes traditional, if not mythical, apprehensions of psychological disorders—perpetuated nowadays by critics who see 'madness' as 'extreme, excess, overwhelming, beyond categories' (Gagneret 2019: 16) and a queerness that the novel likes to delve into.

For the novel indeed deploys a complex and intricate imagery of sexual innuendoes and metaphors which foreground sex in ways that do not necessarily make it easy for the reader to distinguish between the sexual relation, gender constructions and the unconscious dimension of sex. In Lacanian terms, there is a fundamental difference between sex—the sexual organs, or the biological apprehension of sex—and sexuation, which is the result of the symbolic absence of a signifier for two sexes, and which is always problematic for subjects because these are defined by their alienation to language and its signifiers (Lacan 1975). In the novel, sex is first described as that which society condemns and that which defines your place in society, that is, as what helps define masculinities. On the one hand, the repression surrounding sex is made visible in Prior's constant attempts to sneer at sex, as if the subject was bound to shock his therapist, or else as if therapy was the only place where he could account for his sexual drives and ideas. 'That what you Freudian Johnnies are on about all the time, isn't it? Nudity, snakes, corsets' (R, 29). Prior's sarcasm reveals that he knows too much about Freud not to be fooled by the way the 'snake' is going to be interpreted in Rivers's long silence, and to think that what is at stake is the expression of what is silenced usually: 'You want me to say my wife…' (R, 28). Prior tries to (meta)comment on the therapist's job so to speak and his sarcasm derives from the idea that the origin of psychic traumas and symptom formations is always and indisputably attributed to a story of a sexual nature. 'Were there remaining symptoms?'/'"Headaches". He watched Rivers make a note. "It's hardly a reason to stay out of the trenches, is it? *Not tonight, Wilhem, I've got a headache*"' (R, 50). The relation between the war and sexuality, in addition to being the cause of the irony, is also a way of yoking together disparate elements that can therefore be interpreted along the same lines, as based on a logic of contiguity, if not metonymy.

It could be tempting to see the sarcasm as a way of confessing that which cannot be admitted in seriousness. Karolyn Steffens does not seem to question this sarcasm but wishes to take it unambiguously as the novel's attempt to show Rivers as 'denuding the dream of its sexual overtones and rejecting the sexual symbolism for which Freud was so (in)famous' (Steffens 2014: 41). According to the critic, Barker's 'act of censorship speaks to her refusal to narrate certain traumatic experiences that are impossible to describe given her historical belatedness' (Steffens 2014: 52). Notwithstanding the many reasons for debating the idea of 'historical belatedness', which fails to indicate how these 'experiences' could be discriminated from others, what strikes me is the replacement of a symbol by another: Freud was wrong because of his emphasis on sexuality; Steffens is right because she finds something else to explain the sign (something non-sexual and therefore more acceptable?): 'the snake therefore symbolizes not the phallus but simply the familiar symbol of medicine' (Steffens 2014: 40). The symbol of medicine, one might argue, has much to do with a phallic symbol of power, mastery and the law—such as the character of Dr Yelland proves. It is not a major shift from the Freudian reading of the symbol contained in Prior's dream. Perhaps the snake should therefore be considered as a sexual symbol not meant to be simply equated to what its initial sense is, but to be analysed for its signifying effect in terms of Prior's subjective *sexuation*.

Quite a few critics have obviously noted the importance of sexuality in the novel, but not often as a way of re-appraising the logic of repression deemed inherent in the production of symptoms in the therapeutic set-up. Sexuality is approached as a dangerous question that should not be discussed because it could jeopardise social decorum. Critics have stressed gender stereotypes, the relationship between Prior and Manning, between Prior and Sarah and the latent homosexual feelings, if not homosexuality, of Dr Rivers. Barker is even thought to implement a vision of the war symptoms as a result of 'particularly restrictive and repressive ideologies of masculinity' (Brannigan 2005: 98). Gender readings of the novel have indeed flourished. According to Cavalié, Rivers is torn between his ambiguous relationships with his patients, which interrogates his vision of genders, and the father figure he represents (Cavalié 2015: 238). Prior calls him 'a sort of... male mother' (R, 107, qd in Cavalié 2015: 240). These quotes are in keeping with the subtext of male hysteria—announced by Barker's use of Showalter—and Cavalié's close readings of the challenges posed to masculinity in the novels as a result of class and public-school education, ideological representations and the symbolic meaning of stammering (Cavalié 2015: 194; 197; 227). Quoting the 'patriarchal constructions of masculinity' identified by Harris, Vickroy explains: 'Barker portrays a culture that uses violent suppression and accusation to quash traumatic symptoms that attest to the consequences of the war effort' (Vickroy 2004: 48). Barrett sees Prior's pathologised bisexuality as 'the medicalization of dissent' (Barrett 2012: 240). The most consistent analysis of sex remains Ward's contribution: 'while sex is never reproductive in Barker's trilogy, it is occasionally *productive* in an alternatively social sense' (Ward 2016: 320). In particular, Ward is interested in tracing the logic of marginalisation of queer groups 'in national narratives of mourning and redress' (Ward 2016: 321).

The pathologising of sexuality in relation to mental health treatment is one of Barker's subtexts, as indicated in the first pages of the trilogy: 'I suppose it is possible someone might find being locked up in a loony bin a fairly *emasculating* experience?' (R, 29). Men behaving as women are expected to, falling into the category of hysteria, inevitably call for a reappraisal of masculine identities: 'They won't *let* you make a martyr of yourself, Sass' (R, 7). But Barker's text is much more convincing, because much less demonstrative, when it focuses less on prejudiced interpretations of gender as a norm, and more on what some would call 'queer' behaviour or a queering of the narrative, and which I would tend to read as the production of symptomatic sexual practices. Symptomatic here should not be understood according to the logic of repression and hysteria, but as a subjective way of knotting together the Imaginary dimension of sex (in which one could include social and cultural representations of the ideal of sexed identities), the symbolic dimension of sex by which subjects are deprived of a signifier to account for two partners, and the real of a *jouissance* that is ineffable because of the operation of language. In other words, because of his unstable place in language which is related to the meaning he ascribes to masculinity, Prior forms relationships with others whose function is to stabilise, if only fleetingly, his sense of self.

The Sexual as the Engine of Fiction

One of the most analysed passages related to the question of sexuality is the opening of *The Eye in the Door* which gives us to see, or witness, a scene of a sexual nature that ties together layers of interpretation that are fathomless: Prior randomly meets Charles Manning, a government official who is also one of Rivers's patients and who leads a respectable, heterosexual life despite having random homosexual sex. This scene has often been analysed as a welcome outing of homosexuality in the army. Ward is interested in the historic/memorial aspect of the lived experience of sex between men (Ward 2016: 332) when he carefully analyses this scene. I, on the other hand, am interested in how Prior offers us a way of apprehending sexuality. Symbolically, his being led into the servants' quarters has been interpreted as the sure sign of a British class system that polices bodies and experiences. I argue that this scene, opening the second volume of the trilogy, is also—and perhaps this is the reason of the saturation of class in the construction of the scene too—key to Barker's gradual giving up of the repressive hypothesis: first of all, the scene is not recounted to the therapist; it is a secret that only readers know about and which results, in part, from the work done in sessions but which is not treated as a 'symptom' in the medical sense. Secondly, it opens the second volume, plunging us into a new apprehension of the body, sex and repression. For repression is no longer a valid motif of the symptomatic usage that is made of sexuality by the characters. Prior emerges from this scene as fairly in command, possessing a way of appropriating other people's desires which points to the function of his own symptomatic formation.

Analysing the place of memory and remembrance within the historiographic economy of the novels, Catherine Bernard says of the body that it is 'a symptomatic palimpsest, to be read and transcribed' (Bernard 2007: 181). The body indeed, in its symptomatic formations which give it a medical relevance, surfaces with iterative regularity throughout the novels. However, not all of the characters' bodies have the same function in the text. It is the case of Prior that I want to focus on because it serves a particular function which cannot be entirely subsumed in the question of the symptoms' meaning and/or original meaning now lost and having to be recovered. In other words, the 'palimpsest' is perhaps not the metaphor I would use, but I would say that the body is the site of a writing that will never cease to remain unwritten.

Prior's body, in other words, functions as the recipient of an excess he is alienated to and which he cannot fully grasp in his talking cure because it is produced by his very subjective (or singular) way of relating to others. Prior's body is both his symptom in the sense of that from which his dissatisfaction stems and the site of his finding a solution to keep the real at bay. His dissatisfaction with intercourse runs through the novels, as can be seen in the final scene in which his experience is graphically described but nothing approaching satisfaction is conveyed: 'Nothing particularly attractive about him—dead white skin, splodgy freckles, curious flat golden-brown eyes—not that it bothered me. After two months without sex I'd have settled for the pigs' (GR, 247). The scene symmetrically responds to the opening one and contains many similar features. The lack of attraction of the partner, in this case a German soldier, is the condition for Prior's bodily exchange and what remains after the encounter is less the coupling than the fissures that find their ways into his own body, signifying its excessive *jouissance*: 'And then we parted. And I've been neurotically running my tongue round my lips feeling for sores ever since' (GR, 248). This in turn serves the idea that there was a transformation through therapy, the effects of which can be witnessed in the rest of the novel. His symptom operates as an instrument of his relationship with the Other, and particularly as embodied by Rivers. The first to notice it is Rivers himself who, comparing patients' relationships with their fathers and with their therapists, situates a core of opacity in his relationship with Prior, which intrigues him: 'Mercifully, doctors are also opaque to their patient. Unless the patient happens to be Prior' (R, 106). Appreciating Prior's special place in the series of his patients, Rivers leaves unnamed and unthought the actual product of the special relationship he notices. He treats it as joke, an oddity he observes but to which he does not attribute a potential therapeutic effect to be translated and inscribed in Prior's *jouissance*. The key might be given indirectly when another case is discussed. Sassoon, who was the case that started the trilogy, is evoked by Rivers's accomplice and mentor, Head, thus:

> 'Do you think [Rivers] still thinks Sassoon went back because of him?'
> Head hesitated. 'I think he knows the extent of his influence.'
> 'Hmm,' Ruth said. 'Do you think he's in love with him?'
> 'He's a patient.'
> Ruth smiled and shook her head. 'That's not an answer.'
> Head looked at her. 'Yes, it is. It has to be.' (E, 227)

The dialogue and narrative stop here. This allows the reader to ponder what the nature of the relationship was indeed, and we are invited to set this in parallel with Rivers's special relationship with Prior.

In the second novel of the trilogy, the first scene sets the tone of a programmatic narrative strategy that foregrounds the body and Prior's relation to others as a symptomatic formation. This means that his relationship with others, via his body's reactions, is to be seen as a subjective solution to the lack of being through which he experiences meaninglessness. Even if Prior is first shown trying to 'fumble with the fly buttons of middle-class morality' (E, 5), the text will no longer be about repression as much as it is about subjective creations in which what is at stake is to 'tie a knot in it [rather] than have to live with that image' (E, 5). In the opening scene, Prior tries to force himself on a girl he had intercourse with the weekend before. It is probably one of the few scenes in English literature to allow the author, in the very first page, the privilege of unzipping the generic fly of novelistic conventions and 'giving her free play with his cock and balls' (E, 4). The sexual meaning prevails in the text, being out in the open and uncensored. The scene displays the many equivocal entanglements of this romantic affair which is neither romantic, nor an affair: both lovers lied to each other, and they are unwilling to repeat an act that was licentious and undesired. Their sexual relationship is devoid of any romantic feelings, and they separate immediately; the author plays with our readerly expectations and perhaps also with a reversal of our prejudices about hetero-normative sexual practices. The body however is 'read and transcribed' tirelessly by the narrative, in its most appalling, disgusting and repulsive aspects if one looks at it from the perspective of morality: the sordid trunk of the tree, the stench of the trenches and smell of civilians, the foreplay that ends up being a fiasco, all point to the most repellent aspects of a physicality that is inescapable. And yet, Prior knows how to avoid many pitfalls: he refuses to drink or be drunk, tries to stay away from women and does not allow himself to be violent with Myrta. The absence of the transference scene in which this would be recounted to Rivers suggests that Prior is handling his life rather well, on his own, and he endeavours to knot together various dimensions of his being which his body is the site of: sexuality, identity, class, drives and emotions. It also means that Barker's narrative strategy has evolved from the therapeutic, fact-based context that dominated her first novel, and we now see Prior at play, so to speak, without the prism of therapy and the question of being cured.

The restlessness of Prior's body—which needs sex and sees the potential for sex in all the passers-by—is yet attuned to other bodies—something made remarkable when he notices discreet signs of another person's sexual drives: 'some unconsciously registered nervousness in the other man's voice,' which makes him look up (E, 8). Above all, his sexual urge is presented as meaningful on various levels: it is connected to his upcoming return to the front (a structural feature returning later in *The Ghost Road*), the absence of his girlfriend, his being rejected by the inconsequential partner that Myrta is. However, it is most interesting to note that Prior's sexual drive is presented as irrepressible and hardly focused on an object: Myrta, the girl who plays with his genitals, is not described, and the description of the man who soon is going to be his lover is guided by the fact that Prior thinks he recognises him, more than his lust. The man and Myrta are used as examples in a series of sexual partners with whom the same question of Prior's subjective place returns and recurs. Quite ironically, the question of place is that of where the sexual act could take place, but this also literally signifies the absence of sexual place and location for Prior.[4] In other words, his sexual being has no habitat, something confirmed by his open bisexuality—which is not interrogated or presented as something strange—and his habit of 'not paying' prostitutes.

The collusion of sex and paying, in addition to threatening the bourgeois morality that is already impaired in the first pages of the novel, situates the bodily transaction in the lack of symbolic exchanges or at least a dysfunctional one. Barker's subtle note that this was an episode he had told Rivers, although initially based on the necessity for her readers who

---

[4] This has been the object of many comments the present chapter takes for granted and does not revise, concerning the meaningful evocation of 'place' from a sociological point of view and the inflections of Prior's voice (GR, 109).

132 N. P. BOILEAU

may not have read *Regeneration*, to *place* Rivers, proves extremely fruitful for Prior's functioning and to signify the structural place of sex in Prior's subjective attachment to others: Prior does not see prostitutes because he does not pay, in the same way that he does not have therapy because he does not speak. The interpretations given in the text for his motto, 'I don't pay', certainly stress Prior's imagining of other people's reactions, but it also points out what the nature of his relationship with the other is: 'he knew exactly how the payer looks to the one he's paying' (E, 8). Money, like words, belongs in the symbolic order of the exchange which Prior refuses to take part in, because he needs to make sure that it is the other that is lacking: the girl who will take him without getting money, the man with a funny leg, Rivers's failings. 'Prior smiled. "Now that is lucky, isn't it? Lucky for you, I mean. Because if your stammer *was* the same as theirs you might actually have to sit down and work out what it is you've spent fifty years trying not to say"' (R, 97). By pinpointing what Rivers does not see as his own symptom, Prior refuses to *place* the analyst in the position of the one who is supposed to know and makes sure it is the therapist that is lacking. The gender of his partner matters less than the insurance that he is not the one losing in on the transaction, something which the talking cure was threatening to do and which medical treatment enacted. His body somehow is the site of this intense negotiation between the real of a *jouissance* that cannot be avoided and the symbolic aspect of his relationships with others.

What is striking is Barker's revelling in the details of sexual intercourse: fellatio and penetration are recounted bluntly in a language that verges on (Northern) slang. This contaminates the whole narrative since Prior 'coins a phrase': 'he was bloody nithered' (E, 11)—significantly using here the same word Myrta had used to his face (E, 4). The signifier, a coinage only insofar as Prior borrows it from someone else, links both sexual encounters and somehow gives indications as to the symbolic function of this coldness in Prior's being, the lack at the heart of his sense of being. It is noteworthy that interpretations regarding the attitude of his partners proliferate in the scene, but Prior's own judgement is not related to the question of the pathological: when Manning asks him if he used to be neurasthenic, Prior replies that it is asthma that gets in the way of his fully recovering as a soldier (E, 15), even if he no longer is considered to be on sick leave. This means that he is aware of the symptomatic function played by his relation to others and his body. More crucial perhaps both in terms of the character's development and in terms of literature's conventions, his bisexual activity with Manning is not questioned or interpreted as something he should feel guilty about—just like Manning refuses to change despite encouragements from the police to do so.

The person displaying the medical symptoms is Manning—'noting the MC ribbon, the wound stripe, the twitches, the signs of tension, the occasional stammer' (E, 11). These are indicative of a nervousness that could be related to the long-term stigmas of the war or the short-term nervousness of the situation. Prior notes the signs but refuses to interpret them or elevate these signals to the function of symptoms. Instead, he makes sure the sexual act is not delayed any longer by first taking off his top and secondly starting to perform oral sex—both denials of the alleged obstacles to the sexual relation that the multiple doors, broken hatches and warped keys evoke. Despite the narration's details, the whole scene is neither erotic nor clinical: it is said to be 'playful' and to evoke Prior's reflection: 'He was thinking how impossible it is to sum up sex in terms of who stuffs what into where' (E, 13). Burns's and Prior's traumas, like Carol's murder, resist any form of dialectical re-inscription in the symbolic order. If the function of narrative and, even more so of art, is 'the utterance of the unutterable in utopian fashion' (Bernard 2007: 183),[5] then Barker's work also acknowledges that representation, to remain paradoxically true to itself, must 'peer into the darkness', must also stand face to face with what defies linguistic re-cognition (Bernard 2007: 183). The narrative itself is defeated in the game of interpreting the sexual act: the list of feelings supposedly attached to the act (lust, resentment, sympathy, envy) is abruptly stopped by suspension marks which could express the long, silent list to come or equally the vain, sure to fail perspective of emotional decoding. What the narrative does is return to the imaginary level of what happens: 'And a growing awareness that while he had been looking at Manning, Manning had also been looking at him' (E, 13). Yet this again reshuffles the place of the object which Prior desires, enabling the exchange that is constitutive of the subjective experience. In another scene, Prior is shown looking at Beattie's file and Spragge's reports when 'he looked up, puzzled by the sense of something unfamiliar in the room. He stared round him, but could see nothing different, and then he realized that the change was in himself' (E, 44). Equipped with a certain language that disrupts his symbolic and imaginary representations, Prior finds a way of functioning without the battlefield and the therapist, by inscribing his sexual body into an intersubjective exchange. This is performed through a symptomatic

---

[5] Birus, Hendrick, "Adorno's 'negative Aesthetics'?" in Sanford Budick and Wolfgang Iser, eds., *Languages of the Unsayable. The Play of Negativity in Literature and Literary Theory*, Stanford: Stanford UP, 1987, 140–64, 149.

relationship with an other—be it sexual partner or therapist—who enables him to speak.

At first, the body in *The Eye in the Door* is dissected and turned into disjointed pieces like the vision of Prior's genitals in the first page. Later on, other descriptions will saturate the narrative: Scudder's legless drunkenness for having been treated with EST (E, 169) or the landlady's fascination (if not jouissance?) for the Ripper's victims' states (E, 194) and so forth. All echo the dead and corpses of the trenches, but they also evoke loss and failure, while Prior's body will somehow retrieve a semblance of unity. If the 'spectre of the symptom... short-circuits materialist understanding' (Hitchcock 2002: 15), reading that spectre turns it back to being 'a link, a signifier' (Lanone 1999: 266) in a causal, discursive chain (Bernard 2007: 181). Barker's realist perspective is therefore defeated by the symbolic inscription of the body which negates the possibility for the body to tell a story. It is not endowed with imaginary meanings but reduced to drives that function for the subject: 'No such things. It's a bit like medieval trial-by-combat, you know. In the end moral and political truths have to be proved on the body, because this mass of nerves and muscle and blood is what we are' (E, 112).

This is how I want to reinterpret Barker's self-confessed fascination for silence. Barker is equally concerned by the failure of communication ('You have to indicate that communication is being impaired' (Stevenson 2005: 176)) as she is by the enigmatic function of the stammer, which she does not reduce to the question of impaired communication: 'Rivers himself was from a generation of stammerers. There are two kinds of stammers: one, a reaction to shock, was almost universal among officers of the First World War, and the other was the lifelong stammer, where there's a troubled background of some kind' (Stevenson 2005: 177). Lacan's work on the other hand has consistently consisted in using linguistics to show how communication was not at stake in the psychic structure of subjects, because communication of meaning is impossible. His teaching shows his gradual realisation that language was first and foremost the outlet of a *jouissance* that cannot be contained, and which is deprived of any meaning. After situating language as a function of a *link* between subjects (Lacan 1975: 32), Lacan asserts that 'what is written is not to be understood' (Lacan 1975: 35). He concludes that language is not, as he initially thought when influenced by Saussure, an instrument of communication of meaning because 'the unconscious is not the fact that being thinks... the unconscious is the fact that being, by speaking, enjoys, and... wants to know nothing more about it' (Lacan 1975: 95).

It is therefore interesting to note that therapeutic talking cure recedes in the second volume and disappears in the third. Its presence in the first book derives from the question of how to produce meaning in the context of the meaninglessness of war. Instead, Barker aims for the function of language enjoyment, which she pursues through Prior's diary. Indeed, Barker chooses to work on introspective usages of language, moving back into a comprehension of language as self-satisfaction. The novels open on a play on words that underpins the narrative. Answering Sassoon's provocative question about what he should fear in case he does not return to the front, Rivers's answer is: 'Shut you up in a lunatic asylum for the rest of the war' (R, 7). Of course, he means to be imprisoned in a designated area, but this resonates with another meaning of the phrasal verb. Silence and being shut up are not simply a mode of assignation but also a mode of interaction for some who seek to circumscribe the opaque core of their being by choosing to resist the injunction to speak—and therefore enter a symbolic exchange.

The beginning of *The Ghost Road* prolongs the exploration of the new relation between the body, language and the Other which *The Eye in the Door* contrives to build. Despite the title which indeed relates the novel to a 'trauma novel' (Luckhurst 2008: 87), a scene similar to the beginning of *The Eye in the Door* recurs. Prior meets up with a prostitute but warns her that he will not be paying her. Again, class is at the heart of the construction of the scenes: 'You couldn't go for a walk anywhere in Scarborough without seeing the English class system laid out before you in all its full, intricate horror' (G, 35). More importantly, the fascination for salacious details shows the body in its physicality and materiality while it strips the scene of its modicum of eroticism: the story of a customer's exhibitionist wish (G, 36), the recollection of their first encounter based on the question of money and the symbolic function, the insistence on the stench of the unhygienic bedroom, and so forth. Prior's body's reaction is the focus of the scene, especially when connected to what looks like a traumatic re-enactment:

> He was pulling his half-unbuttoned tunic over his head when he noticed a smell of gas. Faint but unmistakable. Tented in dark khaki, he fought back the rush of panic, sweat streaming down his sides, not the gradual sweat of exercise but a sudden drench, rank, slippery hot, then immediately cold... he told himself there was no reason to be afraid, but he was afraid. All the usual reactions: dry mouth, wet armpits, skipping heart, the bulge in the

throat that makes you cough. Tight scrotum, shriveled cock. Jesus Christ, he was going to have to put a johnny on that, talk about a kid in its father's overcoat. He heard his own voice, awkward, sounding younger than he felt.
'I'm afraid this isn't going to work.'
'Aw, don't say that, love, it'll be al-'
Phoney warmth. She was used to pumping up limp pricks. (G, 38–39)

Symmetrically situated in the text, if we compare it to the scene with Myrta/Manning, this episode replays many of the character's symptoms (evoked again in the beginning, especially the paralytic stammer (G, 11) that has disappeared) but from an internal viewpoint that ultimately strips his vision of any therapeutic, pathological inscription.

What happens instead is the vision of a body with a life of its own, agitated by drives and impulses that the subject cannot control and to which he is alienated but which produces a story of its own Prior is now able if not to control, at least to articulate. The role of the prostitute is akin to that of a therapist who would be guided by the consolidation of Narcissism, the phallic mien given by an apprehension of the subject from the unique point of view of the phallus. Here, however, Prior's 'limp prick' or 'shrivelled cock' are the signs of a subject who is not all caught in the phallic logic. The subjective place of being not entirely absorbed or subsumed in the phallic logic is what Lacan situates on the side of feminine *sexuation*, something which is not based on the subject's biological sex, but which is related to a position towards *jouissance* (Mitchell and Rose 1985: 42–43; Lacan 1975). Mitchell explains this quite clearly when she reviews feminist criticism against psychoanalysis and states that 'by concentrating on the status and nature of female sexuality, it often happens that [female sexuality] is treated as an isolate, something independent of the distinction that creates it' (Mitchell and Rose 1985: 20). Thus, I don't see this confession as a failure of masculinity, or as a reappraisal of masculinity, but simply as the result of Prior's symptomatic way of building relationships, in which the other is situated as the witness of his own failure to entirely fit into the phallic logic.

Conclusion

Thus, this may account for the logic at play in the last volume of the trilogy. Two elements seem particularly relevant: first, hysterical symptoms return and saturate the narrative—as well as the theories that try to make sense of these symptoms; second, the narration from time to time is given to Prior via extracts from his journal. In these, readers are told how he has been able to build his own voice through writing, and they show us that the real presence of other people listening to his account is no longer necessary. His symptomatic relationships only seem to be based on the imaginary and symbolic versions of the other now. Regarding the first point, that is the hysterical symptoms, what is witnessed is that those described take place with no immediate or direct reference to the war. Moffet's hysterical fit, presented 'in one sense' as 'quite simple' (GR, 20), turns out to be the object of medical failure: the jargon (hypnagogic hallucinations (GR, 26), 'paralysis, deafness, blindness, muteness' (GR, 49)) is less telling than the 'dead German standing by his bed' (GR, 26) or 'the 17th century witch-finders [who] used to stick pins in people too' (GR, 48). Doctors remain victims of their own pretension to discover truth in the details of their observation. Following up on Freud's showing 'that there are illnesses which speak' (Lacan in Mitchell and Rose 1985: 64), some practitioners run the risk of 'sheltering under the wing of a psychologism which, in its reification of the human being, could lead to errors besides which those of the physician's scientism would be mere trifles' (Lacan in Mitchell and Rose 1985: 64). Barker's text goes well beyond such psychologism, by first refusing the notion that symptoms derive from a natural cause (GR, 96) or by revealing the discrepancy in the apprehension of Prior's symptoms by other doctors, some of whom 'don't believe in shell-shock' (GR, 99). Rather than linking it to army Medical Boards' refusal to recognise male hysteria, I suggest that what is at stake is indeed the inefficacy of such a diagnosis because of its link to circumstances (the war) instead of the logic of a subjective position (in Prior's case, the fact that he is dependent on and forced to create the intersubjective relation to exist in the symbolic order).

After being offered the job of a clerk, writing reports and minutes, working on his handwriting and the letter, Prior eventually yields to the temptation of a diary, some months after the end of the war. After being fairly articulate regarding the reasons why he felt reluctant to write in it, how he was intimidated by the enterprise, the text he writes starts with Manning, giving him again the structural place of being the one who enables him to function as a responsible man. 'Soldiers who aren't military, pacifists who aren't prigs, and *talking* to each other. Now *there's* a miracle' (GR, 109). It turns out the other soldiers write and read too, finding in the letter a way of entangling their *jouissance* (back) into a signifying articulation. Within this context, Prior becomes quite articulate himself, even acknowledging that which he fantasises about (GR, 175) in connection with nakedness and the body, which he sees as the point of his singularity: 'I feel uncomfortable, and I suspect most of the other officers don't' (GR, 175). The function of the diary is to remember but more importantly, it helps Prior remain steady: he explains that thanks to his writing, none of the conditions in which he would normally break down threaten his well-being now. He comments on this ironically as 'success stories' of the hospital (GR, 200), but through Barker's work on his introspective dialogue and his writing, what we are meant to appreciate is that he, himself, is in fact the story of his own success. 'I realize there's another group of words that still mean something'. (He says after mentioning how he thinks about Sarah all the time.) 'Little words that trip through sentences unregarded: us, them, we, they, here, there. These are the words of power, and long after we're gone, they'll lie about in the language, like the unexploded grenades in these fields, and any one of them'll take your hand off' (GR, 257). This quote enables Barker to show Prior regain command of the imaginary function of language as an instrument of meaning in which the community is restored or at least aimed for while continuing to interrogate the function of language as pure enjoyment outside meaning: the signifiers are presented as travelling agents which force subjects to constant renegotiations because they hold no fixed place among 'tripping' words.

This chapter therefore argues that the relevance of a social reading of the trilogy does not preclude the existence of a form of excess, a core of being that is at times impossible to avert and yet outside the symbolic order. This could be repressed material, seen from a very orthodox Freudian perspective. Or it could be the sign of something that even the Freudian theory of repression cannot account for and which, if we are to follow Lacan, signals the inherent split nature of the subject who is created in a language that alienates them to the phallic signifier. I have endeavoured to show that what appears as secondary in the novel, Prior's relationship to Rivers, and yet which insists throughout, up until the moment when Prior, on his own and back to the front, restores the figure of the therapist. Indeed, Rivers is often mentioned in his diary despite being not there (GR, 177): 'And suddenly I was back in Rivers's room... Rivers's silences are not manipulative. (Mine are. Always.)' (GR, 214). This is the symptomatic formation from which Prior emerges as a stronger character. A reading of the novels from the characters' symptomatic formations strips the interpretative process of its cultural prejudices and preconceptions and enables readers and critics to refrain from blindly accepting the discourse of medicine which, in any case, the patients of the First World War defeated (Micale and Lerner 2001). It enables us to see this precisely in the figure of Rivers, who discovers in practice what Lacan suggests is the role of the analyst, that of operating from the position of the object cause of desire rather than the master's discourse endorsed by doctors. This shift is central to the process of transference:

> the power to heal if you like springs directly from some sort of wound or deformity in him... In fact, for me it's the best thing about him—well the only thing that makes him tolerable, actually—that he *doesn't* sit behind the desk implicitly setting himself up as some sort of standard of mental health. (G, 111)

This enables readers to appreciate the distance between this text and Woolf's satirical representation of Bradshaw in *Mrs Dalloway*. The question does not lie so much in the nature of Rivers's therapy and its success, or lack thereof, but rather in the function he plays in reinstating Prior into language by having him first speak and then write, both ways of exercising, so to speak, one's subjective existence.

BIBLIOGRAPHY

PRIMARY SOURCES

Barker, Pat (1991). *Regeneration*. London: Penguin Books, 2008.

SECONDARY SOURCES

Baker, Charley, Crawford, Paul et al. (2010). *Madness in Post-1945 British and American Fiction*. London: Routledge.
Barrett, Michèle (2012). "'Regeneration' Trilogy and the Freudianization of Shell Shock". *Contemporary Literature*, Vol. 53, No 2, 237–260.
Bernard, Catherine (2007). "Pat Barker's Critical Work of Mourning: Realism with a Difference." *Études anglaises*, 2007/2, vol. 60, 173–184.
Bernard, Catherine (2018). *Matière à réflexion: du corps politique dans la littérature et les arts visuels contemporains*. Paris: Presses Universitaires de Paris-Sorbonne.
Bonikowski, Wyatt (2013). *Shell-Shock and the Modernist Imagination, The Death-Drive in post-World War I Fiction*. Burlington: Ashgate.

Brannigan, John (2005). *Pat Barker*. Manchester: Manchester University Press, "Contemporary British Novelists".

Brown, Dennis (2005). "*The Regeneration Trilogy*: Total War, Masculinities, Anthropologies, and the Talking Cure." Monteith et al. (ed.) (2005), 187–202.

Cavalié, Elsa (2015). *Réécrire l'Angleterre: l'anglicité dans la littérature contemporaine*. Montpellier: Presses Universitaires de Montpellier.

Chesler, Phyllis (1994). *Preface* to Geller Jeffrey L. & Harris Maxine, eds. (1994). *Women of the Asylum, Voices from behind the Walls, 1840–1945*. New York: Anchor Books.

Childs, Peter (2012). *Contemporary Fiction: British Novelists since 1970*. London: Palgrave Macmillan.

Didi-Huberman, Georges (1982). *Invention de l'Hystérie*. Paris: Éditions Macula, 2012.

Foucault, Michel (1963). *Naissance de la Clinique*. Paris: Presses Universitaires de France, "Quadrige grands textes", 2003. For the English version: http://monoskop.org/images/9/92/Foucault_Michel_The_Birth_of_the_Clinic_1976.pdf

Freud, Sigmund (1905a). *Jokes and their Relation to the Unconscious*. London: Norton, 1989.

Freud, Sigmund (1905b). *Cinq Psychanalyses*. Paris: Presses Universitaires de France, 2008.

Freud, Sigmund (1923). "la Disparition du complexe d'Œdipe". *La Vie sexuelle*. Paris: Presses Universitaires de France, trans. Laplanche, 1969.

Freud, Sigmund (1926), *Inhibition, Symptome et Angoisse*. Trans. J. and R. Doron. Paris: Presses Universitaires de France, 1993.

Freud, Sigmund (1931). "On Female Sexuality" trans. "Sur la sexualité féminine", in La Vie sexuelle, Paris: PUF, 1969, 139–155.

Gagneret, Diane (2019). *Explorer la frontière: Folie et genre(s) dans la littérature anglophone contemporaine*. Unpublished PhD thesis defended at ENS Lyon, 22.11.2019, under the supervision of Prof. Vanessa Guignery.

Hitchcock, Peter (2002). "What is Prior? Working-Class Masculinity in Pat Barker's Trilogy." *Genders 35*, http://www.genders.org/g35/g35_hitchcock.html

Lacan, Jaques (2001). *Autres écrits*. Paris: Éditions du seuil, "Champ freudien".

Lacan, Jacques (1975). *Le Séminaire, Livre XX, Encore* (1972–73). J.-A. Miller (ed.). Paris: Éditions du Seuil.

Lacan, Jacques (1991). *Le Séminaire, Livre XVII, Envers de la psychanalyse* (1970). J.-A. Miller (ed.). Paris: Éditions du Seuil.

Lanone, Catherine (1999). "Scattering the Seed of Abraham: The Motif of Sacrifice in Pat Barker's *Regeneration* and *The Ghost Road*." *Literature & Theology* 13: 3, 259–68.

Luckhurst Roger (2008). *The Trauma Question*. New York: Routledge.

Maleval, Jean-Claude (2010). "Comment entendre la voix?", in L. Jodeau-Belle & L. Ottavi Laurent (eds.) (2010), 185–197.

Micale, Mark S. & Lerner, Patrick (eds.) (2001). *Traumatic Pasts, History, Psychiatry and Trauma in the Modern Age 1870–1930*. Cambridge: Cambridge University Press.

Mitchell, Juliet & Rose, Jacqueline (1985). *Feminine Sexuality, Jacques Lacan and the* École freudienne. London: Norton.

Monteith, Sharon, Jolly, Margaretta, Youssaf, Nahem and Ronald, Paul (eds.) (2005). *Critical Perspectives on Pat Barker*. Columbia: University of South Carolina Press.

Paul, Ronald (2005). "In Pastoral Fields: The *Regeneration* Trilogy and Classic First World War Fiction". Monteith et al. (eds.), 147–161.

Ross, Sarah C. E. (2005). "Regeneration, Redemption, Resurrection: Pat Barker and the Problem of Evil." In Acheson & Ross (eds) (2005).

Saunders, Corinne and McNaughton, Jane (eds.) (2005). *Madness and Creativity in Literature and Culture*. London: Palgrave Macmillan.

Showalter, Elaine (1985). *The Female Malady, Women, Madness and English Culture, 1830–1980*. London: Virago Press.

Showalter, Elaine (1997). *Hystories, Hysterical Epidemics and Modern Culture*. London: Picador, 2013.

Steffens, Karolyn (2014). "Communicating Trauma: Pat Barker's *Regeneration* Trilogy and W.H.R. Rivers's Psychoanalytic Method". *Journal of Modern Literature*, volume 37, No. 3, 36–55.

Stevenson, Sheryl (2005). "The Uncanny Case of Dr. Rivers and Mr. Prior: Dynamics of Transference in *The Eye in the Door*". In Monteith et al. (eds.) (2005), 219–233.

Stone, Jon, et al. (2008). "The 'Disappearance' of Hysteria: Historical Mystery or Illusion?". *Journal of Royal Society of Medicine*, 101, 12–18, DOI: https://doi.org/10.1258/jrsm.2007.070129

Vickroy, Laurie (2004). "A Legacy of Pacifism: Virginia Woolf and Pat Barker". *Women and Language*, vol. 27, No.2, 45–50.

Walezak, Emilie (2021). *Rethinking Contemporary British Women's Writing: Realism, Feminism, Materialism*. London: Bloomsbury.

Wall, Oisin (2018). *The British Anti-Psychiatrists, from institutional Psychiatry to Counter-Culture, 1960–1971*. London: Routledge.

Ward, Sean Francis (2016). "Erotohistoriography and War's Waste in Pat Barker's *Regeneration* Trilogy". *Contemporary Literature* 57:3, 320–345.

Whitehead Anne (2005). "Open to Suggestion, Hypnosis and History in the *Regeneration* Trilogy". Monteith et al. (eds.) (2005), 203–2018.

PART II

The Symptom and the Body: Discreet Signs of Psychological Disorders

CHAPTER 5

The Body as Dangerous Jouissance in *The Fifth Child* by Doris Lessing

The first section of the book was focused on finding a way out of the rut that pits psychiatry against psychoanalysis, or against the patients. Our aim was to show that the satire targeting psychiatrists and the psychiatric institution in the fictional works selected is not so much concerned with the ridicule of mental health care as with the possibility of a shift in the way illness and its symptoms are perceived and used both outside and inside treatment. In the wake of Woolf's Septimus Warren Smith's portrayal, the fictions of Barker and McGrath use the debacle of the psychiatrists' treatment to offer another approach to the symptom which becomes an ontology of the subject: defined as alienated by a *jouissance* that cannot be fully articulated, subjects become the peculiar/singular compound of their own experience, the lack inherent in their expression of it and the response they offer to the external world, a peculiarity manifested in symptomatic formations that need to be articulated back into their stories. Literature of madness thereby constantly re-instates the subject against the reification that the scientific method, in its attachment to statistical and countable realities, can only neglect.

In the following section, I'll look at texts less directly concerned with psychiatric treatment itself, but in which the presence of someone afflicted with mental health problems has fictional repercussions that enable us to look at a more specific symptomatic formation, that of the core relation of

© The Author(s), under exclusive license to Springer Nature Switzerland AG 2023
N. P. Boileau, *Mental Health Symptoms in Literature since Modernism*, Palgrave Studies in Literature, Science and Medicine, https://doi.org/10.1007/978-3-031-37630-6_5

a subject with their body, and in particular here with the body as sexed and the question of how to form relations with others—a question that becomes central in these texts. This will enable us to look at new symptom formations, less extraordinary, more discreet and more discreetly noted by the novelists, taking into consideration the progress made by medical treatment as will be seen in Lessing's mid-1980s fictional story and Hollinghurst's twenty-first-century depiction of manic depression.

Doris Lessing's Nobel Prize paradoxically did not lead to a re-appraisal of her work in laudatory terms. Harold Bloom's declaration that her later work was 'fourth-rate science fiction' (Ridout and Watkins 2009: 1) was still less accusatory than critics who lamented her Conservative leanings, a continuing trend since the late 1970s (Showalter 1977: 313). However, Ridout and Watkins argue that these comments are mostly voiced by critics who were disappointed that she did not hold up to her own, initial engagement (Ridout and Watkins 2009: 10), or that she did not entirely fit in the guise of the progressive feminist-Communist-postcolonial writer that she set out to be. For all these negative comments, she is still described as a 'canonical' writer of Africa in textbooks (Innes 2007: 148). Yet, early critics had noted Lessing's uneasiness with terms ending in '-ism' (Knapp 1984: 7–9), a political stance reinterpreted now as the 'starting-point' of any analysis of her work: her 'resistance to categorization and her persistent impulse to cross borders of all kinds in her work and life' (Ridout and Watkins 2009: 2) is what characterises her fictional work and can be said to account for the inconsistent critical reception of her novels. In this introduction, I do not intend to review Lessing's critical reception, but only to give a few pointers so as to stress the originality of my own contribution. I will not be able to include my argument into a broader appreciation of Lessing's *oeuvre*, which ranges from memoir to genre fiction (Herman 1992), from feminist manifestoes and formalist masterpieces to short stories, plays and essays. Such a variety of texts and interests would deserve more than the scope of a book chapter. My own contribution is based on the symptom of illness in a specific short novel by Lessing, *The Fifth Child* (1988), which she published after a decade of second-rate texts which, except for *The Good Terrorist* (1985), had failed to receive the critical attention reserved for her earlier texts—such as *The Grass Is Singing* (1950), *The Children of Violence* series (1952–1969) and *The Golden Notebook* (1962). She had also made a name for herself with more intimate novels exploring madness and the place of the individual in the collective action of the 1970s—*Briefing for a Descent into Hell* (1971) or *The*

Summer Before the Dark (1973) to take but two examples. I follow here Knapp's serialisation of Lessing's work (Knapp 1984: 104–114). I have chosen to discuss *The Fifth Child* because the novel defies logical explanations and is interested in the symptomatic relationship that is developed between a mother and her estranged, 'alien' son, Ben. Because I have chosen to focus on *The Fifth Child*, which was written in England, by a writer who had lived in England for over 30 years, and is set in England, near London, I shall not discuss the postcolonial aspect of Lessing's works which is not central to my argument.

After the heyday of unmitigated critical praise of her work in the 1960s, Lessing's novels were thought to be less attuned to the spirits of the times (Scanlan 2001: 75): Showalter sees this 'shift'—from an early work marked by a strong Communist ideology to a work less politically engaged— as a consequence of Lessing's pessimistic view of the future of civilisation, which rendered feminist and gender issues irrelevant (Showalter 1977: 308). It is true that interest in her work dwindled, despite her prolific career. Lessing's attitude, which consisted in bluntly expressing her views against Communism and feminism in essays published or publicised in the press (*The Guardian* 2001), infuriated many, among whom Showalter who, like with Woolf, continuously criticises Lessing's feminist engagement: in *The Female Malady*, she clearly sees Lessing as an advocate of Laing's anti-psychiatry and models her analysis of Lessing's work on the parallels she can draw between Lessing's novels and Laing's theory, concluding: 'Lessing's novels were no longer at all concerned with the schizophrenic journey as a woman's exploration of the self; and Watkins's male adventure story is less interesting and complex than Anna Wulf's memories, dreams and fictions' (Showalter 1985: 241). Notwithstanding the essentialist subtext such a comment infers, I would like to stress that few feminist scholars[1] have looked at Lessing's work beyond the 1970s in spite of her being a 'feminist icon' (Scanlan 2001: 75). If Winterson's reaction to Lessing's final criticism of feminist forays were polemical in the wake of Lessing's Nobel Prize, Raman's very recent work is valuable in trying to take some distance with these now established feminist responses because of her intention to sound them again some 50 years after Lessing grew out of favour: taking issue with the idea that Lessing's feminism should be seen as an initial mistake made by critics which her later, reactionary works are said to have contradicted (Raman 2021: 3–6), Raman contextualises

---

[1] With the exception of Rahimnouri and Ghandehariun (2020).

148   N. P. BOILEAU

Lessing's feminism as based on a refusal of essentialist visions of both men and women, and as straddling various eras (from the Victorian education of her mother to the 1970s' women's liberation movement) and various spaces (from her natal Africa to the England she lived in until her death) (Raman 2021: 8–10) to account for a plurality of feminisms. Raman thus advocates a reading of Lessing's fiction not simply as a return to conservatism or a gradual disinterest in the gender question, but as a continuous exploration of women's roles in society and a repeated deconstruction of fixed identities. This is why Lessing still features in the corpus of feminist critique (Rundgren 2016).

Within this critical context, Lessing's *The Fifth Child* seems to stand alone both in Lessing's overall critical historiography and in feminist readings of the text. Interestingly, Raman does not retain it in the corpus of novels she chooses to analyse: the novel does not focus on the early themes that characterised Lessing's work: racial conflicts or political action and sex (Schlueter 1973: 126). However, class is still touched upon in some passages, as when the narrator notes the differences between Harriet and David (FC, 23; 24; 87); its length aside, the novel's format does not show any evident attachment to experimental or aesthetically defined forms of storytelling; its theme conventionally focuses on the demise of a family and condenses into less than 200 pages the encounter, wedding and 15 years of a marriage that begets five children, one of whom, the last one, is abnormal, even if the family doctor refuses to translate this into a medical diagnosis (FC, 87). The novel was written in the 1980s but is set a decade before (late 1960s up until mid-1970s), placing it in an odd situation of being written after the Women's Liberation Movement of the 1970s, when the Conservative backlash in England was at its apex, while describing a period preceding such engagement.[2] Although the narration is external, most of the action is seen from the perspective of the mother, Harriet, who is the first to witness the difference of her son—as early as in the first few months of her pregnancy—and will be the only one who tries to bond with him, or at least save him from the planned death David, his father, and the rest of the family have imagined for him by sending him to an institution. The novel was so successful among the public that it has constantly been re-edited and Lessing was talked into producing a sequel, *Ben, in the World* (2000), by her German publisher (Hilson 2012: 18). Finally, the novel stands aside from the rest of Lessing's production

[2] For a specific exploration of the Thatcher influence on the novel, see Yelin (1998): 91–93.

because in it she explores the situation of a woman who seems to fully embrace or endorse the Conservative, or Thatcherite (Brock 2009) ideology and traditional roles of motherhood and domestic life, to the point of physical and mental exhaustion.

For the novel presents itself as a domestic novel, or a story of 'domestic terrorism' (Rowe 1994 qd De Vinne 2012: 17): Harriet leads the life of a housewife and has to go through five pregnancies in a very short time, being exhausted physically as well as mentally by the strain of having to raise children, entertain large family gatherings and being the only one in charge of the household. Quite rapidly, the fifth and last child, Ben, is the agent of a change in the family's happiness which had, so far, outlived all expectations. The novel interestingly approaches the body as a source of both pleasure and pain, strength and weakness, and a psychic rather than physical reality for the woman and mother, Harriet. When Harriet gives birth to her fifth child, her family is already marked by opprobrium—why have so many kids when contraceptives exist?—and excess, but the fifth child will inevitably come to stand for the punishment they must face for indulging in the excessive pleasure of begetting and parenting. As opposed to the works discussed in the first section, the 'anomaly' of Ben is barely treated from a medical or psychiatric point of view: even the institution where he is sent seems to be a place of agony and legalised murder, rather than a place of therapy (FC, 95–100). The stress is placed not on the question of fixing the child's abnormality, but on the function his apparent symptoms play in revealing his mother's own subjective position in the world, up until then hidden behind the normative discourse of society. I explore the partnership between mother and son not as pathological but on the contrary, as the condition for each of them to survive and perhaps even for Harriet to exist. By locating her son's symptom at the place where she fails to be a mother, that is, by noticing the excessive appetite he has for life when she is drained of energy, Harriet ensures that even more than her other children, Ben should be regarded as the epitome of the *jouissance* she craves for: an unbridled body marked by no self-consciousness and which is a real object, that is one that she cannot relate to. It is a body that constantly escapes her grasp, signifying her never-ending role as mother.

As can be seen in this short summary of the novel, there is no apparent trace of Lessing's being 'a keen satirist of the personal shortcomings of political idealists and the poses and postures of the public meeting' (Scanlan 2001: 75). However, the novel does continue a 'familiar part of

Lessing's landscape', that is, her interest in madness (Scanlan 2001: 81), or what others have called the shift from 'the politics of the left' to the 'politics of madness' (Pickering 1980 qd in Knapp 1984). Because of this shift in the 1970s, many commentators have analysed Lessing's work in relation to madness and psychiatry. There have been analyses of Lessing's close relationship with Laing's anti-psychiatry: Showalter says that 'the eleventh vignette in *The Golden Notebook* paraphrases R. D. Laing's hypothesis in *Sanity, Madness and the Family...*' (Showalter 1977: 312), in which the British psychiatrist explains that the 'most "normal" member of a family' is the one 'who is really sick' (Showalter 1977: 312 quoting Mark). The most consistent analysis of the close ties between Laing and Lessing is Rigney's chapter on *The Four-Gated City* (Rigney: 67–89), the book being a Laingian reading of Brontë, Woolf, Lessing and Atwood. Laing's work led to an extremely influential cultural movement in the 1950s-70s in England and can be summarised as the idea that 'madness, particularly schizophrenia, was not only intelligible but actually a reasonable, if not always rational, reaction to an impossible social situation' (Wall 2018: 19). It is not difficult to see why a former Marxist like Lessing could have been tempted by Laing's theory: his much publicised wish to make do with the institutionalisation of patients, his democratic or peer-approach to psychiatric treatment, based on creating a community competing with the stifling society that causes madness, especially in relation to the anti-psychiatrists' work towards promoting a counter-culture (Wall 2018: 90–120), leaves little doubt as to the appeal such a theory could have had for Lessing in connection with her later mysticism. Insanity was seen by Lessing more as a symbol than a medical condition; it was 'a reaction to a violent society' (Knapp 1984: 17).

Focusing on Laing, however, may make us overlook other possible links between her novel and psychoanalytic theory or mental health treatment. Lessing's obsession with and reliance on the fictional effects of dreams and the subconscious is so blatant that the author herself often commented on it. The most obvious reference is Freud (Freud 1899), all the more so as Lessing's early novels were written at a time that was the most influential for psychoanalysis for both writers and critics: Freud is quoted by some, especially in relation to Lessing's awareness of the 'limitations of story-telling and the simultaneous realization that the story must nevertheless be told' (Danziger 1996: 1). His relevance is crucial in *The Fifth Child* because the novel is often described as a fantastic tale calling forth Freud's theory of the *unHeimlich*, otherwise called 'uncanny' in English (Freud

1919). The concept is repeatedly used as a way of paying tribute to the idea—often used quite vaguely and commonly—on Lessing's narrative strategy. When some want 'to reflect on the uncanny prescience of this claustrophobic little book' (Brock 2009: 7), others use it in their titles without necessarily delving into the reference: 'The Uncanny Unnamable in Doris Lessing's *The Fifth Child* and *Ben, in the World*' (De Vinne 2012). Together with the uncanny, the 'repressed' is another such term that belongs in the critical vocabulary used for Lessing: 'the gothic convention of the return of the repressed' (Brock 2009: 7)

Lastly, secondary psychoanalytical voices can be heard. Jung is a strong reference when Lessing's use of the subconscious and Communism is ana-lysed (Casablancas-Cervantes 2010; Berets 1980; and Rubenstein 2009). Here again, the cultural dimension of Jung's subconscious goes hand in glove with Lessing's own interest in the social implications of race and class conflicts, and the primitivity of Ben, the fifth child of the novel. Scanlan cites an extract from *Documents*, in which Lessing explains that for the inhabitants of a repressive planet called Sirius 'anyone who tries to use language accurately to describe what is in fact happening vanishes into torture rooms and prisons, or diagnosed as mad, into mental hospitals' (Lessing qd in Scanlan 2001: 81). This gives me an opportunity to add Lacan as a potential thinker whose work could have interested Lessing, although there is no element to confirm that she may have read his work or was familiar with it. Her idea that language that is 'accurate', that is, language that is correct and corresponds to reality, is a sign of madness for society befits a Lacanian idea, so to speak. This corresponds to what Lacan argues about the schizophrenic for whom all the symbolic is real (Lacan 1966: 390). When Lacan says that words are real for the psychotic subject, he means that language does not operate in its symbolic function of filling up the emptiness of non-existence and of cutting the subject off from what language, by its operation, makes inaccessible. Language is taken for the thing itself, or rather *mis*taken for the thing instead of being regarded as an operation that designates the thing which, in turn, becomes lost—this operation of language is what underlies Lacan's revision of the Freudian concept of castration, which he calls symbolic castration. This aspect of insanity is based not on deficiency or lack but on an experience of excess, because the real that is not grasped symbolically, a real that is not struc-tured on a lack that makes its naming forever unsatisfactory, cannot be fended off by language and overwhelms the subject (Maleval 2019: 51). This resonates with Ben's experience of life, in which language is almost absent, and Harriet's more and more blatant absence of articulation when confronted with a reality that she cannot name. Both testify to this level in which the 'symbolic stops making sense and stops making a narrative: the symbolic is at the level of noise where everything can be heard' (Miller 2007 qd in Maleval 2019: 24).

For the novel, as I argue in this chapter, is an exploration of the body as an experience of a real, a *jouissance*, that fails to enter the symbolic order, which Lessing gives us to witness through the complex skein of relationships between sexual partners, parent and siblings. The arrival of a child that cannot be named in his odd symbolic place, other than by being numbered, brings to the fore this bodily experience that is untamed. Hsieh keeps referring to Ben in the sequel as 'the creature' (Hsieh 2010) and Brevet calls him a 'traumatic, semi-human creature' in the first line of her article on *The Fifth Child* (Brevet 2011). They endorse the label given by most characters in the text in turn, without taking much distance. The reference to Frankenstein in various critical works also comes to signify the opacity of Ben's identity, which blurs our notions of fixed categories, as Lessing herself sought to do: it 'bears the deep imprint' of 'the terrible class system of castes and pigeonholing people, which is characteristically British' (*Conversations*, 194 qd in Brevet 2011). In the following chapter, I show that the novel is not a fantastic tale about a dream-like figure but the account of another kind of symptoms, lodged in the subject's body as that which cannot be named and which obsessively surfaces in the life of Harriet to signify the excessive *jouissance* of her own body and the dangerous, sickening *jouissance* of an Other she begets but is incapable of controlling.

'Playing with the Conventional Structures of the Novel'

The first 'symptom' that can be spotted in the novel is the social symptom that looms large over the family from the beginning, namely the conservative family values around which the couple of David and Harriet hinges and which drives them to have many children, despite their lack of money, and in an urgency that defies the logic of common sense. As I argue in this first part of this chapter, the family bliss sought through having children is based on the lie of an ideal which Lessing constructs in order to reveal its sham foundations. It would be too easy to regard Ben as the only one suffering from an illness or mental symptoms, just as much as it would be reductive to think of Harriet as being the only one suffering from the vision of her son. What I will argue is that both form a couple that is a symptom of their subjective outlook to the world.

Lessing's career initially sparked interest because of her (feminist/feminine) ability to de-centre western perspective in her novels. Throughout the 1950s and 1960s, her writings focused on or were related to Africa, especially South Rhodesia (now Zimbabwe), where she spent her childhood and young adulthood, before moving back to London permanently when she was 30 years old. The beginning of *Martha Quest* focuses on racial prejudices and detailed descriptions of the Rhodesian countryside (Lessing 1952: 18). In addition to offering a 'novel' setting and speaking from a position of marginality, stressing the experience of women and working-class people (May 2010: 201–203), Lessing's first novels manage to both continue an aesthetic of social realism which corresponded to the Marxist and leftist dominant ideology in academia and present readers with some new experimental ways of telling stories, notably in the precocious yet durably popular *The Golden Notebook* (1962), 'Doris Lessing's real breakthrough' (Ridout and Watkins 2009: 1). The first decade of her production is thus marked by great novelistic experimentation in themes. The *Children of Violence* series is particularly striking in that respect. It starts with a fairly conventional first volume owing much to the Victorian Bildungsroman, albeit with greater concern for descriptions of sexual practices and traumas, *Martha Quest* (1952); and it ends with a more abrupt denunciation of Communism in *The Four-Gated City* (1969). This political, feminist engagement was noted and praised and remains attributed to a marginal position linked with her origins (Innes 2007: 180). Yet Lessing's interest in form is more or less ambivalent: although she never chooses conventional stories or conventional storytelling, as can be seen in the quasi-absence of novels without any formalistic intentions, she always considers that literature fails so to speak, at least that her own voice should not be lost in the superficial effects of an aesthetic achievement: 'Only in *The Golden Notebook* and *Four-Gated City* does she attempt anything radical in form, and considers her effort in the former novel to be a failure, especially since most reviewers understood her intentions' (Schlueter 1973: 126). Before Ridout and Watkins offered a vision of Lessing's works as potentially seeking to 'embody, in a creative process of border crossing, the dynamic relation between supposedly opposing ideas' (Ridout and Watkins 2009: 12), her work was considered by some to be too difficult to categorise while lacking in novelistic experimentation. One may note that her dislike of Woolf is based on her alleged bourgeois vision that lays too much emphasis on aesthetic considerations. If some like Rigney (Rigney 1978) and Showalter (Showalter 1977: 310–311) have likened Lessing to Woolf, it seems to be based more on the two authors' similarities in themes than in style. Both critics emphasise the points of connection between Lessing's interest in madness and *Mrs Dalloway*, but Brevet argues that *The Fifth Child* owes more to *To the Lighthouse* in its depiction of a woman imprisoned in her feminine, domestic role (Brevet 2011).

The Fifth Child seems to have attracted mostly generic evaluations, but with little consensus other than its fairly conventional or generic conformity: for some it is a 'a fairy tale turned sour' (Raschke 2003: 10) while others regard it as part of Lessing's science fiction works. Saiful sees it as 'part horror story, part fable' (Saiful 2013: 276) and De Vinne calls it an 'uncanny tale' (De Vinne 2012: 15). Doris Lessing, explaining how much she disliked writing it, described it as a 'horror story': 'it seems to me it's a classic horror story' and she did not understand why the critics called it a 'moral fable' (Rothstein 1988). (Generic) conventions are indeed given pride of place in the beginning of the novel, especially in relation to domestic roles and family life—perhaps also a sign that Lessing had mainly worked on science fiction in the previous years. The novel opens on a romantic setting that more or less adheres to the most conventional love stories: a party during which two singletons fall in love at first sight, attracted to each other by the insurance that they both have conservative views. In what is redolent of postmodern narrative strategies, Lessing leaves no doubt as to the fictional nature of such a scene: 'The famous office party became part of their story' (FC, 10). It is both a story that happened and a story that was meant to be given a symbolic function. The author playfully uses the pronoun 'they' all the time as if their union was inevitable and had created a new being, 'Aiming, like all their kind, at an appearance of unconformity, they were in fact the essence of convention, and disliked any manifestation of the spirit of the exaggeration, of excess. The house was that' (FC, 18). The first part of the novel is impressive in its density in terms of both action and descriptions: within only 20 pages, the couple meets, buys a house, faces the opposition of their family and is pregnant with their first child. This also contributes to highlighting the conventional aspects of this novel, or rather how much Lessing was sure to rely on the readers' knowledge of the well-trodden paths of such love stories, giving it both the safe feeling of the well-known and the eerie quality of an excessively dense account which, as the title points to, will abruptly end its conventional course with the fifth (and last? the reader may wonder) child. The birth of the child, announced in the title, cannot but be anticipated from the start. Such urgency in the way the story is delivered also explains the final instability of the genre, as the initial romance is quickly replaced by a domestic novel told in the uncommon tone of success, before turning into a horror story: instead of stopping when they married and lived happily thereafter, Lessing chooses to first linger on their happiness in order for us to see it end too.

The novel is said to be 'a critique of the confluence in the Britain of the 1980s of defensive family values and fear of social unrest' (Brock 2009: 7). The argument goes that Lessing wrote it in the 1980s, when Thatcher's conservative politics led to a strengthening of family and domestic values in the public opinion, in keeping with the idea that Thatcher did less for the feminist cause than men could have done and in a context of the AIDS epidemic that posed a threat to sexually liberated mores. The conventional family model and the notion of a domestic bliss are so outdated for Lessing that she decides to set the story 20 years before, not long enough for readers to feel entirely disconnected from the timeline but at a time sufficiently remote to suggest that this, like romance, is now over. Thus, even the unconventional divorce of David's parents is treated with distance, as something destabilising the notion of family but not putting an end to David's desire to have one: 'He joked, far too often, that he had two sets of parents' (FC, 12). David's joking is a way of taking some distance vis-à-vis a situation that was then very infrequent, but the narratorial remark suggests an excessive irony that perhaps defeats the initial purpose. All in all, conventions seem to be the key word of the two main characters' lives and the narrative suggests that these principles cannot be trusted, that there are rents in the fabric of social conformity. In a manner that Lessing would have disputed (Rothstein 1988), Yelin argues that when the youths Ben befriends invade the space of the house, 'what was once the quintessence of England becomes a travesty of postcolonial, postmodern, transnational commodity culture, represented in the array of multinational fast foods they consume' (Yelin 1998: 103). The book is thus perceived by some as showing a war of civilisation, pitting one norm against another. However, from the beginning of the novel, the realism or naturalism of the story is evidently undermined by the ideal nature of the situation.

One could object that David and Harriet also offer a vision of conventional sexual roles that cannot but attract the attention of those who come to Lessing thinking she writes about women's social and cultural independence. Casablancas points out that the story's action coincides with the publication of Adrienne Rich's *Of Woman Born: Motherhood as Experience and Institution* (1976), which is not entirely true since most of the action has already happened by 1976. Robbins also thinks the novel echoes the long-lasting influence of Friedan's *Feminine Mystique* (Robbins 2009: 97). However, it is true that the action takes place in the midst of the second wave of feminism, which adumbrates the social context in which Harriet becomes a woman. The least that can be said is that she seems to have been impervious to the changes brought about by the feminist movement. If both David and Harriet are 'freaks and oddballs' (FC, 9), it is because they refuse the dogma of sexual liberation: David, in traditional fashion, despises the women he had sex with out of wedlock, while Harriet has remained 'a virgin now, her girlfriends might shriek: "are you crazy?"' (FC, 9). This is certainly noted by contemporary readers as being the sign of conservative views, but the way Lessing presents these characters' resistance to evolving gender roles is almost too hackneyed not to sound slightly wrong or false: it is almost as if she played with the readers' expectations, at a time when sexual liberation was a given and the domestic bliss of marriage no longer corresponded to the majority of cases. This is what Ellen Pifer for other reasons calls 'the subversion of the pastoral' and what De Vinne translates in the following terms: 'the imagined family paradise has imploded' (De Vinne 2012: 19). Domesticity is certainly worshipped but it is also that by which the characters are doomed. Lessing gives us all these clues in the first pages.

The distribution of roles—David as bread-winner; Harriet as housewife—is a picture that fails to convince and the two protagonists' insistence that they be seen like this almost evokes the symptomatic formation of a couple who has discovered in one another something unnamed that they camouflage with principles: 'They talked as if talk were what had been denied to them both, as if they were starving for talk… close, talking until the noise began to lessen in the rooms across the corridor. There they lay on his bed holding hands and talked, and sometimes kissed, and then slept' (FC, 11). The narrative does not linger on what they talk about: meaning matters less than the enjoyable function of the talk and how this is the condition for some form of attachment between the two protagonists. What is relevant is the excessive *jouissance* of a talk in which they complement each other, or unite, as can be seen in their bodily gestures and the safe place they feel to be in when they fall asleep. Sex has been substituted by talk, with the same libidinal outcome, but the overflow of words of that first night is a pact Harriet is entrapped in: 'she was breaking the rules of some contract between them: tears and misery had not been on their agenda!' (FC, 45). The first children are born into a family that already is based on the 'lie' of the conventional story: 'When he bent to kiss her goodbye, and stroked her head, it was with a fierce possessiveness that Harriet liked and understood, for it was not herself being possessed, or the baby, but happiness. Hers and his' (FC, 24). The illusion of a common appeal and common experience emerges from a couple defined by their forming one, which incidentally makes the couple possible where it had failed in David's parents. Yet the sentence finishes with a clear-cut separation between the two, 'Hers and his', in an isolated phrase which is ominous of the gradual separation of the pair when they encounter their fifth child.

The model of the traditional family is presented as incompatible with the 'spirit of the times, the greedy and selfish sixties' which 'condemn[s] them', isolating and 'diminish[ing] their best selves' (FC, 29). This may be the reason why so many critics evoke the tale-like, imaginative tone of the text, such as Casablancas who considers that the novel has 'a dreamlike atmosphere in which reality and imagination merge' (Casablancas-Cervantes 2010: 1). The general impression given by the beginning is on the contrary that of a 'distant' fairy tale (Brevet 2011), the story being vaguely familiar but definitely uncommon. This is symbolically evoked by the house chosen by the couple: it is too big to house a family of the 1960s, too bourgeois for their means, too old and decrepit for a young couple, and yet they stick to it as if it were the pre-condition for their happiness and as if they sought a shelter from the disapproving look of everyone else. The house is not just a backdrop, it is an engine for them, already marked by excess: it helps them make their first decisions, it becomes David's *raison d'être* ('What he was working for was a home' (FC, 13)), it is also, like their family, that which alienates them as well when it becomes clear they cannot get rid of it, and it is invaded by other people, not only their relatives but also Ben's marginal companions (FC, 152–153).

The function of houses and places in Lessing's fiction has been analysed elsewhere: 'We may view the threshold in the novel as a literalisation of the Lovatts' obsessive *territoriality*, conceived in Peter J. Taylor's terms, as 'a form of behaviour that uses a bounded space, a territory, as the instrument for securing a particular outcome' (Brock 2009: 8). For Hilson, it is more specifically the table that concentrates social expectations and the ideal of a model family for the Lovatts (Hilson 2012: 21). For Yelin, it represents

England, 'simultaneously stand[ing] for the nation … and stand[ing] in opposition to a morally bankrupt national culture' (Yelin 1998: 101). As early as in the early 1980s, Knapp had noticed that the symbolic role of the house was prevalent in Lessing's fiction: the 'motif of rooms and houses in Lessing's work … symbolizes the limited possibilities of separating the individual from the environment' (Knapp 1984: 6). Just before *The Fifth Child*, Lessing had written the story of a small group of Communists living in a squat that Alice, the main character, tries to refurbish (*The Good Terrorist*). The 'vulnerable and temporary' essence of the house (Knapp 1984; 7) does not stop David from trying to secure a safe space for his family. He is only too aware of the vulnerability of houses because he had the experience of two households as he was growing up and of his father's decision to be without a conventional home he would return to after travelling around with his new wife: David, when he argues with his mother, tells her: 'My room—that was home' (FC, 37). The confusion between the house and home seems to be the logic behind the choice of a house where everyone would have a room, but which David fails to work towards turning into a home: it is an excessive literalisation of the metaphor of the room.

When Dorothy, Harriet's mother, wonders why the couple insists on displacing the young children to separate rooms every time a new baby is born, David's answer leaves no doubt as to the symbolic and signifying functions space and rooms have: 'It's important', said David, fierce; 'everyone should have a room' (FC, 31). Finally, David insists that the couple's bedroom is what is responsible for their fertility—'the baby maker' (FC, 40). Once Ben is born, David's contribution to managing the child is to lock him up in his bedroom to avoid his violence—like another Bertha up in the attic (FC, 68; 78)—before he seeks to institutionalise him: David's response to his lack of place in the world is to try and find shelter or stay away from dominant society. This drive towards a room where one is encapsulated is a symptomatic sign that without it he feels prey to being overwhelmed by something that he does not name. In any case, his fifth child challenges this strategy by making the other enter the house. Time and again, the others look at the couple as if they were mad, often in side-comments designed to be understood in various meanings: '"It's crazy!" said Dorothy. She was flushed with the hot tea and with all the things she was forcing herself not to say' (FC, 42). The story also follows how the house which kept them away from these looks becomes open to everyone's gaze.

Despite being heavily conceived as endowed with a symbolic meaning, the room David imagines for himself and his children fails to have the symbolic function he would like it to hold: first, the rooms he attributes to his children rapidly are dissolved in the number of children which forces him to constantly shift them on, leaving them with virtually no time to be contained within one space; they hold a room only in relation to their place in the family count. David never seems to talk about his children as individuals but he counts them, not because they count but because their number means he has to work more to sustain the family, he has to make room for them. De Vinne has shown that all of their children, save Ben, have very traditional Christian names: Luke, Paul, Helen and Jane (De Vinne 2012: 16). They are not marked by a form of singularity and in the first part of the novel, they are very likely to be treated as one whole: 'the children', an especially ominous turn of phrase when one thinks of how many of them there are and the possibility for them to be treated as individuals. By pointing at the sinister aspects of family values, the novelist suggests an interpretation of what causes violence at all levels of society, that is, the loss of individual freedom through group mentality. Virginia Tiger claims that Lessing's fiction of the late eighties such as *The Making of Representative for Planet 8*, *The Good Terrorist* and *The Fifth Child* are 'cautionary' texts because they 'challenge political extremisms, championing ... individual independence, moderate iconoclasm in the face of ideologies' (Tiger 1990, 89, qd in Brevet 2011).

Excess and Overgrowth: Two Key Words of the Family's Shared Symptoms of Displacement

This presentation of the Lovatts' family life is more or less in keeping with the ideals of domestic bliss and traditional values designed to ensure economic and perhaps national stability, especially as the novel indicates that the world out of the house is becoming more and more criminal and the TV or newspapers often report the wrongdoing of young delinquents. And yet, the family is only regarded so if one overlooks Lessing's many indications, prior to Ben's arrival, that this is only a façade that cannot be taken for granted. The novel underlines constant outbursts of passion and laughter; the family's emotional state is always described in heightened terms; there are but very few pauses in the narrative itself that unfolds the story of this couple as if it was precipitated. Some ironic comments—'it was their attitude to sex! This was the sixties!' (FC, 9)—right from the beginning suggest as well that there is a subtext to the conventional story told, even though that subtext remains opaque.

The opacity of the couple and their relationship is remarked by other people's and especially their relatives' judgement which time and again serves to mark them as behaving oddly, against all expectations. 'Then the frown appeared on their faces that Harriet dreaded, waiting for it: she knew it masked some comment or thought that could not be voiced' (FC, 73). What was bearable before the arrival of Ben—the couple was often laughed at for making decisions that did not conform to social expectations anymore—has become impossible to cope with now. The overall ironic strategy that Lessing resorts to consists in opposing two moments: the moment preceding Ben's birth, when the whole family disregards the couple's choices in an upfront manner; the moment after Ben's birth, when the whole family disapproves of Harriet's choices but refuses to tell her so. When social expectations were only slightly deviated, it seemed acceptable to express opposing views. Now that the couple's family is beyond social expectations, nothing can be said anymore. Thus, even before Ben, there is a suggestion that Harriet's subjective position may be marginal: 'As far as I'm concerned, you are both rather mad. Well, wrong-headed, then' (FC, 18). Harriet's reactions and attitudes are often treated as unreasonable and illogical. When she imagines that the birth of her sister's daughter with Down's syndrome should be some divine punishment for her sister and her sister's husband's constant bickering ('Sarah and William's unhappiness, their quarrelling, had probably attracted the Mongol child—yes, yes, of course she knew one shouldn't call them mongol' (FC, 29)), David thinks this is 'silly hysterical thinking: Harriet sulked and they had to make up' (FC, 29). Later on, Harriet has retained this epithet as being hers when she asks David for confirmation of what he may think of her: 'Would you say I was an unreasonable woman? Hysterical? Difficult? Just a pathetic hysterical woman?' (FC, 59). The many questions come down to one and the same idea: as woman, Harriet's way of thinking is insensible, volatile and lacks coherence. But one wonders whether Harriet is questioning David here or simply herself: are these questions that she addresses herself in relation to the opacity which she represents for others? She notices how David is pitied and she never is: 'Sometimes, rarely, poor Harriet… More often, irresponsible Harriet, selfish Harriet, crazy Harriet' (FC, 140).

The assumption that Harriet may herself be 'different' certainly seems to guide her apprehension of her most peculiar son, Ben. I do not mean to suggest that the key to understand the novel is to place Ben as the consequence of Harriet's alleged madness, perpetuating thereby a stereotypical vision of mothers as always responsible for their child's ill being. I will not follow in the Winnicottian reading offered by Yelin when she evokes the '(not-)Good enough mother' (Yelin 1998: 92). In order to avoid falling into that condescending view, some critics have over-emphasised Harriet's positive role, saying of her that she 'has matured into a mother willing to take a lonely stand with the child who needs her most' (Raschke 2003: 16). The novel invites us into an uncomfortable zone in which it is unclear whether Ben is afflicted with an illness, or a social condition, or assigned to a place of abnormality that bears no relation whatsoever to reality. Lessing wanted her readers to face that conundrum without clearing it up: 'We don't like things that are complicated, that perhaps there isn't a solution to. And there's no solution to the problem of this book; there's no right way to behave. Maybe people get upset by that. I don't think we like dilemmas. We like to think we can solve everything, but we can't always' (Rothstein 1988). Harriet is constructed as opaque, difficult to read and understand.

Like for Ben, Harriet's oddity is lost in the absence of social or medical diagnosis, which prevents her from being placed. No cause is ever clearly established and Lessing certainly borrows much from her Laingian influence when she describes the medical profession as people whose action stigmatises instead of caring. Harriet's conclusion—'For by now she knew that people understood very well—that is if they weren't experts, doctors' (FC, 110)—draws attention to the defeat of the medical discourse in its alleged position of authority and leaves no room for the readers' interpretations. The vague sensation that the foetus is too active is immediate and this sensation becomes a point of certitude: she never calls him her baby as she does with the others, but 'the being crouched in her womb' (FC, 53). Ben is never perceived as a child, but he comes as the ultimate being in a series that had left Harriet exhausted and unable to cope. For the novel does not focus only on Ben. Right from the beginning Harriet is presented as 'oddball', in a manner that goes well beyond the social inaptitude that she shows and the conservative views she has about marriage and sex. Among the ironic comments of 'chilly contempt' that women of her generation might say of her for being too prudish, the one that stands out, being placed at the end of a list and a paragraph, seems to lay the emphasis on something else that just an attitude or principle: 'it must be something in her childhood that's made her like this. Poor thing' (FC 10). The phrase is redolent of pop-Freudianism, based on the intuition that a symptom is always linked to a trauma in the past but it also indicates a structural subjective position that Harriet is able to relate to: instead of denying the others' judgement or suffering from their lack of comprehension of who she is, Harriet endorses the status of 'misfit', which is how she defines herself: 'She had sometimes felt herself unfortunate or deficient in some way' (FC, 10). This sets her in parallel with Ben, who is also called '*Poor* Ben' (emphasis mine) and treated like a misfit, setting mother and son in a mirror relationship that raises many questions left unanswered in part because Harriet never seeks help or therapy. She suggests Paul should see a psychiatrist, she wants Ben seen but she remains a blind spot of her therapeutic tyranny.

This strong identification to the misfit, which is never negated, leads her to seek perfect conformity to a degree that attracts the attention to a disorder known as transitivism (Maleval 2019: 100–140). As Maleval remarks, many psychiatrists and philosophers have worked on the question of identification, noting that identifications are operative only in as much as they are then dropped. 'The individual is not only threatened by a diffuse and unsteady identity, but also by the rigidity of an identity, sclerosis, in other words by an over-identifying identity' (Kraus 1998 qd in Maleval 2019: 101). In psychoanalytic terms, this means the (partial or total) failure of the symbolic operation, by which a subject is no longer a 'being' but becomes a subject in language and action and is marked by a diffraction of the self's image: either the subject is incapable of forming a sense of enduring identity despite change—in which case, these subjects tend to compensate for that by imitating their peers, often an elected subject whom they copy in style, behaviour and choices—or they conform so much to social identities that they are drained of the possibility of having a sense of self of their own. This vision of the subject's image goes against ego-psychology or the prevalence of the self, which is noted, for example, in Casablancas: the critic sees Harriet's determination to 'embody the established cultural prototype of the mother' as only a 'fantasy' (Casablancas-Cervantes 2010: 2). The reason for this is that Casablancas considers 'mother' as being endowed with an intrinsic positive value. Furthermore, she considers that identification is a process that needs strengthening, which is a way of improving a subject's life, something which Maleval disputes (Maleval 2019: 87). Casablancas highlights the failure of identity construction but she attributes it to the overwhelming presence of subconscious fantasies.

I argue that Harriet is constructed in the text as a subject who fails to build identifications (and not identities). Even the mother that she becomes is an identification that is rigid and stifling and which causes her great pains: for all that can be said about Harriet's alleged conformity, the one domestic queen in the story is in fact Dorothy, while Harriet is gradually seen as wanting to stick to her role as hostess but indeed failing to perform any of the domestic tasks associated with it. It must come as more than a surprise for readers to see that when Harriet's sister has a child with Down's syndrome, Dorothy remains with Harriet, instead of sharing her time between the two daughters, or even dedicating most of it to the disabled child and her family. 'Do you realise that I might just as well be the mother of the others when I'm here?' (FC, 84–85). Harriet's motherly role is an ideal that no longer holds but to which she clings in the symbolic order.

However, Harriet seems to be unclear about her relation to Ben, as if in speaking of him, she was really speaking of herself: 'I'll give you a sedative', he said. For her. But she thought of it as something to quiet the baby.... She begged tranquilizers from friends, and from her sisters' (FC 49). Even though Ben seems to be more of an animal than a human being, he has the characteristics of both, which makes him ambivalent and makes our attempt to classify him inefficient. To Harriet he is 'the nasty little brute' and when she says that she doesn't 'want to kill' him (FC, 67), it is hard not to think that she is in denial. She alternates between wanting his death and attempting to see him as a fragile baby she could cuddle: 'A little child, ... our child' (FC, 90). The readers' impression is that Ben is never quite where he is expected to be: 'Ben... stood watching them, in his usual position, which was apart from everyone else' (FC, 89). Throughout the novel, the description of his physical restlessness and prowess makes us picture Ben as much older than what he is. When it is time for him to go to school, the reader may have had the impression that Ben was already a teenager. Before the age of 6, Ben has already been institutionalised and brought home; he has killed a dog (FC, 84), and frightened the family; and despite being the last child, he does not occupy the 'baby's room' (FC, 115), where he belongs; on top of everything else, Harriet leaves him to a group of young delinquents with whom he spends all his days until he starts school. The narration hammers home the point that Ben is not the fifth child, but the odd child out, which Luke summarises when he says: 'They're sending Ben away because he isn't really one of us' (FC, 93), recalling the 1932 *Freaks* film phrase in which a number of misfits commune, whereas the family here refuse to welcome Ben in.

This 'misfit' nature of Ben recalls Harriet's in the sense that it is difficult to specify it outside social considerations and the text's assertiveness that treats it like a point of certitude that suffers no argumentation. For if one looks closely at the diagnostic signs of his difference, what one notices is that Ben is not completely inadequate: he is capable of learning many skills that are said to be social: he is not physically disabled, can eat on his own, he learns at school in a way that does not worry the teachers too much, and when he leaves for the day with the group of boys, Harriet never worries about his well-being. She notes it at some point: 'He did know a lot of things that made him into a part-social being' (FC, 117). After he returns from the institution he had been sent to, a similar behavioural remark is expressed: 'He had unlearned all the basic social skills that it had been so hard to teach him' (FC, 108). While Sarah's daughter is called the 'defective child' (FC, 34), Ben is never named in his difference. Yet his presence makes the whole group crumble: the other children have to lock themselves in their room at night, they soon decide to leave for boarding schools and David sometimes sleeps over in London; the house that was excessively filled and big in the beginning has become an empty space that only marginal people can strive on, which cannot be interpreted but in social terms as a pessimistic vision of the future of society after the oppressive politics of the right with its excessive trust in the ideal of family life brings about individual demise. Lessing's interest in the dynamics of the group and the various fractures that threaten its cohesion is rooted in her own experience of life as a colonial in Rhodesia and she explored this as early as in *Martha Quest*:

> And each group, community, clan, colour, strove and fought away from the other, in a sickness of dissolution; it was as if the principle of separateness was bred from the very soil, the sky, the driving sun; as if the inchoate vastness of the universe, always insistent in the enormous unshrouded skies,... bred a fever of self-assertion in its children like a band of explorers lost in a desert, quarrelling in an ecstasy of fear over their direction, when nothing but a sober mutual trust could save them. (Lessing 1952: 61)

After Ben has been seen as violent and crying, the trust referred to here is out of the window and Harriet is held responsible by everyone for bringing him back from the hospital without being able to tame him. Harriet's certitude that her son is not normal fails to be acknowledged by the others. When she asks them '*What* is he?' (FC, 66), all she gets as an answer is silence. David's rejection, often quoted, is a gregarious reply that leaves Ben's essence unnamed: 'He may be normal for what he is. But he is not normal for what we are' (FC, 79). Lessing's technique of raising questions that are impossible to answer is here blatant.

Harriet never stops trying to interpret that 'extraordinary' creature, refusing to let him go and 'be murdered' (FC, 140) while admitting to her 'repugnance' at having to look after him. The teacher who first sees Harriet about Ben is benevolent and kind, and suggests that he might be 'hyperactive, perhaps' (FC, 121), adding 'of course this is a word that I often feel evades the issue'. Yet, this diagnosis fails to convince because it places the emphasis again on questions of behaviour when Harriet feels the roots of his problems are far deeper, finding no one to lay at rest her fear that he may not even be human and is more connected to other forms of life. 'And as Harriet left, she saw how the headmistress watched her, with that long troubled inspection that held unacknowledged unease, even horror, which was part of "the other conversation"—the real one' (FC, 121). This 'real' conversation that never occurs guides us towards the *jouissance* identified by Lacan as the rest resulting from the operations of language and the imaginary, two dimensions that in Harriet and Ben's relationships fail to be given an efficient function in order to protect them from the surfacing of the real.

THE BODY, APPETITE AND JOUISSANCE

The idea that the 'other conversation' is happening not in what is said but in the saying—the word 'unacknowledged' together with the concept of 'other' cannot but evoke psychoanalytic theory—is quite revelatory of Lessing's writing technique in this novella. She operates a shift from the frontal confrontation in keeping with political engagement that was central to her first writings, by stressing the role played by dialogue in the naturalistic representation of human relations in *The Golden Notebook* (Danziger 1996: 74). This almost disappears in *The Fifth Child*, which is mediated by the voice of a narrator who has two roles: first, they keep a certain distance vis-à-vis the situation, which makes the horror of certain scenes, such as the ones when Harriet goes to the institution where Ben is secluded, bearable; second, they mediate Harriet's story, preventing the reader from identification or empathy. This enables Lessing to point out the logical place of Harriet's symptomatic forms of excess in relation to her uncontrolled access to a real which is never acknowledged and precipitates her downfall. The real is not an 'underlying reality' waiting to be discovered—to say it with other critics (Danziger 1996: 3)—but something which is here all the time and which needs to be tamed lest it becomes overwhelming and threatening, two epithets that could work well for Ben. Ben comes at the very place where Harriet would like the unbridled *jouissance* that overwhelms her named, and therefore lost. His existence as she perceives it makes him an obstacle to her own excess: his arrival empties the house in the same way that she had tried to keep it filled to the brim before. Although she brings him back from his place of seclusion, she makes sure he is away most of the time.

Her subjective solution consists in identifying fully to Ben's lack of place or marginality, thereby enacting her own misfit position. 'Now he was locked into his room each night, and there was heavy bars on the door as well. Every second of his waking hour, he watched. Harriet watched him while her mother managed everything else' (FC, 78). The apparatus—pinpointing Ben, watching him while he watches—assigns Ben to a place of contemplation suggestive of wonder and puzzlement. One should almost say that it is very important that Ben should not be designated as something else than the other who accounts for Harriet's own otherness. 'Harriet sat waiting—as she had done, it seemed to her, far too often in Ben's short life—for some kind of acknowledgement that here might be more than a difficulty of adjustment' (FC, 120). Thus, unlike in other works studied so far, the failure of the medical discourse should not fool readers into believing that Harriet's despair only comes from other people's refusal to categorise Ben. It would be fairly hypocritical to regard the medical profession, which is often criticised for doing the exact opposite and pathologising excessively, as this time round being excessively non-normative. Harriet's idea about Ben's origins, translated by Dr Gilly as 'a throwback' (FC, 127), seeking to embrace the notions that he might be from another world, another planet, not human and so forth, reflects her incapacity to name Ben's difference and perhaps also the logical place of uncertainty where she wants him to be. The failure of the medical discourse to cater to her needs, 'I want it *said*. I want it recognized. I just can't stand it never being said' (FC, 127), invites us to think about the symbolic function Ben has for Harriet: she seems to hold on to the labelling and naming of her son's condition as a solution to her puzzlement. Her certitude makes her interpret every person's reaction as an unnamed admission of his abnormality, but she is not happy with any attempt made to name him either.

Thus, we may come back to Harriet before Ben, since so much of the novel's critical reception is based on her with him. 'Harriet's emotions … control her response to the child, are all embracing, but are also perhaps merely idiosyncratic' (Robbins 2009: 98–99). In that respect, it might be worthwhile to note that the number five is often a symbol of dislocation and dissolution in Lessing's fiction, making Ben an operative symbol too: 'He held her hair close around her throat, so that it slightly choked her, and said that she would marry a good city father and become very respectable and have five nice, well-brought-up children' (Lessing 1952: 242). Her initial introduction is not unrelated to some emotional state that is difficult to describe and perhaps impossible to apprehend without experiencing it: 'Both had reflected that the faces of the dancers, women more than men, but men too, could just as well have been distorted in screams and grimaces of pain as in enjoyment' (FC, 8). One is immediately reminded of the statue 'The Ecstasy of St. Teresa' by Bernini as described by Lacan to illustrate the mixture of pleasure, pain and all sorts of excessive passions that *jouissance* provokes (Lacan 1975: 70–71). Many characters indeed tend to feel horror at other people's bodies and repugnance: 'The trouble was that he was distressed by physical disability; and his new daughter, the Down's syndrome baby, appalled him. Yet he was very much married to Sarah' (FC, 32). Other people's bodies are therefore presented as essentially causing wonder and bafflement. The veil of propriety is expected to keep it away from view but Lessing's text discloses and forces us to see the solutions that need to be found when this is exposed.

Harriet's own body is marked by similar aspects that could cause feelings of disgust in others: 'Her appetite was enormous, insatiable—so bad she was ashamed and raided the fridge when no one could see her' (FC, 54). The presence of Ben within is almost as painful to her as his presence without: her apprehension of her body during the pregnancy is in keeping with her later role as mother without the signifier of her *jouissance*: 'Her whole body energetically denying the pain' (FC 51). And yet, it would be reductive to attribute this to Ben only, because right from the beginning, there are indications that Harriet's pregnancies cause her a kind of mingled excitement and horror that she is not more articulate about than the doctors are about her son: if 'this pregnancy, like the other one, was normal' (FC, 25), she says as if to reassure herself, because they are all marked by a body that changes into an outpouring of fluids and excessive consumption of food; she feels sick and tired and starts thinking that she'll need more than three months between various pregnancies. With Ben, her bodily experience manifests in the fact that she requests to give birth in hospital, against her doctor's and husband's advice. Besides, the manifestations of her body become unacceptable for others: 'Her husband and her mother knew she was being sick. Which they were used to. But they were not used to ill-temper, tears, fretfulness' (FC, 44). Through her pregnancies, she experiences this excess which is both painful and enjoyable and to which she allows herself to be subjected: 'The creature with whom she was locked in a struggle to survive' (FC, 53). Most of Harriet's choices come to a subjective structure that ensures she is entrapped with an unnamable other: the other of family ties; the other children, Ben as the other, the maternal other, even David and so forth. It is no wonder that she should have been extra careful before not to encounter such aspect of life, when she refused to play by the rules of sexual liberation: the men would 'take her refusal as much as evidence of a pathological outlook as an ungenerous one' (FC, 10). Couples, like other relationships, are very problematic.

One of Lessing's feminist objects is her exploration of singular responses to women's condition, which she envisages through activism (e.g. through Martha Quest and Alice Melling), through women's gender roles but more importantly perhaps through women's experience of motherhood. Birth, giving birth and being born are terms that Lessing gives us graphic descriptions of in her fiction, and which serves as a mode of exploration of *jouissance*, in the sense of that rest of the linguistic operation which is unnamable and ungraspable, and therefore even more terrifying for that very reason:

> Then there were those who said it was the birth itself which set Martha on a fated road. It was during the long night of terror, the night of the difficult birth, when the womb of Mrs Quest convulsed and fought to expel its burden through the unwilling gates of bone (for Mrs Quest was rather old to bear a first child), it was during that birth, from which Martha emerged shocked and weary, her face temporarily scarred purple from the forceps, that her character and therefore her life were determined for her. (Lessing 1952: 13)

As early as in 1952, Lessing connects birth with the 'fate' of her character, but she focuses on the child's destiny and their inability to cope with what is presented as an original trauma, beyond words and signification. Robbins recalls the fact that 'birth itself is figured as a monstrosity' in Yeats's poem 'The Second Coming' (Robbins 2009: 93) in order to evoke why structurally this aspect is repressed, to ensure that women may still want to bear children. In *The Fifth Child*, I argue that the focus is shifted to the mother or 'the mother/child story' which offers a corrective vision that modifies the cultural ideal (Robbins 2009: 95). The sequel, *Ben, in the World*, is almost like a hackneyed sequel that reveals the absence of attention Ben receives in the first novel, contributing to the opacity of his being and of his mother's reaction. Surprisingly, the five births are almost skipped by the narrator, despite the suggestion that Harriet's was not made for easy births: 'It goes without saying that the doctor had wanted Harriet in hospital' (FC, 24). In the middle of a scene described as perfect—everyone weeping with joy—this negated phrase seems to infer that there were causes for worry. In 1966, there were still 25% of home births in England.[3] Is Lessing commenting on Dr Brett's medical outlook or Harriet's condition? For Harriet is said to be '*bone* tired', 'indeed worn-out' (FC, 27), something which is not explored fully but sill expressed. Jane's birth is not even commented upon, in 1970, as if birth itself did not account for Harriet's mood swings. 'The fourth baby, Paul, was born in 1973, between a Christmas and an Easter. Harriet was not very well: her pregnancies had continued uncomfortable and full of minor problems—nothing serious, but she was tired' (FC, 30). Interestingly, these are noted by the narrator but not developed and they do not converge into a community of experience. Dorothy, whose name suggests a divine presence, Molly, whose name is 'pet form of Mary, the archetypal Christian Mother' (De Vinne: 17), Sarah and other members of the family are mothers but Harriet is the only one who seems to go through these births feeling exhausted and yet incapable of stopping them: there is an excess that she is not capable of voicing, articulating, comprehending, sharing and which drives her to a place where Ben, in all his difference, comes to stand for the supreme disorder of her life.

[3] https://www.ons.gov.uk/peoplepopulationandcommunity/birthsdeathsandmarriages/livebirths/bulletins/birthcharacteristicsinenglandandwales/2017#home-births-more-likely-among-women-after-having-their-first-child

Hence, her aggressive feelings and her reliance on the most esoteric causes to account for a reality that no discourse seems able to name. Commentators of the novel have looked into the possible origins of Harriet's theories concerning her child, which range from a genetic problem to an extraterrestrial being she would have given birth to. The logic of all these explanations remains the same: she names the extraordinary and odd nature of her son because science has no name for it. The proliferation of metonymic significations is directly linked to the obstinate absence of terms, medical or otherwise, that would encapsulate her experience of him. There is a difference between what he is—her first question—and what his existence does to her. She is said to be 'longing for him to say something else. What? *An explanation*' (FC, 46), but going to see Dr Brett had always, instinctively, seemed to be 'beside the point' (FC, 47). The only patient in the story is Harriet. Not simply because of the patriarchal system that assigns women to a certain place where they cannot stop short of representing the ideal of motherhood. This is certainly seen at play in her encounters with Dr Brett, but she insults him behind his back— 'You bad-tempered *cow*' (FC, 46)—which shows that she is barely subjected to this patriarchal system. What is more interesting is how this 'creature' in her body triggers off a reaction that is outside the symbolic system, irretrievable in language. She experiences the excessive enjoyment produced by the foetus, who unrealistically 'demands' something from her in the first weeks of the pregnancy, because she becomes subjected to the demands of her own body which, like the house, is emptied.

CONCLUSION

As pointed out in the beginning, this novel contains very few characteristics of Lessing's writing: it is very short, contains few dialogues, does not have any science-fiction or social-realist features (Maslen 1994: 1), and it is not even part of a long series of books, like most of her earlier fictions. In accordance with Harriet's own emptiness, the book is empty of the traditional literary features that the first pages invite the readers to imagine. The romance that the book starts with soon finishes; the stereotypical gender roles are never really criticised or changed; the family itself seems to be the point of interest and yet, one finds oneself at a loss as to characterise the other children, save Paul who, again, is defined by his own deficiency—David insists that he be seen by a psychiatrist to great effect (FC, 330), a solution that surprisingly is never considered for Ben, or Harriet.

All in all, most themes come down to a very basic storyline and like the trajectory of this family suddenly coming to a halt because of Ben's arrival, the fictional story-line seems to be stopped in its development: 'The literary experience of maternity, whether as glory or as abjection—and more likely a mixture of the two—is filled... with generic instability' (Robbins 2009: 9).

The house (of fiction) is thus progressively emptied, making readers and characters lose their bearings. There are at least two episodes of sheer horror in the novel: one is the description of the institution Ben was sent to (FC, 94–101); the other is the description of the riots in England when Ben is thought to partake of the acts of violence (FC, 148–154). In the first case, Lessing is sure to have been inspired by Laing, and the many accounts of such institutional violence made public by Mary Barnes, Jennifer Dawson, Janet Frame, Sylvia Plath and others throughout the 1960s and 1970s (see Baker et al. 2010). And yet, it can be argued that she almost pays lip service to such a tradition and uses the horrific vision not as a traumatic event for Ben—even if for a while Harriet tries to manoeuvre him by evoking the institution he could return to—because the episode stands on its own and is not developed into something new. In the second episode, the riots are only referred to, enough to give readers a sense of looming danger and potential disruption, but fairly disconnected from the political engagement of Lessing's previous texts and the precise exploration of political action such as what she had done in *The Good Terrorist*, the year before, for example.

The novel ends with Harriet's futuristic vision of the outcome of Ben's life, seeing him as 'searching the faces in the crowd for another of his own kind' (FC, 159), lost in fact in the relentless question that she could never find a solution to: what is he? Which she translates as, where does he belong? When Harriet explains that they are going to sell the house and Ben shows no sign that he will regret it, she wonders: 'was his identification with this gang of his now so great that he did not think of this as his home?' (FC, 153), revealing that identification is Ben's only chance of survival but also explaining why the house is now redundant, perhaps as redundant as literature itself. Some critics have seen in Lessing's rejection of her traditional narrative modes a sign that she wanted to strip her text of any emotional empathy: 'It could well be the case that we are asked to read the novel with the same lack of emotional affect with which Ben... experiences his world or in the same way as his mother experiences her relationship with him' (Robbins 2009: 96). It is certainly true that none of the ideals of gender, maternity and family life are saved or preserved and everything is presented as based on emptiness (Robbins 2009: 104).

More crucial perhaps is the absence of epiphany-like passages, such as the ones that happened in her earlier fiction (see Lessing 1952: 68 for an example), which likened her work to Woolf's Modernism: this is the sign that the evolution of mental symptoms throughout the twentieth century calls for a reconfiguration of the articulation of experience. What was once regarded as deviation, an extraordinary manifestation in which truth emerged from the chaos of the world and could be shaped back into something meaningful, no longer holds as a promise for future stability. With Lessing's *The Fifth Child*, literature has ventured into the chaotic, meaningless situation of an experience that cannot be communicated because it is outside communication: thus, silence has become the discreet sign of the absence of relationship with others, which this story illustrates. The whole novel is based upon the excessive nature of a desire that cannot be named, even in its most horror-inspiring version, namely a child who is so odd that he defies all knowledge. Lessing's invention of this absence of communication central to the relationship between mother and son, with an Other that barely speaks, constitutes a shift in the location of the subject's crisis from the Modernist moment, but remains Woolfian in her taste for storytelling as a way of articulating something of the experience all the same.

BIBLIOGRAPHY

Secondary Sources

Baker, Charley, Crawford, Paul et al. (2010). *Madness in Post-1945 British and American Fiction*. London: Routledge.

Berets, Ralph (1980). "A Jungian Interpretation of the Dream Sequence in Doris Lessing's *The Summer Before Dark*". *Modern Fiction Studies*, vol. 26, No.1, Spring 1980, 117–130.

Brevet, Anne-Laure (2011). "'The shadow of the fifth': Patterns of Exclusion in Doris Lessing's *The Fifth Child*". *La Clé des Langues, Lyon, ENS Lyon, DGESCO (ISSN 2107–7029), December 2011. Last 27/04/2022.* http://cle.ens-lyon.fr/anglais/litterature/litterature-britannique/the-shadow-of-the-fifth-patterns-of-exclusion-in-doris-lessing-s-the-fifth-child

Brock, Richard (2009). "'No Such Thing as Society': Thatcherism and Derridean Hospitality in *The Fifth Child*." *Doris Lessing Studies*, vol. 28, No. 1, 7–13.

Casablancas-Cervantes, Anna (2010). "Creating Oneself as a Mother: Dreams, Reality and Identity in Doris Lessing's *The Fifth Child*." *Forum*, Issue 11, Autumn 2010. http://journals.ed.ac.uk/forum/article/view/653/937

Danziger, Marie A. (1996). *Text/Countertext, Postmodern Paranoia in Samuel Beckett, Doris Lessing, and Philip Roth.* New York: Peter Lang.

De Vinne, Christine (2012). "The Uncanny Unnamable in Doris Lessing's *The Fifth Child* and *Ben, in the World*". *Names*, vol. 60, No. 1, March 2012, 15–25.

Freud, Sigmund (1899–1930). *The Interpretation of Dreams.* trans. J.-P. Lefebvre. Paris: Seuil, 'Essais', 2010.

Freud, Sigmund (1919). *L'Inquiétante étrangeté et autres essais.* Paris: Gallimard, 1985.

Herman, Judith Lewis (1992). *Trauma and Recovery, From Domestic Abuse to Political Terror.* London: Pandora, 2015.

Hilson, Mica (2012). "'The Odd Man out in the Family?' Queer Throwbacks and Reproductive Futurism." *Doris Lessing Studies*, vol. 30, No. 1, 18–22.

Hsieh, Meng-Tsung (2010). "Almost Human but Not Quite?: The Impenetrability of Being in Doris Lessing's *Ben, In the World*." *Doris Lessing Studies*, vol. 29, No.1, 14–19.

Innes, Catherine L. (2007). *The Cambridge Introduction to Postcolonial Literatures in English.* Cambridge: Cambridge University Press.

Knapp, Mona (1984). *Doris Lessing.* New York: Frederick Ungar Publishing Co.

Lacan, Jacques (1966). "Le Stade du Miroir comme formateur de la fonction du Je telle qu'elle nous est révélée dans l'expérience psychanalytique" (1949). *Écrits* I. Paris: Éditions du Seuil, "Essais Points", 1999, 92–99.

Lacan, Jacques (1975). *Le Séminaire, Livre XX, Encore* (1972–73). J.-A. Miller (ed.). Paris: Éditions du Seuil.

Lessing, Doris (1952). Martha's Quest. New York: HarperPerennial, 2001. Part of the *Children of Violence* series (1952–1969).

Maleval, Jean-Claude (2019). *Repères pour la psychose ordinaire.* Paris: Navarin Éditeurs, 2019.

Maslen, Elizabeth (1994). *Doris Lessing: Writers and their Work.* Plymouth, UK: Northcote House.

May, William (2010). *Postwar Literature 1950–1990,* London: York Press.

Rahimnouri, Zahra & Ghandehariun, Azra (2020). "A Feminist Stylistic Analysis of Doris Lessing's *The Fifth Child* (1988)". *Journal of Language and Literature*, vol. 20, No. 2, 221–230.

Raman, Ratna (2021). *The Fiction of Doris Lessing: Re-envisioning Feminism.* London: Bloomsbury.

Raschke, Debrah (2003). "*The Fifth Child*: From Fairy-Tale to Monstrosity." *Doris Lessing Studies*, Vol. 23, No 1.

Ridout, Alice & Watkins, Susan (eds.) (2009), *Doris Lessing, Border Crossings.* London: Continuum. https://doi.org/10.5040/9781472542403

Rigney, Barbara Hill (1978). *Madness and Sexual Politics in the Feminist Novel, Studies of Brontë, Woolf, Lessing and Atwood*. Madison, USA: the University of Wisconsin Press.

Robbins, Ruth (2009). "(Not Such) Great Expectations: Unmaking Maternal Ideals in *The Fifth Child* and *We Need to Talk about Kevin*". A. Ridout and S. Watkins (eds.), 92–106.

Rothstein, Mervyn (1988). "The Painful Nurturing of Doris Lessing's *Fifth Child*." in *The New York Times*, https://archive.nytimes.com/www.nytimes.com/books/99/01/10/specials/lessing-child.html?_r=1

Rubenstein, Roberta (2009). "Doris Lessing's Fantastic Children". A. Ridout & S. Watkins (eds.), 61–74.

Rundgren, Heta (2016). "Vers une théorie du roman postnormâle: Féminisme, réalisme et conflit sexuel chez Doris Lessing, Märta Tikkanen, Stieg Larsonn et Virginie Despentes". unpublished PhD thesis Paris 8, France and Helsinki, Finland.

Saiful, Islam Muhammad (2013). "Anticipating Apocalypse: Power Structures and the Periphery in Doris Lessing's *The Fifth Child* and *Ben, in the World*". *Romanian Journal of English Studies*, 278–292, doi: https://doi.org/10.2478/rjes-2013-0027

Scanlan, Margaret (2001). *Plotting Terror, Novelists and Terrorists in Contemporary Fiction*. Charlottesville: The UP of Virginia.

Schlueter, Paul (1973). *The Novels of Doris Lessing*. Carbondale: The Southern Illinois UP.

Showalter, Elaine (1977). *A Literature of their Own, British Women Novelists from Brontë to Lessing*. London: Virago Press, 1982.

Showalter, Elaine (1985). *The Female Malady, Women, Madness and English Culture, 1830–1980*. London: Virago Press.

Wall, Oisin (2018). *The British Anti-Psychiatrists, from institutional Psychiatry to Counter-Culture, 1960–1971*. London: Routledge.

Yelin, Louise (1998). "Reading Doris Lessing with Margaret Thatcher: *The Good Terrorist*, *The Fifth Child*, and England in the 1980s." Yelin, Louise (1998). *From the Margins of Empire, Stead, Lessing and Gordimer*, Cornell University Press, 91–107.

CHAPTER 6

AIDS, Manic-Depression and the Symptoms of the 1980s in *The Line of Beauty*

The Line of Beauty, Alan Hollinghurst's 2005 Booker Prize–winning 'masterpiece' (Mathuray 2017: 1), seems to be a far cry from the influence of *Mrs Dalloway* and Modernist representations of madness. Its connection to Doris Lessing's *The Fifth Child* is perhaps even more puzzling. All things considered, the theme of madness has never been discussed in academic publications and reviews of the novel, despite the presence of a character diagnosed with bipolar symptoms, who becomes the agent of the story's closure when she reveals to the press that Gerald, her father and an ambitious Conservative MP, is having an affair with his secretary and that he houses a gay man whose promiscuity is an embarrassing revelation concerning his private life, given that he wishes to be in the limelight as one of the best representatives of Thatcher's Conservative views. The reason for the relative neglect of Catherine is that the main story is about Nick Guest, a self-confessed aesthete who becomes a lodger in the London family home of an Oxford friend soon after their graduation. There, over the course of the Thatcher years (1983–1989), 20-something Nick discovers the idle life of the well-off, notwithstanding the subdivisions between the aristocratic stock of Rachel Fedden's family—whose members are lords and ladies with country mansions and art hanging on the walls—and the *nouveaux riches* of Wani's family, as well as gay love and sex. Nick spends his time claiming to write a PhD on the style of Henry James, but

© The Author(s), under exclusive license to Springer Nature Switzerland AG 2023

N. P. Boileau, *Mental Health Symptoms in Literature since Modernism*, Palgrave Studies in Literature, Science and Medicine, https://doi.org/10.1007/978-3-031-37630-6_6

at the end of the decade and the novel, his accomplishments consist in editing the issue of an art magazine only made sustainable thanks to his friend's fortune, *Ogee*, and probably destined to remain the one and only issue. What adumbrates this, however, is Nick's name, placing him forever in the position of marginality to the family and to the world of fiction. This is a point of connection with Catherine, together with their sexual lives. For Nick's greatest success is the long series of one-night stands and boyfriends, which, at the beginning of the novel, Nick presented as an achievement in itself when reviewing the love life of Catherine, the daughter of the family. 'Nick ... felt a certain respect for her experience with men: to have so many failures required a high rate of preliminary success' (TLB, 8). Catherine's attractive power impresses Nick because his definition of romance at that stage is first and foremost intercourse, as suggested in his use of private ads to meet wannabe sex partners.

Yet, Nick's passion for James, which mirrors Hollinghurst's self-confessed interest (2004, 2004b; Terzian 2011: 1), explains why many critics have so far read the novel in the light of its influences and its place within the British canon (Hannah 2007: 87–90; Johnson 2014: 11; Rivkin 2005). When readings do not focus on queer theory and the question of gay writing (Yeager 2013), which surprisingly are not the most numerous by far, they are still indebted to Hollinghurst's reputation for 'finely-wrought sentences, the elegance and precision of his narrative, the subtle rendering of interiority and the impeccably measured mimesis of apprehension and understanding, his arrangement of sophisticated dialogue, and so on' (Mathuray 2017: 2). As a result, most academic articles focus on the aesthetic questions of beauty and the meaningful associations of the line metaphor in the novel (Su 2014; Kim 2016): the line is that of cocaine, of aesthetic contemplation, of the legacy of class, knowledge and power, amongst other fruitful images. Other critics are interested in the vision of history the novel offers, in particular the representation of the Thatcher years (Su 2014; Gutleben 2015). Although Roberts's essay on *The Line of Beauty* delves into the critical conundrum of excavating 'influences' which 'run[s] the risk of twisting the novel into a mere exercise in metafictional game playing' (Roberts 2017: 111), a risk typical of the study of postmodern fiction further on described as having the novel 'fall into a grid as "an historical novel of 1980s Britain", or "political novel"' (Roberts 2017: 126), many essays focus on the metafictional and metatextual echoes in the novel, in what seems to be an attempt at placing the novel within a tradition and smoothing out another blatant feature of Hollinghurst's writing, namely, the presence of many graphic sex scenes (Letissier 2007, 2019; Johnson 2014). Inevitably perhaps, but still, Woolf and *Mrs Dalloway* are quoted, first because 'substantial collections of Proust, Woolf, Nabokov and Waugh' are to be found on Hollinghurst's library shelves (Terzian 2011: 1); but perhaps more convincingly because of the themes explored by both authors: 'It is not difficult to be reminded of Virginia Woolf's *Mrs Dalloway* (1925a, 1925b) as the family of a Conservative MP continue to worry and wait for the arrival of an important figure of state in *The Line of Beauty*' (Johnson 2014: 13). Although the reference is here reductive for both works because it focuses on the story more than on the writing, I think *Mrs Dalloway* may still be used as a point of reference because of the structure of the work: there is a similar interest in both novels for the ruling political class and the looming presence of those that are assigned outside of power: the gay, the mad, the ill, the poor and so forth. These people are tolerated until they pose a threat, while the world of fiction revels in their presence and representation to suggest ways in which they find their solution to a world that is hostile to their presence.

However, one cannot start discussing illness in the novel without first giving pride of place to the major health issue touched upon in *The Line of Beauty*, which is the 1980s AIDS epidemic within the gay community, a fact made evident by the chosen context, the gay men's lifestyles explored in the novel, and the fact that two of Nick's lovers—Leo and Wani—eventually die of the illness/syndrome. At the end of the novel, Nick is contemplating the prospect that after all these years his HIV test, this time round, will be positive (TLB, 500). And yet, some have noted that in spite of being overtly gay in its themes, Hollinghurst's fiction barely places AIDS as a central preoccupation, even in the one novel which focuses on the decade of the epidemic: up until the end, Nick remains immune to the illness which he does not seem to worry about or take many precautions against. If Hollinghurst wrote an MA thesis on 'the creative uses of Homosexuality in the novels of Forster, Firbank and Hartley' (Terzian 2011: 9), he confesses to having had trouble finding the right time and the right format to question AIDS: 'I also wanted to write about AIDS at last, not as something that dictated the architecture of the whole novel, but as an element in a larger historical picture' (Terzian 2011: 18). Taking his distance from the 'historical novel' that presided over the 1990s (Bernard 2018), Hollinghurst states: 'I never do research. I don't like it, really, and I mistrust its prevalence in contemporary fiction. It often so clearly flags itself as research in the finished product. I think imagination is much more important than information' (Terzian 2011: 20).

This echoes the work done by Pat Barker in the *Regeneration* trilogy because the novels' intermingling of facts and fiction has been hailed as one of the few successful contributions to the function of fiction as a mediator of truth which, thanks to her work, can be regarded as achieving what historical facts alone cannot. Hollinghurst's 'homosexualisation of the novel' (Hollinghurst 2006: 15, qtd in Letissier 2007: 199) is both blatant—if only in the graphic sex scenes and slang sex terms used throughout his novels and in particular in *The Line of Beauty*—and complex: Letissier argues that it fails in many ways because of the persistence of strict and long-lasting structural, fictional elements of the British (straight) tradition: 'Hollinghurst hardly breaks new technical ground in the realm of novel-writing… [His style] re-instates psychology, where Firbank did not go beyond mood and sensation' (Letissier 2007: 210). Alderson also shares the vision that the gay theme hardly leads to queer fiction (Alderson 2017: 138). One way of specifying what Hollinghurst does that is new in writing is precisely to avert the eyes away from the most blatant themes and plunge into the symptomatic formations of Catherine, which rubs off on Nick and his boyfriends.

In this chapter, I intend to look at a secondary character, Catherine Fedden, who, like Septimus, functions both as a character in her own right and as the revelatory agent of a psychotic subjectivity that pervades in all the other characters. Her handling of her manic-depressive symptoms offers a counterpoint to the way homosexual disease, as AIDS was then often called, is approached in the novel. Where gay characters are given no respite or comfort and die in almost generalised oblivion, Catherine's comfortable home alienates her to her symptoms, forcing her to live on despite causing much more havoc than promiscuous gay men. My focus on Catherine enables me to uncover the symptomatic subjective appropriation of a body that is libidinal and agitated by uncontrollable drives, before we look at Catherine's own failure to construct a solid knot from which she could function as a social being in the world, something which the protection of money conceals in her case while, symmetrically, it is shown as inefficient in Wani's case. Throughout the chapter, it will be necessary to carefully distinguish between the effect of an organic disease and the symptoms of a psychic illness, and therefore keep away from the neurological hypothesis that psychic diseases are also somatic. The symmetry between Wani and Catherine has been noted by others, such as

Hannah who thinks they form with Nick a community of marginal guests: 'Wani, as the son of a Lebanese immigrant, and Catherine, as the daughter of an obliquely misogynistic Tory, are, like Nick, privileged guests, in the social world of their peers' (Hannah 2007: 89). However, I think the very mode in which they comply with their place as, or function as, marginal beings need to be studied carefully. The symptoms they complain about are the way into understanding how they handle their condition as subjects. Thus, we are first going to look at Catherine's liminal or marginal place within the social context of the novel, before looking at the function of the subject's body when stripped of its meaningful attachments in order to finally see if Catherine is an example of a solid use of symptoms or rather the symptom of a psychiatric institution that trusts in medication to the point of obliterating the subjective experience.

Social Understanding of Illness: Inside, Outside, Marginal

As with all the novels discussed in this book, the most obvious storyline of Hollinghurst's *The Line of Beauty* is the exploration of social classes in Britain. To a certain extent, the novel owes much to the comedy of manners of Forster's and the heritage films by Ivory (referred to TLB, 486). In particular, the extensive use of dialogue with humorous, when not simply satirical, narratorial observations, reminds us of Austen and Forster's ironic narrative voices. One example of this is when Sophie, Toby's girlfriend, realises her boyfriend took her to the wrong place to buy a wedding ring: '"I knew we wouldn't find my ring," said Sophie, with the crossness that hides a sweetness that hides a softness' (TLB, 114). Such an aspect of Hollinghurst's novelistic strategy came to full fruition in *The Stranger's Child*, his following novel, in which each remark uttered is the object of the narrator's mocking comment. The social comedy of *The Line of Beauty* is predetermined by the structure of the plot: the story has to do with the presence of an outsider within and unfolds according to the subsequent questions posed by making sure there is a difference between what is private and what is public, what is inside and outside, what is acceptable or not and so forth. The lodger of the house is given too much place in a world where he does not belong, despite naively feeling 'in possession' or 'in charge' on many occasions—as he remains in charge of the focalisation despite Hollinghurst's choice of an external narrative voice.

Nick feels at home throughout the novel, in spite of being often rebuked by everyone else but the Feddens and even when it becomes clear that he has outstayed his welcome: 'Trembling with the contagion of madness Nick said the thing he'd come to say, but in a tone of cheap sarcasm he'd never intended to use: "Well, you'll be devastated to hear that I'm moving out of the house today. I just dropped in to tell you."/And Gerald, furiously pretending not to have heard, said, "I want you out of the house today"' (TLB, 482).

The novel offers itself as a string of social embarrassment and mishaps: Nick allows himself to be invited to birthday and political parties, private and more public affairs, the French holiday home and so on, even when it seems clear to the readers the invitations he received are perfunctory. The social comedy is enhanced by the plot's setting, which is extremely homogeneous in time and place, adding some theatricality to the events taking place, with recurring characters sketched as social types. The neighbourhood of the house is barely ever left, only to visit similar estates in the countryside or in France or to go to nearby pubs and cruising places, where middle-class life might be glimpsed at, but never fully embraced. However, that situation is made modern by the strong influence of the 1980s' Zeitgeist which Thatcher's politics, money worshipping and drug abuse represent: 'What also exonerates *The Line of Beauty* from Brannigan's elegiac suspicion is its contextual and referential emphasis on the reality of gay life and political intrigue in the 1980s' (Gutleben 2015: 4). Thatcher herself will be one of the 'Guest[s]' in the novel, a fictional character who enables Nick to shine fleetingly when he invites her to dance (TLB, 383–85). There are moments when the novel dwells on Nick's own ambiguity regarding class, turning the novel into a coming-of-age story which sees him reject and re-embrace class divisions: Nick's lover, Leo, is lower class and Nick feels ashamed of him, while Wani is an outrageously rich hero who looks down on Nick. Furthermore, Nick's family is treated as secondary to his social climbing process: he sees them as parochial, respectable but slightly conservative, and his ambivalence towards them is revealed when Gerald Fedden meets them on his tour to be re-elected. Throughout the novel therefore, Hollinghurst raises the question of the visibility of those who do not belong in a specific class and questions social mobility by setting it in parallel with another aspect of identity, gay-ness, which, in the 1980s, is both made visible by the AIDS epidemic and the recent decriminalisation of homosexuality, and invisibilised as a social fact: '*The Line of Beauty* seek[s] to map out alternative understandings of public membership, foregrounding heteronormative deployments of a rhetoric of repression and exposure in the monitoring of queer private lives on the public stage' (Hannah 2007: 73).[1]

Within this strong structural subtext, Catherine's place duplicates the questions raised by those that are marginal to the social norms of the 1980s but from the angle of behavioural symptoms that she inscribes on her body, and which are monitored by the family through medication. She indeed offers an example of the visible daughter that the family wants unseen, the feared who is firmly situated inside the family; she rapidly stands for the one aspect of the Feddens' life that they want out of view, an anomaly in a family characterised as being intent on showing it all, almost. This division between the public and the private, the visible and invisible, showing and concealing is inscribed in the novel through the intertextual references to Henry James, whose 'style', Nick explains, when asked about his PhD project, 'hides things and reveals things at the same time. For some reason this seemed rather near the knuckle' (TLB, 54). Hollinghurst makes sure that Nick experiences Catherine as a slight anomaly, as in the very first scene in which the two of them find themselves alone in the house. When Catherine has been in the kitchen of her own home, Nick thinks 'there was a vague air of intrusion' (TLB, 10) as if she did not belong in the house. It turns out that Nick is capable of sensing the signs of her loss of mind because the mess she created in the house at that point seems to have been the result of an irrational moment during which she tried to harm herself, or was tempted by self-mutilation again. This early scene in the novel, when the rest of the family are summering in France, is described from the divide between the visible and the invisible.

This might have been inherited from the Feddens' own ambivalent attitude with regard to their own home. Whether it be the objects of art that are displayed in the large house or the notable affluence of the couple, the Feddens like to show anyone around their homes, even lower-class people like Leo who, for all Gerald's reluctance, is still welcomed in. The gardens' key is an object of great pride for the neighbours, but Gerald does not care, as he does not seem to care about intrusion or burglary. It is only when, at the end of the novel, journalists threaten to trespass that the key is requested back. There are only two things that the family refuse to see: sexuality and mental health issues—two issues that reek of a very

---

[1] On top of this, an issue about race could be discussed, linked to Leo and Leo's family, but this would need a development in itself.

backward, Victorian moral stance in keeping with Gerald's being a member of the Conservative party. Nick is thus never suspected of having bad intentions despite clearly belonging to another world: he is invited as a guest, however meagrely, taken on holiday and to birthday parties and so on, feeling part of the family (TLB, 4) as if the Feddens did not care for his presence at all, or did not feel the need to be left alone.

In contrast with this apparent open-mindedness, Catherine is only tolerated: her 'manic depression' and self-harming habits are mentioned straightaway, like Nick's being gay, and this seems to be the reason why both are ostracised from spending the summer in France with the rest of the family. They are 'paired', we are told initially (TLB, 16), and the first manifestation of this is their stroll in the communal gardens which Yeager has so brilliantly analysed as a foundational space in the novel for homosexual identity to be situated (Yeager 2013). 'His initial task—"Looking after the Cat" in the family phrase—disguises as pet care his response for the manic-depressive daughter Catherine' (Rivkin 2005: 289–90). The joke is on Catherine, but the phrase hides, at the same time and as much as it reveals, the very reason why the 'cat' needs looking after. And yet, this takes place in the very first pages of the novel, contributing to the association between Nick and Catherine, which takes place by magic or chemistry, but instantaneously and without explanation; in the rest of the novel, this association will never be disputed. It is noteworthy that Catherine's 'odd' behaviour is first presented in the epanorthosis mode, that is, as a long list of unsatisfactory terms to describe her 'madness': Toby defines his sister's illness first with the superordinate term 'mad'—a term that recurs on several occasions (TLB 59)—before talking of less worrying 'ups and downs', her being 'pretty volatile' and having 'these moods' (TLB, 6). The reader is thus made to feel the discomfort of a brother probably as much worried by his sister as he is perplexed by what makes her different: the stylistic effect of his choice of words is soon going to be underlined by the narrative voice when it is said that, in this new world Nick discovers, 'in six months' time, he would know, he'd have sorted out the facts from the figures of speech' (TBL, 35). For now, the language is not yet decipherable and the figure of speech acts as a smokescreen which is not without appealing to Nick, whose 'queer' behaviour would equally be defined as somewhat different: it is not the language of medical symptoms that Toby uses, even though Catherine is medicated and therefore has been diagnosed with a condition, about which the family is made knowledgeable through the reading of her therapist's book (TLB, 413). The narrative remains vague as to whether the symptoms are caused, attenuated or enhanced by the medication. 'She used to, you know, cut her arms, with a razor blade' (TLB, 6). Toby voices out what he is uncomfortable telling Nick and the absence of further explanation is likely to produce what Nick feels about the present day: curiosity ('he found himself glancing tensely at her arms' (TLB, 6)) and polite distance; in other words, Catherine indeed falls prey to the social question of visibility and invisibility, which in turn is interpreted, if not experienced, as that which is accepted and that which is repressed.

It is difficult not to feel slightly uneasy that the character that shows signs of psychological instability should be one of the few female characters in Hollinghurst's fiction, because it could be said to perpetuate the stereotypical gendered notion that a woman is moody and whimsical, instead of giving her case more substance. Roberts seems to have even looked down on Catherine's attitude from the point of view of morality, as if her actions were somehow to be judged according to their 'beauty', another unfortunate association: 'One of the first things we learn about the less appealing side of Catherine's cyclotropic personality is that, as her brother notes, 'she used to, you know, cut her arms, with a razor blade' (TLB, 6–7) (Roberts 2017: 116). Although Roberts later on sees her 'downswings' as part of a 'straight' nihilistic mindset that is structural in Hollinghurst's novel (Roberts 2017: 113–16), he still makes a reference to Catherine's self-harming as an act that he would prefer not to know about. And yet, as critic, it is precisely this symptom, in its relation to writing and letters, that will be central to my analysis: we must look at Catherine, since so many significant others avert their eyes from the 'pattern of right-angled scars that you couldn't help trying to read as letters; it might have been an attempt at the word ELLE' (TLB, 7).

Even if no character asks her why she does this or what she meant when she did it, the interpretation offered here, like the psychiatrist's interpretations in *Mrs Dalloway*, *Regeneration Trilogy* and *Asylum*, cannot fail to influence the reading of Catherine's character as basically structured around the question of femininity suggested both by the word chosen and by the fact that she offers them to people's gaze as a result of the erotic sleeveless tops she wears. As Letissier remarks, 'it is through their interpersonal relations that the predominantly male characters of Hollinghurst's fiction are presented: they are detached from economic activity and public space, and their existence revolves around their affects and libido. Thus, the novelist accomplishes a literary anthropology of masculine intimacy'

(Letissier 2007: 5). It is therefore noteworthy that a female character should be placed in this position of exceptionality, a fact that is made especially relevant because she performs or overdoes femininity. Not only is she a female character, but she pushes to the extreme the traditional feminine features: she seduces all men; she often takes on the role of social matchmaker; she is dressed provocatively but always remains at home with her parents; she is both strong-headed and soft to the point of weakness. The word *Elle* that she attempted to write on her arm could thus refer to the fashion magazine and infer the sense that Catherine's psychic disorders have been caused by the mediatic norms of femininity; but the word also is the French for 'she': thus, the word, as well as the 'metaphoric lines' which some critics have analysed at length (Hannah 2007: 89), can therefore be seen as pointing to what leaves her perplexed, the sexual dimension of her psyche. What we do discover in the first pages of the novel is that, contrary to what Toby thinks, Catherine, who wears dresses that 'seemed hardly a garment at all' (TLB, 11), continues to be tempted by, if not to perform, self-harm and mutilation (TLB, 12), a revelation she wants Nick to know about and which justifies that she asks him to stay close to her, even though he is otherwise engaged with a possible date, and thereby she forces him into a heterosexual love that he is of course impervious to. The medication seems to be unable to correct this.

Self-mutilation aside, Catherine's symptoms are first and foremost behavioural, that is, linked to a certain idea of social composure and made manifest in a certain attitude towards norms and cultural expectations. Hence the fear repeated by the family that the medication would stop to work and that she would embarrass them if she did not take the right amount: '"Oh, she's fine," said Gerald, breezily; and then, seeing some use in the idea of being worried, "she's had her ups and downs, hasn't she, Nick—the old Puss? It's not easy being her. But you know, this thing called Librium that she's on has been an absolute godsend. Sort of wonder drug…".' (TLB, 278). Gerald gets the name of the drug wrong, and he uses phrases that leave Catherine's ailment entirely unspoken or undescribed so much so that it is clear that he is only interested as long as Catherine's attitude remains under control. Catherine is anything but fine and the medication is envisaged as the only solution, something she must stick to for the collective good, while all the other expressions are hackneyed, almost ways of not saying that which concerns her. Nick himself is embarrassed at various points by Catherine's tendency to shock her family and their relatives and friends 'through "inappropriate" forms of sexual

explicitness that implicate him' (Alderson 2017: 133). This is quite ironical given that Nick himself does not hesitate to bring over Leo and have
sex with him in the communal gardens where the Feddens could see them
if they happened to go on their balcony. Nick's own interest in Catherine,
after the first episode, consists in making sure she keeps taking the medication—'looking after' means making sure she is made appropriate and fit
for society. He barely ever goes beyond the hackneyed, phatic questions of
how she is and the cliché attitude that a surrogate brother may take on as
a chivalrous act of protection: 'I mean she's quite steady at the moment,
but it would just be disastrous if she came off this medication again' (TLB,
260), says Nick in a mock-version of a brother towards his sister's boyfriend, something which Jasper notes when he responds by laughing.
What this disaster entails, for her or for the whole family, is unclear. 'It was
hard work living with someone so helpless and negative, and much worse
if you'd known them critical and funny. Well, sometimes, perhaps, it made
your own problems look light; at others it amplified them, by a troubling
sympathetic gloom' (TLB, 412). And yet, up until the end, Catherine
never is seen endangering the family other than by refusing to stick to one
boyfriend, being fairly promiscuous and getting involved with men of different social classes; in other words, most of her symptoms seem to be
summarised in her ability to get out of her way to ensure that her parents
will feel social awkwardness and that she will not conform to the image or
role of the Conservative upper-class daughter.

Again, the repressive hypothesis concerning social interaction in British
society seems to explain the attitude of Catherine's relatives, the Feddens
being masters in the art of hiding and camouflaging what they think. '*The
Line of Beauty* provides plausible instances of the variety of such repression
in the fact that it also represents 'the "obsolescence" of the Freudian
model of subjectivity' (Alderson 2017: 132). Alderson's idea is of paramount importance because it lays the stress on the necessity to take stock
of the question of the repressive model, inherent in the Oedipus paradigm
set by Freud, while at the same time, it invites us to re-appraise the formation of subjectivity as not entirely constructed on repression. Clearly,
Alderson concludes that 'Catherine's rebelliousness' must be comprehended along symbolic lines and it is interesting in that respect to see the
imbalanced response she receives from her parents. Her attitude, Alderson
goes on to explain, 'is her peculiar inheritance: her feminine, liberal sensi-
tivity is matched with a masculine determination to cut through the crap
in a way that results in naively vulgar left-wing outbursts (which also

remind us of Helen Schlegel)' (Alderson 2017: 138). The critic, who analyses the role played by influence in Hollinghurst's fiction, quite naturally here lays the stress on the origin of her very singular affects, which in turn are imposed upon the social scene. However, Catherine should also be seen as a fictional laboratory for something else in the economy of Hollinghurst's novelistic formats.

Her father's response to Catherine's condition (Rachel, her mother, is rarely seen describing or worrying about Catherine) is a distinctive feature of right-winged politicians: 'Gerald frowned faintly, to deny any interest in the women, and Nick realized his paradigm for this inspection was some difficult encounter with his own parents, who would have blushed at the sexualised style of the whole magazine, and called it "daft" or "rubbish" because they couldn't mention the sex itself' (TLB, 99). However, there does not seem to be much behind these passing remarks other than Hollinghurst's social comedy skills and his ability to rend through the veil of appearances in order to underline his characters' pretence. It is almost as if Hollinghurst only paid lip service to the Freudian model of family romance, and his vision of Catherine's psychic symptoms may thus, at times, be used for sheer mockery:

> In the back window of the car shiny white cushions were neatly aligned; he couldn't see the number plate but the thought that it must be BO something made him smirk—he pressed the smirk a little harder into a ghastly smile of admiration. One of Catherine's neuroses was a horror of maroon; it outdid her phobia at the *au* sound, or augmented it perhaps, with some worse intimation. Nick saw what she meant. (TLB, 247)

Catherine's medical symptoms are not fully developed because she is not the centre of Nick's attention and she gradually recedes into the background, when Nick's life among the Feddens does not require the subterfuge of the daughter's mental instability that he is expected to care about on behalf of everyone else. Her medical condition is used as comic relief, light-hearted small talk:

> 'Yes, well, I don't think any of us are triskaidekaphobes, are we?' said Gerald. They were all very up on the names of phobias, since at various times Catherine had suffered from aichmo, dromo, keno, and nyctophobia, among a number of more commonplaces ones—it was a bit of a game with them but it cut no ice with Elena, who stood there biting her lip. (TLB, 121)

When her medical condition is discussed, it is always rather vague:

> She said she couldn't concentrate on a book, or even an article. Sometimes she acted in her quick pert way, but it was a reflex: she observed it herself with bewilderment and kind of longing. Mostly she sat and waited, but without any colour of expectation. Nick found himself talking with awful brightness of purpose, as if to someone old and deaf; and it was more awful because she didn't find it condescending. (TLB, 413)

Yet, more importantly, Catherine's social and behavioural symptoms are presented as possible keys to those that Nick suffers from, although he often remains ignorant of them since he is the observer rather than the observed: 'He had groaned over Dr Edelman's style and corrected his grammar to protect himself from a superstitious fear that the book awoke in him: of finding the symptoms in himself, now he knew what they were. They certainly seemed to be present in all the more volatile, the more irascible, or oddly lethargic people he knew' (TLB 413). Once again, the language used is certainly not the language of medical treatment, but the generalised vision of unfit people cannot possibly exclude Nick himself, forcing him to envisage that his association with Catherine be a symptomatic formation of sorts, something helping him go through the beginning of his adult life. All that can be said about Dr Edelman's language is that it is a language that is presented as unfit for the thing it seeks to depict—the grammar is incorrect, the style is wrong and the epanorthosis returns—but the description associates Nick and Catherine in the same social stance and situation: they are queer characters who threaten the non-volatile people they meet every day. The equivocation in English between drug as prescribed medicine to heal (Catherine) and drug as (in the 1980s) chemical substance with hallucinatory effects (Nick) further contributes to the parallel view of both Nick and Catherine. 'Hollinghurst's novel consistently emphasizes the fragility of the aesthete's detachment from heteronormative surveillance [:] (...) scenes of exposure, scenes that stage the movement from private concealment to public display as a kind of "coming out" structurally underpin *The Line of Beauty*' (Hannah 207: 86). Yeager also engages with questions of private and public spaces and community from the point of view of queer narratives and theory: 'In such a community, Hollinghurst can situate Nick's process of sexual discovery in social terms' (Yeager 2013: 311). The question remains of how Catherine may serve the purpose of situating other characters and interrogating the social link between them at a time when romance is dead and replaced by what appears at first as unbridled consumption of bodies and sexual liberation gone wrong, something which the AIDS epidemic came to stand for as retribution for those that dared indulge in their libidinal drives.

'Proper Romance Is a Sham' (Alderson 2017: 141)

The novel therefore knits together the social implications of behavioural inaptitude with the personal consequences of the unregulated market of bodies, bodies that are reified or commodified at an age in which the ideology winning over throughout the 1980s was the capitalist free-market: the 1980s seem to be a decade of loosening mores and sexual liberation, growing hegemony and growth, and the Feddens find themselves in a situation in which they have to adapt to the young people's new ways of drug and sex while adjusting to putting up with the limited recreational enjoyment these substances provoke or lead to. Catherine is only a secondary character, it is impossible to set her in parallel with characters like Septimus or Prior, and what pervades the novel rather than the question of madness is the body of young Adonis-like men whom Nick craves for (see in particular the beginning of the second part and its title 'To Whom Do You Beautifully Belong?'): 'Hollinghurst's aestheticization of Leo's and Wani's bodies also facilitates the criticism that the novel commodifies and thingifies the male body' (Kim 2016: 171). Perhaps this is less something to deplore than to embrace because it also poses the question of how sex is consummated in the 1980s and what it reveals of the place given to the singularity of subjectivity. Through sex and the body, Nick and Catherine are associated in ways that their marginal social situation is not sufficient to account for. Catherine's character is not developed fully, and one could argue that she is only perceived from an external point of view that makes any attempt at defining her *sinthome*, that is, the singularity of her handling the symptoms she suffers from, likely to fail. Yet, I would like to relate the sketchy nature of Catherine in the text as basically the effect of her symptom: in other words, it is because she fails in handling her symptom towards subjective satisfaction that Catherine is interesting to the critic and constructed as incomplete by Hollinghurst. Her discreet presence is the sign of a new modality of madness, one that is controlled by medication but hardly cured.

Catherine's psychological, subjective symptoms offer a significant point of reference to understand some of the questions that the narrative raises about gay social comedy and the lived experience of illness with which Nick is confronted, all of which are encapsulated in the romantic stories of the novel—and romance here only refers to the experience of love as constructed in the gay stories. Nick is seen with two lovers: on the one hand, Leo, with whom he discovers sex and for whom he will keep a long-lasting tenderness, despite their relationship being short-lived; and Wani, the Lebanese-French golden boy, of the kind that was hailed by society back in the 1980s, and with whom Nick lives a mostly secret, unofficial affair. Kim reviews the critics' tendency to despise Wani and look down on him as a target to disparage a certain attitude which they attribute to the depravity of Thatcher's London (Kim 2016: 166). Nick is never Wani's exclusive partner, but he is significant enough that he inherits a substantial part of Wani's fortune after Wani dies. None of these characters are pinpointed as having psychological or behavioural disorders, but the reader may have an inkling of something awry in Wani's sexual practices. I will try not to do what Mathuray has noted about critics: 'Certain reviewers and critics seem to work hard to "sanitise" and often to "de-gay" his texts' (Mathuray 2017: 2). On the contrary, it is by looking at ways in which both Wani and Catherine use or abuse their own bodies that perhaps the function of her symptom can be better comprehended. Wani's sexual practices are characterised by excess (in the sense that he has multiple partners but also seems to think about sex for the most part of the day). In a very hackneyed conversation centring upon the state of the youth, Wani and Sally end up agreeing on the following proposal: '"sort of sex-mad, isn't it, the world we live in," said Sally, as if that was their general conclusion. "I know", said Wani' (TLB, 340). The phrase seems insignificant, but resonates as particularly true in Wani's case.

With Wani, it is not so much the promiscuity that interrogates as his constant, inescapable need for seduction and sexual satisfaction, as exemplified by his habit of turning on porn videos on his TV set as background to his own sexual practice, or backdrop to his life. He does not seem to enjoy anything other than the promise of having sex while being drugged and he is ready to break all social codes for his own satisfaction: cruising, sex in the upstairs toilets when invited at a civilised party, sex in the garden shed and so on. Whenever Nick takes him to places, he sets up plans that entail an onlooker, a third part, the presence of another person or couple for his sexual encounters, while at the same time, his sexual leanings are camouflaged: Wani presents himself as straight, having a girlfriend who turns out to be a paid cover girl. The apparatus designed by Wani to ensure his satisfaction is often one that Nick himself is uncomfortable with and that he wishes Wani would not need—it clearly evokes the pervert's set protocol (Castanet 2012). The examples abound, which makes us ponder the nature of the relationship between Nick and Wani: when one is an art connoisseur, who claims to enjoy beauty and style, the other goes on a European tour with the sole intent of getting as much sex as possible, hence the guide book of gay hotspots (called '*Spartacus*') that they take with them as a sort of queer Forsterian Baedeker. Where Nick seems to have found a way of sublimating his libidinal drives into the exploration of beauty and art, Wani's forms of enjoyment denote a lack of sublimation, and a tendency to relish in disposable pleasures, as if there was no barrier for him to channel these drives.

One particular example, central to the novel and to this argument, brings Catherine, Nick and Wani together and points to a structural analysis of their subjective place. Nick and Wani are holidaying in the Feddens' French summer house, being presented as family friends even though they are secretly sexual partners. Since Wani also knows Toby, there is nothing to make people doubt this version, until Gerald finds a used condom in the pool-house and Catherine finds out the truth. In the central section of the novel, Hollinghurst constructs a scene replete with symbols of the summer holiday—liberation, illicit behaviour, heightened sensual experiences—but breaks its effect with an unusual scene that verges more on the erotic, if not pornographic, novel than on romance. Both Wani and Nick are titillated by Catherine's current boyfriend, Jasper, especially because the straight couple are far from prudish and are more than happy to show themselves in amorous acts beside the swimming pool, as if they wanted to arouse the people around them or were confident that the exhibition of their relationship should satisfy other people. At one point, on one of those hot afternoons of a long summer, Wani and Nick have sex to the sound of Catherine and Jasper 'going at it' in their own room. Hearing the creaks of the bed and the slow murmur of the sexual intercourse, Wani is turned on, perhaps through the help of coke, as if he was looking at the scene and as much as he, in other parts of the novel, is when he watches uninterrupted X-rated videos. Wani directs Nick's hand and mouth towards his sex while he can overhear the next-door couple, but Nick's reaction is not as enthusiastic as Wani's: 'Nick laughed but was embarrassed too, almost shocked to hear them at it (which he never had before) and at it so promptly and so fast. No wasteful foreplay there—it made him wonder if Catherine was liking it, if Jasper wasn't being a brute with her, when surely, she needed such careful handling' (TLB, 257). As Wani gets into a fantasy that works wonders, Nick 'felt awkward, pulled in to service a fantasy which he couldn't quite share—he tried again, he'd jerked off a few times about Jasper already, but Catherine was his sister, and on lithium, and, well... a girl' (TLB, 258).

The scene is particularly interesting because it seals the comparisons between Catherine's behavioural difficulties and lack of symbolic place, and Nick's social marginality, through the lived experience of her body and in particular the sexed body. As Nick himself is placed in a situation of discomfort, he projects the same discomfort onto Catherine, without noticing that what he mentions is as much his as it is supposedly hers. 'When surely she needed such careful handling' strikes us as fairly naïve and potentially sexist on the part of a man who agrees to many sexual practices he does not particularly want. Catherine may be on 'lithium'; she may have difficulties observing the norms of society and saying the correct things when needed; she may have 'ups and downs'—none of this, lest we be judgemental and think of ourselves as authorities in the field of correct behaviour and sensible ways, should make us prejudiced as to what kind of sexual practices she enjoys and whether the absence of foreplay is necessarily Jasper's responsibility—again, a fairly sexist prejudice to have. In other words, the question of whether Catherine likes it or not is valid if Nick asks her, but the way it is formulated here suggests that Nick has already made up his mind that she does not. And yet, what matters is whether the fact that she agrees to it, whether she likes it or not, can be traced back to a subjective logic. Lithium is used in psychiatry as a mood regulator, an agent to stabilise mood swings, not as medicine against fragile beings. Her manic-depressive symptoms do not entail a subjective weakness—it is not the sign of an illness as such—but a singular way of responding to the world. And yet, Nick may also underline that he perceives her acceptance of rough intercourse as (self-)harm, a sort of extension of Catherine's taste for harming herself, by her own means or through dysfunctional relationships. For Catherine's enjoyment undeniably dovetails with what she seems to find repulsive: '"Fortunately I won't even have to look at you eating it," said Catherine, though she did quickly peer at it with a kind of relish of revulsion' (TLB, 120).

This revulsion corresponds to one of the meanings of Lacanian *jouissance*, which, in the last stage of his teaching, becomes the starting point rather than the consequence of subjective experience, that is, a disjointed, disintegrated real which is mortifying and against which the subject tries to set up protections in the form of language, identifications and so forth (Miller 1999). Catherine's attraction for that which is tasteless and shocking has much to do with Wani's uncontrollable sex behaviour, which he knows puts him at risk of AIDS, but which he cannot not try and accomplish. Sontag's analysis of AIDS as not an illness but a condition is helpful to draw a parallel with manic depression: 'Strictly speaking, AIDS ... is not the name of an illness at all. It is the name of a medical condition, whose consequences are a spectrum of illnesses' (Sontag 1989: 104). What Sontag suggests is that the virus itself is not the illness, in the same way that the symptoms of manic depression, such as mood swings, are not in themselves an illness, but become so when they impede the subject's life. The infection will make patients likely to catch illnesses, but what matters more is that they are in fact subjected to a condition which in turn defines them:

> The illness flushes out an identity that might have remained hidden from neighbours, job mates, family, friends..../The unsafe behaviour that produces AIDS is judged to be more than just weakness. It is indulgence, delinquency—addictions to chemicals that are illegal and to sex regarded as deviant. (Sontag 1989: 113)

AIDS is therefore not only an illness but the site of a process of identification to a community. Sontag prefers to use the term 'condition' that resonates with the social implications of the consequences of being diagnosed. What I would like to underline in Sontag's analysis is also the fundamental role played by *jouissance*, that is, here defined as morally reprehensible behaviour, excessive and yet discomforting, illegal and yet desired. She also suggests that there is a similar access to *jouissance* derived from drugs and promiscuity, a sort of heightened state of emotions that signifies the lack of control of any repressive method *and* the destructive risk taken by those that indulge in it. A similar argument could be made about mental illnesses that are in fact mental conditions reflecting the subjects' relations to their own *jouissance*, equally marked by social opprobrium and other people's puzzlement. Sontag's cultural analysis in this respect silences the physical effects of the virus for the sake of comprehending the social value the virus gives to those afflicted with it.

Wani's liberated sexual practices turn out to be the sign of a condition that precedes his illness, so to speak. They are not conducive to happiness but rather to a life of dissimulation, family conflicts, lies and eventually self-harm. In parallel, Catherine's own sexual practices show us that she is perhaps no more fragile than anyone else, but more attuned to the *jouis-sance* that she cannot control and to which she finds herself alienated. In any case, she is named ill and therefore expected to have symptomatic practices, while Wani, who isn't yet ill, is not presented in a pathological fashion. The parallel sex scenes do not lead to formalistic innovations, writing prowess or structural upheaval, but they discreetly destabilise the fixed, traditional narrative modes identified by Letissier (Letissier 2007). The scene is so discreet in fact that the episode remains a sort of parenthesis since Catherine and Jasper will never know, nor any other character. Besides, the narrative resumes almost without further ado, except for Nick asking Jasper to look after Catherine, but social comedy is not interrupted, reproducing therefore in the text the division between the conscious and unconscious processes, making us see what is usually unseen. The need to return to social comedy is blatant, as if Hollinghurst was conscious of breaking so many moral codes he had to re-instate structure and order to his narrative. However, the scene sets a paradigm between the characters and enables us to start forming the logic of their self-harming progress.

What the scene opens up to is a shift in perspective. It is now Catherine who, in a sort of mirrored relationship with Nick, wonders if he is happy in his relationship with Wani when she finds out after a used condom was left in the garden shed:

> 'You'd fall in love with someone just because they were beautiful as you call it.'
>
> 'Not anyone, obviously, that *would* be mad.' He resented her way, now she'd gained access to his fantasy, of belittling the view.
>
> 'People are lovely because we love them, not the other way round.'
> (TLB, 349)

This passage is also commented upon by Kim, who concludes that this is the sign that Nick and Wani's romance does not entail the involvement of their subjectivity in the relationship (Kim 2016: 182). According to Lacan, it is precisely because subjectivity cannot be avoided—that is, human beings exist only as subjects because of their entrance in language—that there can be no relationship (Lacan 1975: 9), but there can be love, which is another term for the way in which a relationship may be substituted for that which misses. Here, Catherine's reflection indicates that subjects are signifiers for other subjects: she sees other people as having a function and no intrinsic definition or value. 'Beauty', which is central to Nick's concern and which resonates with his taste for art, his wish to enter the tasteful world of the powerful and his own romantic experiences, refers to the artful, that is, creative aspect of romance, in which both partners are involved in pairing or coupling with a subject who may lay their *jouissance* at rest. The shift is also perceptible in the fact that Catherine in the first scene was the agent of Nick's failure to go to his date with Leo, whereas here she is worried that Nick may not be mating with Wani in the correct way. Given the parallel suggested by the narrative between Catherine, Nick and Wani, there comes a way to review why Catherine is regarded as ill, while Nick and Wani are only presented as singular, different beings that seek to grow into adults.

CATHERINE'S SINTHOME (LACAN 2005)

The Line of Beauty, as such, does not linger on the question of madness and manic depression. However, the presence of such a character raises the issue of the place they are given and the solution they can find to fall back into a socially acceptable way of functioning in the world. What is worthy of analysis is that Catherine's fits and depressive moments are never described: they always have already happened. Catherine is found in a state, but she is never shown getting into that state, making the origin of her symptoms lost. The narratorial strategy of Hollinghurst in handling Catherine almost evokes tragedy, when, as in *Hamlet, King Lear* or *A Streetcar Named Desire*, the tragic flaw has already happened: readers, like Nick, witness the aftermath of her depression, the consequences that she is unable to face. More importantly, Catherine seems to remain unaware of these moments herself. It is as if she was not there: 'After her break- down last year she had gone with her parents to Venice for a tense attempt at recuperation, which she now claimed scarcely to remember' (TLB, 303). This is another 'line of beauty' that the novel explores and seeks to follow, but which has attracted less attention than others, notably drugs, writing and influence.

The reason why the 'line' is also a metaphor to be kept for the analysis of Catherine's character is that the novel shows her trajectory from the silenced, sinful nature of her practice and behaviour to the more open, in- yer-face acceptance of the very oddity that is situated at the most intimate junction of her being. 'You look such old wrecks lying there, she said, and crackled in the "mad" style that she now allowed herself' (TLB, 301). If she allows herself to show her madness, it is first and foremost because she also sees madness everywhere else, especially in the heart of her own family, who are either useless or masters in the art of dissimulation. As stated above, Catherine is never taken into account as a subject with difficulties, but she is treated as a patient monitored by drugs. This results in the family being clueless as to what she feels or experiences: 'Gerald hesitated, peering over his raised wine glass but took his daughter's part. "I think I'd say she's just very soft-hearted," he said; which it seemed to Nick was just what she wasn't' (TLB, 335–6). The misunderstanding about Catherine is reiterated throughout the novel, as if she was meant to remain an enigma, or perhaps forced into a place where she stood for the riddle in a family that otherwise controls every aspect of life: culture, politics, economics, leisure and pleasure: '"When he came in, I just thought, yes, I'm in the right place, this is enough."/Catherine said, "I think that's awfully dangerous, Nick. Actually I think it's mad."/"Well, you're an artist," said Nick, "surely?"' (TLB, 349). I am interested in the fact that in this argument, Nick and Catherine think in terms of imaginarised places—identifications to the lover/the artist/the supposed 'danger' of being thought what you are not—but also in terms of symbolic places—where one feels they belong, where one feels at home. It turns out that Catherine is assigned a place by Others with an authority—such as her father, her psychiatrist and now her carer, Nick—and as a result, she is stripped of her own subjective choice. She keeps returning to this notion of placelessness by shattering through the veil of propriety and imposing her 'truthful' talk and details which shock. Why would Nick call her an artist when precisely she seems to be more prone to smash things and bodies and relationships than to create? This is precisely because she demonstrates the singularity of her voice and point of view. These are also the signs of her 'artist's view', that is, her singular vision of the relationships between people and the creative aspect of her life.

Catherine therefore demonstrates the problems inherent to/ in? a therapy based on the erasure of symptoms and the normalisation of bodies and practices: they leave no room for the creative usage of subjectivity:

> The book [*A Path Through the Mountains: Clinical Responses to Manic Depression*] had helpful facts in it, but it left Nick with an imaginative uncertainty, as to where Catherine was when he looked at her and spoke to her:

not in the black and shiny place of her old depressions, but in some other
unfeatured place, policed by Dr Edelman's heavy new dosage of lithium.
(TLB, 413)

Again, the question of the symbolic place of Catherine returns as a
question mark in Nick's apparently simplified logic and everyday speech:
Where is Catherine is a question that leaves him perplexed and we see how
the medicine is no longer perceived as a helpful tool, but as an authoritarian regime of enjoyment in a society that would like to erase subjectivity
and replace it with 'unfeatured' places of consumption. It is quite amusing
that another Edelman should be referred to in analysing this question of
symptomatic formation: Kim refers to Lee Edelman's concept of 'sinthom-
omesexuality', which she defines like this:

> Lee Edelman calls 'sinthom-omesxuality' [Edelman 2003], a term combin-
> ing the Lacanian word *sinthome* and homosexuality. Defined by Edelman as
> 'stupid enjoyment' (Edelman 2003: 231) and 'the access to unthinkable
> *jouissance* beyond every limit of pleasure' (Edelman 2003: 232), *sinthome*—
> and its implication of sinfulness—is entailed in homosexuality. (Kim
> 2016: 166)

Edelman's Lacanian reading of the *sinthome* and homosexuality is
grounded in his exploration of nineteenth-century fiction, with examples
taken from Charles Dickens and George Eliot, but Kim refers to it about
The Line of Beauty because she sees in this vision of homosexuality a
response to *jouissance* a way of turning the character into 'an ethical site of
expanding thoughts on beauty' (Kim 2016: 166). This reference is evidence that the novel indeed is interested in how symptomatic formations
may be meaningless effects of an unknown *jouissance*. Hollinghurst does
not seek to explore the meaningful echoes of Catherine's symptoms but
works on placing them within the economy of generalised *jouissance*, an
excess of exchanges, transactions, communication-less intercourse which
was valued during the Thatcher years and justified the unbridled consumption, deregulated social mores and other symbolic, liberal measures
taken. Under cover of liberating society and giving them access to things
otherwise forbidden, this policy led them to become alienated to the possession of objects and identifications.

The second reason why Edelman's term works well for my argument is
that it combines the notion or function of *sinthome* with sexual practices

and self-definition, a compound that shows the way in which these various aspects are knotted together into a whole that is forever fragile, as indicated in the persisting hyphen. Catherine's identification is with the madness that her family attributes to her, irrespective of her actual condition: '"She's frightfully *up* at the moment", Rachel said. "You've no idea what she'll do". "Isn't she taking the pills?" said Lionel, firm and vague at once.' (TLB, 448). As the novel comes to a close, Rachel's remark strikes us as 'frightfully' undeveloped: she talks of her daughter with the same aloofness she had at the beginning, ten years before. Catherine leaves everyone perplexed for good. There comes a time when this becomes not only her symptom but her *sinthome*, that is, the mark of her suffering is also that to which she is assigned a place in the family and that to which she responds by using the terms that others use to describe her: '"Oh, how are you, Cathy?" said Sally Tipper. "Still mad!" said Catherine' (TLB, 315). The reflection is not underlined by the narration or the narrative structure: this is followed by the arrival of Gerald and Rachel who draw away all the attention and Sally's reaction is not told us, making Catherine's answer echo throughout the page and the rest of the text as both an accusation and the recognition of a condition that she is assigned through language. Is the absence of Sally's reaction a way for the narrator to suggest that despite the blunt phrase, this would be no surprise indeed? Furthermore, there is something striking in the fact that this affirmation comes after Sally's use of the short name 'Cathy', when no other character is the object of such instability with the act of naming: the character is always called Catherine by the narrator, who incidentally calls Nicholas, Nick, Tobias, Toby, but she is rarely called like this by her family: she is the Cat, hence 'the old Puss', Cathy, Catherine, and often darling for Nick, among others. What this suggests indeed is that the writing of Catherine into the symbolic order is a challenge many grapple with.

CONCLUSION

Throughout the novel, Nick is meant to be writing a PhD he never quite completes and articles about art that he never gets round to actually write. In other words, there is in Hollinghurst's text a reflection about the obstacles of writing, the intimate relationship for Nick between the written word and the meaninglessness or carelessness with which his life is lived, with no attachment. When Leo, his first lover, dies of AIDS, Nick's immediate reaction is that he should write to Leo's mother. By some 'deep

convolution of feelings' (TLB, 411), which can be interpreted as unconscious processes, Leo's mother is placed alongside his own mother, who
was the 'one person who really suffered for his homosexuality'. The letter
that is written on an urge will never be sent. The failure to send the letter
suggests that indeed Nick's argument that he seeks to console Leo's
mother is in fact being written to an Other figure he conceives as impossible to please and satisfy. He writes one sentence and thinks: 'there, it
existed, he'd hesitated, but written it, and it couldn't be unwritten' (TLB,
411). This is immediately contradicted by the text that unwrites it so to
speak by making it un-sent. Henry James's phrase about the death of Poe
comes to his rescue: '*The extremity of personal absence had just overtaken
him*'. The phrase resonates on many levels: Poe is the author of the
'Purloined Letter', a story of a letter that although written has stopped
existing; James's sophisticated language creates a plurality of meanings
and defeats Nick's attempt to console: 'He felt the limits of his connois-
seurship of tone' (TLB, 411). What Nick fails to realise at this point is that
his knowledge of writing does not preclude the failure of his own production of writing: he may be a good analyst of James's style, but this says very
little of his own attachment to writing. This is verified in his failure to
write of death, to write about death, something which again takes us back
to Hollinghurst's self-confessed admission that for a long time, he could
not write about AIDS. The sophistication of Nick's language enables him
to reflect upon the obstacles to any form of writing about the real, how it
always escapes and keeps being written again and again. This is also what
Sontag suggests when she reflects upon her own enterprise:

> The purpose of my book was to calm the imagination, not to incite it.
>   Not to confer meaning, which is the traditional purpose of literary
> endeavor, but to deprive something of meaning: to apply that quixotic,
> highly polemical strategy, 'against interpretation', to the real world this
> time. (Sontag 1989: 102)

Hollinghurst manages to do this as well: the highly sophisticated text
he writes is a very discreet way of stripping it of meaning by making the
latter so plural, so extensive that it becomes impossible to interpret.
Catherine is like the unconscious drives in his novel: lurking in the background, discreetly undermining the dominant discourses, she makes the
readers realise the vacuity of the descriptions given and brings out the only
question worth raising, which is how to account for the lives lived at the

margins, and, as pointed out in this book so far, how to write the unwritable and mobile place of the subject in the symbolic order. Hollinghurst finds in Catherine a way of rending the veil of literary propriety and the traditional template of the comedy of manners—with which Woolf also had to grapple—in order to question how a subject can be overwhelmed when they are assigned to an identification that is so strict, it is mortifying. The question thus raised is how to find one's voice, in writing as well as in life, as shall be seen in the last section of the book.

BIBLIOGRAPHY

PRIMARY SOURCES

Hollinghurst, Alan (2004). *The Line of Beauty*. London: Picador, 2005.
Woolf, Virginia (1925a). *Mrs Dalloway*. Oxford: Oxford World's Classics, 2009. Introduction by David Bradshaw (2000).
Woolf, Virginia (1925b). *The Common Reader, First Series*. New York: Harcourt Inc., with an introduction by Andrew McNeillie, 1984.

SECONDARY SOURCES

Alderson, David (2017). "Attachment and Possession: The Romance of Family, Politics and Things in *The Line of Beauty*". M. Mathuray (ed.), 129–149.
Bernard, Catherine (2018). *Matière à réflexion: du corps politique dans la littérature et les arts visuels contemporains*. Paris: Presses Universitaires de Paris-Sorbonne.
Castanet, Hervé (2012). *La Perversion*. Paris: Economica-Anthropos.
Edelman, Lee (2003). "Sinthom-osexuality". in P. Matthews & D. McWirter (ed.). *Aesthetic Subjects*. Minneapolis: U of Minnesota P., 230–248.
Gutleben, Christian (2015). "Serious Play: The Representation of the Thatcher Years in Malcolm Bradbury's *Cuts*, David Lodge's *Nice Work* and Alan Hollinghurst's *The Line of Beauty*." *Études britanniques contemporaines*, 49:2015, doi: https://doi.org/10.4000/ebc.2705
Hannah, Daniel K. (2007). "The Private Life, the Public Stage: Henry James in Recent Fiction." *Journal of Modern Literature*, vol. 30, No. 3, 70–94.
Hollinghurst, Alan (2004b). "The Middle Fears". in *The Guardian*, Sat. 4 September 2004.
Johnson, Allan (2014). *Alan Hollinghurst and the Vitality of Influence*. London: Palgrave Macmillan.

Kim, Soo Yeon (2016). "Betrayed by Beauty: Ethics and Aesthetics in Alan Hollinghurst's *The Line of Beauty*". *Texas Studies in Literature and Language*, vol. 58, No.2, summer 2016, 165–188. Doi: https://doi.org/10.7560/TSLL58203

Lacan, Jacques (1975). *Le Séminaire, Livre XX, Encore* (1972–73). J.-A. Miller (ed.). Paris: Éditions du Seuil.

Lacan, Jacques (2005). *Le Séminaire, Livre XXIII, Le Sinthome* (1975–76). J.-A. Miller (ed.). Paris: Éditions du Seuil.

Letissier, Georges (2007). "Queer, Quaint and Camp: Alan Hollinghurst's Own Return to the English Tradition". *Études anglaises*, 2007/2, vol.60, 198–211, 10.3917/etan.602.0198

Letissier, Georges (2019). "L'œuvre romanesque du romancier Alan Hollinghurst: contre-épopée anglaise et généalogie d'une culture alternative". *Itinéraires*, 2019, 2 & 3. 10.4000/itineraires.7020

Mathuray, Mark (ed.) (2017). *Sex and Sensibility in the Novels of Alan Hollinghurst*. London: Palgrave Macmillan.

Miller, Jacques-Alain (1999). "Les Six Paradigmes de la Jouissance". *La Cause freudienne* No. 43, 7–29.

Rivkin, Julie (2005). "Writing the Gay 80s with Henry James: David Leavitt's *A Place I've Never Been* and Alan Hollinghurst's *The Line of Beauty*". *The Henry James* Review, vol. 26, No. 3, 282–292.

Roberts, Adam (2017). "Ogee: The Line of Beauty". In M. Mathuray (ed.), 111–128.

Sontag, Susan (1978–1989). *Illness as Metaphor* (1977–78) and *Aids and* Its *Metaphors* (1988–89). London: Doubleday.

Su, John (2014). "Beauty and the Beastly Prime Minister". *EHL*, vol.81, No3, Fall 2014, 1083–1110.

Terzian, Peter (2011). "The Art of Fiction No.214: Interview of Alan Hollinghurst". *The Paris Review*, Issue 1999, Winter 2011.

Yeager, Myron (2013). "The Topography of Gay Identity: Alan Hollinghurst's 'The Line of Beauty'". *CEA Critic*, November 2013, vol. 75, No. 3, 310–319.

PART III

Voices, Contemporary Symptoms and Social Cohesion

Voices, Silence and the Body: Cusk's Modernist Explorations of Symptomatic Encounters in the *Outline* Trilogy (2014–2018)

After looking at the therapy scene and witnessing how writers look away from the medical gaze into a different approach to the symptom as that which constitutes the core of a subject's singularity and needs to be written into the symbolic order to become operational, I have focused on the effects of biomedicine in reducing symptomatic manifestations to discreet signs. This has led us to appreciate the role played by secondary characters in bringing to the fore the subjective logic, without necessarily seeking to re-establish or restore or even unveil meaningful relations of cause and consequences. In the third and final section, I want to look at something that was touched upon before but hadn't acquired yet a status as prevalent as in the following two works studied: the importance of voices and silence as explorations of contemporary modalities of psychic symptom formations. In other words, contemporary works have to make do with a new therapeutic reality: the biomedical approach has furthered the pathologisation of many practices and behaviours, transforming the plurality of identifications into even stronger injunctions to identify to a community, to name who we are, to expect everyone to recognise themselves in and conform to accepted identities. The only site of resistance can therefore be the intimate level of the subject's interiority, once again. The body's

© The Author(s), under exclusive license to Springer Nature   203
Switzerland AG 2023
N. P. Boileau, *Mental Health Symptoms in Literature since
Modernism*, Palgrave Studies in Literature, Science and Medicine,
https://doi.org/10.1007/978-3-031-37630-6_7

management via biomedical drugs and hygienic physical activities have contributed to splitting the subject once again, and so have the technological devices allegedly made to connect people. What is the place of literary works if humankind is now defined by its hyperconnection to objects? Surprisingly, a few contemporary British writers have decided to return to introspection and stream of consciousness techniques, which they present as ways of contradicting the temptation to silence that is felt by the tension there is between hyperconnection and disconnection. In particular, Ali Smith and Rachel Cusk have invented a new mode of narration in which interior voices, silences and body-free modes of expression surface in everyday speech, rejuvenating the contemporary refashionings of the Modernist aesthetics, since voices become the point of connection for a relation to the Other, which is first presented as made impossible, or at least almost so. This will enable me to conclude by analysing new modes of enjoyment (*jouissance*) and new symptoms in which the story one tells matters less than the core of enigmatic, opaque behaviour these new symptoms are able to produce.

Rachel Cusk Is quite articulate about the ambiguous effect of writing, which led her to be tempted into total silence, something which she interprets as a symptomatic formation. 'Without wishing to sound melodramatic, it was creative death after *Aftermath*. That was the end. I was heading into total silence—an interesting place to find yourself when you are quite developed as an artist' (Kellaway 2014). Here is how Cusk describes her own rebirth into literature in an interview following the publication of *Outline* (2014), a novel which is now part of a trilogy with *Transit* (2016) and *Kudos* (2018).[1] *Aftermath*, an autobiographical essay on the end of her marriage, had been published two years before and in what has now become customary in Cusk's career, it had caused more outrage than praise (Chancellor 2011 qd in Gallagher 2011; Derbyshire 2012). Like *A Life's Work* (2001) and *The Last Supper* (2009), the latter quickly went out-of-print after some legal proceedings due to some people who disapproved of Cusk's depiction of them in the text, her third openly autobiographical text was misunderstood by critics and readers alike (Kellaway 2001), who got confused as to what the work was trying to achieve: its innovative format, intermingling fiction with essayistic reflections, was regarded as stylistic flaws that made her point all the more unclear and debatable.[2] That she may have been heading towards complete

---

[1] In this chapter all references to Cusk 2018 will be to O for *Outline*, T for *Transit* and K for *Kudos*.

[2] *Coventry* has since been published to more favourable reviews.

silence after that is very paradoxical because this artistic depression engendered three novels replete with chatter, small talk and every possible mode of endless conversation and uninterrupted monologues.

Cusk's trilogy inscribes her in a Modernist, experimental ethos that foregrounds the crisis of identity and failure of meaning and communication that writing tries to stitch up. Inevitably, Woolf scholars will find in Cusk's reflection about the aftermath of *Aftermath* a reminder of Woolf's similar anxiety about and drive towards silence. The opening quote evokes the much-quoted sentence of Woolf's first novel: 'I want to write a novel about silence, the things people don't say. But the difficulty is immense' (*The Voyage Out*, 232). Bringing these two authors together is not infrequent (Boileau et al. 2013), but the trilogy makes the analogy explicit. For example, the character says he had considered entitling his book *A Shed of One's Own* (T, 97), a direct reference to Woolf's canonical feminist essay. In another episode, the narrator tells an interviewer that she remembers the description of her house where 'most of all you could hear the bells that rang unendingly from the town's many churches, striking not just the hours but the quarter and half hours, so that each segment of time becomes a seed of silence... The conversation of these bells, held back and forth across the rooftops, was continued night and day' (K, 62). This cannot but echo the role played by Big Ben in *Mrs Dalloway*, already identified as a source text for *Arlington Park* (2005) (Latham 2016), with only the variation that in the contemporary world of the collapse of grand narratives (Lyotard 1984), the monumental time (Ricœur 1984) has exploded into subjective, microscopic units of time. In this context, Cusk explores the failure of marriage and forms of contemporary unions. Her characters cannot find a substitute to alleviate the suffering of their solitude. Could the trilogy's entanglement of silence and excessive talk be regarded as a symptom of Cusk's (Neo)Modernist endeavour to articulate meaning against contemporary forms of social disconnection? Is there an argument to be made that Septimus's silence, which resonates with all the works studied so far, and Woolf's influence may account for Cusk's choice of a new format in which silence and voices are the objects of new novelistic echoes?

Few writers have evolved as much as Cusk over the course of their career. Her early novels, including *The Country Life* and *Arlington Park*, were more conventional satires of the tolls of interdependence and family life, based on conventional plots in which the characters evolve or face existential crises. Then came her biting memoirs, *A Life's Work: On*

Becoming a Mother and *Aftermath: On Marriage and Separation*, 'which raised hackles by bucking against society's bias towards domesticity' (McAlpin 2018). With *Outline*, Cusk set off on a new path, shifting to a sort of serial, stripped-down first-person storytelling that sometimes evokes podcasts-on-paper (McAlpin 2018). I intend to draw the 'outline' of Cusk's new fiction by tracing back the source of her experimentation before showing her rebirth into the modernist techniques that she claims to have found in D.H. Lawrence (his work is highly praised by one of Faye's students, O, 208–210), that she explicitly refers to by quoting Beckett (O, 234–35) and for which, everyone else sees Woolf! Cusk's reflection will strike any reader as paradoxical on many levels, the first of which being that the three novels rest on a radical change in style: the author was hailed for having found a new voice, which I think also partakes of a Woolfian tradition of constantly swinging between works of self-fiction and works of fiction, outlining an ever-changing, iterative knotting of life and language. In so doing, she also circumscribes new forms of enjoyment and *jouissance* in language, which manifest in contemporary symptoms of disillusion and depression, using the heteronormative couple as the paradigm of the demise of the self.

The three novels problematise silence, in the sense that the characters talk about their wish to avoid speaking and communicating altogether. At the same time, the novels are repositories of apparently never-ending chatter, confidences, conversations that blur the distinction between what is said and what isn't said, what is significant and insignificant, what is imagined and real, and, most importantly, what makes readers oblivious of the fact that all these voices are never the narrator's, who remains conspicuously in the background: it is as if the voices of others penetrated into her very silence where she could found a new language. Lives, experiences and disillusions are exposed to an almost complete stranger, in what is largely a long, metonymic, obsessive unfolding of apparently unsolicited, uninterrupted confessions, central to which are the character's failures and perplexity towards their own lives. The narrator's own voice is only heard implicitly, in between these reported fragments of conversation in which the waffle of small talk surprisingly gives rise to an unprecedented chamber of echoes and reflections of a philosophical nature on marriage, contemporary symptoms of ill-being and the function of writing (Messud 2017). Her voice, when heard by other characters, is often caught in the complex tension of attraction and repulsion, just like her body: Paula, the neighbour from downstairs, says Faye's voice 'makes her feel sick' (T, 159), a reaction that Paula does not have for the builder's, for example. The quality of voice had already been explored in *Arlington Park* (2005), which starts with Juliet being warned by her host that she sounds 'strident', an epithet that makes her feel extremely angry (AP, 10). Although mental health is not evoked directly in the trilogy, the confessions heard throughout evoke the disconnection central to contemporary modes of social enjoyment, the therapeutic effect of talking, and they resound with a feature of Cusk's novels that has been remarkable since the very beginning: the presence at the heart of her fiction of some event or person that is not represented but whose influence structures the whole text (Tang 2013).

The novels are 'fantasies in which the infinitesimal openings of small talk eventually drill down to the centre of the earth' (Lockwood 2018). In other words, the risk of silence that Cusk experienced in real life gave way to verbose novels, novels which seem to be filled with spoken words, reported speech, endless conversations and confidences. As I want to show in this chapter, what she unravels by delving into the things that people say and therefore don't say, is to position herself as a silent interpreter of the modern-day delirium of yore—like the one of Septimus Smith, for example. Or, to connect it more to a Modernist stance, one could say she returns to the conflict of intimacy, between the individual and the couple, in which she finds a paradigm to observe the disconnection at the heart of contemporary society, resulting as it were in a new question posed to the possibility of commonality and sharing experience.

This cannot but evoke a Renaissance of modernist aesthetics (Latham 2016), even if the latter has become multiple and plural (Childs 2012), but the act of 'repeatedly stag[ing] the failure of signification and meaning' (Alfandary and Nesme 2011: 10) gives pride of place to the multiplication of voices and discontinuous experience of language, all of which inevitably points to its reverse, that is, absence, silence and the many failures of communication. Cusk reiterates the modernist, Woolfian gesture of digging up the unconscious, the language of which all the characters speak: she reflects a world of disconnection, in which failures of communication amount to the creation of new, contemporary, psychic symptoms. Everyone seems to complain that they find it difficult to speak and articulate their experience because it does not make any sense or they can't find the way to express it, but by giving shape to it in her tale, Faye, the narrator who is also a writer, intends to alleviate them of the necessity to find a structure by replacing that necessity with the act of writing and by reconnecting it to the symbolic order. In other words, in addition to 'show[ing] perhaps four great preoccupations: with the complexities of its own form, with the representation of inward states of consciousness, with a sense of the nihilistic disorder behind the ordered surface of life and reality and with the freeing of narrative art from the determination of an onerous plot' (Bradbury and McFarlane 1976: 393), Cusk manages to represent outward states of consciousness both voiced and lost, both articulated and pointing to the risk of silence they seek to avert; she focuses on the suffering caused by the operation of language on experience and new modes of passing this on, even if ineffectively or incomprehensively, and thereby she also raises the question of the subjective experience of the body central to contemporary psychoanalytic theories.[3]

Contrary to Ali Smith's, Cusk's work remains ambiguous regarding how it fits in with a political agenda and political implications. And yet, in the third volume, Faye is sat next to a passenger who brings up the issue of Brexit. This is the opportunity for her to reflect the time-honoured feminist motto that the personal is political into its opposite suggestion that the political is personal: 'I said it was true that the question of whether to leave or remain was one we usually asked ourselves in private, to the extent that it could almost be said to constitute the innermost core of self-determination' (K, 12). The relation between lovers is elevated to the paradigmatic organisation of society, and Brexit comes to signify not so much the political manoeuvring of a Conservative party intent on keeping the upper hand against UKIP but a signifier of the conflictual experience of one's relationship with the other, one's experience of commonality: leaving or remaining are renegotiated at the subjective level of how to form couples, hence how to form a community with others, while Faye and Cusk seem to marvel at the exposure of such questions on the public scene: 'writing comes out of tension, tension between what's inside and what's outside' (O, 47). Despite their apparent attachment to speech, the novels really are about writing, therefore about love and connection.

---

[3] In recent years, Quarto has published a special issue, 126, dedicated to the body ('Le Corps, cette guenille qui nous est si chère') in December 2020; Issue 75 of Letterina is also dedicated to the body in 2020: 'L'écrit des corps, Douleurs, jouissance'; Jodeau-Belle, Laëtitia and Truchet Yohan (eds.) (2019), Corps et creation: Perspectives psychanalytiques, Rennes, PUR; Zenoni, Alfredo (2018), Le Corps de l'être parlant, Rennes, PUR and in English, The Speaking Body, special issue of Scilicet, 2015.

FINDING ONE'S VOICE AND MAKING THE READERS HEAR VOICES

After a fairly respectable career of publishing novels that were sometimes derided for being excessively well-made—Cusk 'overwrites... at her worst, she seems to approach novel-writing as a composition exercise in which marks are awarded for periphrasis' (Tayler 2005)—Cusk fell prey to critics influenced by her middle-class upbringing and Oxonian education. It is possible that what she calls 'the book of repetition'[4] may have been misinterpreted as essentialising women back into their domestic roles. She surprisingly became influential through the publication of an autobiographical essay on her experience of motherhood, which fostered a new direction in her style and her politics of feminism, based on much rewriting and reformatting. This led to the 2004 publication of *Arlington Park*, a rewriting of *Mrs Dalloway* that was not a pastiche (Latham 2013, 2016), based on an explosion of viewpoints and the plight of domestic queens. Soon followed *The Bradshaw Variations*, whose title precisely reverts to the well-known rapprochement between music and literature that was so central to Forster's, Proust's (Lucey 2022) and Woolf's Modernist explorations among others. The novels became international bestsellers and *Arlington Park* was made into a film in France, *La Vie Domestique*. Her novelistic explorations fumbled through the question of 'connection', and the way in which communities are constructed, and perhaps end up only a sham (Boileau 2015).

This creative decade was closed by the publication of *Aftermath*. In it, she addresses the way her divorce led her to rethink her feminist stance, her engagement and her beliefs without clearly suggesting what the outcome of this reflection is or what sort of feminism she advocates: 'I started to worry that the defining feature of the "feminist principle of autobiographical writing" might be lack of clarity. There's no point telling the truth if no one can understand you' (Biggs 2012). *Aftermath* was commercialised with a cover showing a jigsaw puzzle with one piece not

---

[4] The basis for this expression is Cusk's 'Shakespeare's Daughters', an article that draws on various feminist legacies, such as Woolf's and Beauvoir's, to delineate the experience of womanhood. Cusk talks about the 'book of repetition', her expression for 'women's writing', which, according to Tang, can be understood as a reaction to and against feminism: 'Twenty-first century female culture', writes Cusk, 'barely acknowledges its debt to feminism', and today's woman writer is likely to be 'careful not to show any special interest in today's woman' (Cusk 2009).

fitting, which could not but evoke the general impression given that the book is a puzzle, lacking direction. This book almost put an end to her influential voice—throughout the noughties, Cusk had become a regular contributor to the *Guardian,* writing opinion pieces that furthered her association to Woolf, in which she developed challenging views of feminism, notably by requesting that domestic work in your own home be paid (Cusk 2009). Within the context of an imbalanced production, made of significant and insignificant pieces, calling forth our deep-rooted tendency to classify, honour and dishonour, canonise and desacralise writers as well, *Outline,* soon followed by *Transit* and *Kudos,* dramatically changed Cusk's literary status and took many by surprise (Messud 2017).

The titles of the novels straightaway elicit a metadiegetic meaning evoking the reduction of the plot to its sketch-like, draft-like, fleeting nature: Faye, the narrator, is a creative writing teacher and novelist who professionally travels to Athens, or central Europe, to attend literary festivals; she refurbishes a 'bad house in a good street' (T, 4); she goes to have her hair cut or dyed; or is invited for dinner. These 'so-called novels' (Woolf, MB: 83) are an *outline* of fiction which renews the ways of representing the solitude and loneliness of women's experience, their states of mind and conscious or subconscious feelings, about which Cusk has consistently written since the beginning of her career (Latham 2016: 168). In addition, Cusk also renews a certain interest in subtle or 'discreet' signs of psychic imbalance—not to use disorder—with which everyone seems afflicted, from separated partners who have never quite recovered from the shattering of their marriage to teenagers caught in the contemporary symptoms of addiction, disconnection and disinterest, in single families or in the freedom granted by the privilege of having disengaged parents. These signs of madness are not great manifestations, but they loom in the background of the stories Faye is told. The monologues of her transient/ transiting partners (K, 53) point to the silence they seek to deal with, theirs or that of others, and the narrator's own, while the constant shifts between direct and indirect speech revisit one of the dominant stylistic features of Modernist language, its interest in reported speech and interior monologue (Cohn 1978). 'Much of the narrative is… recounted after the fact, in the "he said", of the simplest narrative voice' (Valihora 2019: 24), to which one is tempted to add that the simplest verges on the tautological: 'as I say, she said' (O, 188). In our contemporary world, Cusk suggests, the barrier between private and public subjectivities has collapsed: '"It just makes it obvious that you've got something to hide."/I said that seemed preferable to having what you wished hidden on public display' (T, 62). The stream of consciousness is out in the open, disclosed: the voices of her characters are heard in and out of the inverted commas, creating unimpeded fluidity between the reported and the voiced, and enabling Cusk to accumulate voices and create a resounding chamber of echoes in which the utterer is at times lost (T, 4).

The text is like voiced monologues that men and women alike confess to her and it is never sure whether she is there, considered, or if the confession really is interior monologue that Faye happens to hear: 'I listened to this confession, if confession it was, in silence' (O, 174). Cusk, through her alter ego Faye—like her, a middle-aged, middle-class creative writing teacher and writer—becomes the witness and repository of this constantly changing world that never fully manages to be articulated into language, or rather whose incessant talk is the sign pointing to the risk of silence the talk is aimed to fight. The first volume of the trilogy finishes with a woman talking about the barrier of languages being impassable, the writing of plays that she is blocked with and the realisation of the end of her marriage through a telephone call: '... it was immediately apparent, when she spoke to him on the phone that day, that he did not share her view.... *Polar opposites* was the phrase that had, during those difficult moments, popped into her mind' (O, 235–36). The function of these confessions is therefore unclear. She places them on the same footing as her lack of linguistic production connected with the end of her marriage. All the characters seem to try and come to terms with an experience that they find puzzling and enigmatic, to the extent that their assertions about who they are and what they did turn out to be 'explanations', designed perhaps to ensure a solid place in discourse because the general impression shows the opposite, namely, that talking means infinite, meaningless babbling: 'What they failed to recognise... was that a fence or a sign has a meaning that is clear to almost everybody, whereas a human individual... has to explain himself' (K, 89). The explanation that is referred to is perhaps what the novels try to achieve by multiplying confessions and allowing each of the characters the time to patiently evoke their pasts and present.

The novel's *outline* is given to the readers in the first pages: fleeting connections with strangers or recurring people form Faye's community. It is no longer characters who hear (disincarnated) voices, like Septimus in *Mrs Dalloway*, but readers, as the text is almost never a narrative: voices people this house of fiction that Faye literally refurbishes in the second and third volumes, after we have seen her homeless and travelling, in exile from a reality no longer accessible, for the first time in her work outside the United Kingdom—*The Last Supper* also deals with foreign experience but it owes much to the English tradition of travel writing (Rannou 2013). These voices, which are hardly ever connected to bodies and which come and go fleetingly, resemble in many ways, not least stylistically, the stream of consciousness of Cusk's influences. The monologues are only interrupted by flimsy accidents, contingent thoughts and encounters, which suspend reflections of an essential nature in mid-air, like the interpretative interruptions of a therapeutic session: 'Faye's interest in this man and his story constitutes another form of repetition [the critic compares it to Freud's *Fort/Da*], yet with a difference; it is in an almost therapeutic form, like a controlled experiment' (Valihora 2019: 25).

As a result, the novels seem to be an attempt at harnessing the overflow of conversation and confessions, as established from the beginning with a scene that cannot but be interpreted at the metadiegetic level of the novel-in-the-making: 'We were strapped into our seats, a field of strangers, in a silence like the silence of congregation while the liturgy is read' (O, 4). In a world bereft of any god-like figures, silence like small talk is overwhelming and there's a wish for bodies to be strapped, deprived of what animates them usually. *Transit*, in particular, evokes the question of language overflowing the subject, the negative risk of being blocked, the circulation of ideas and speech, and the balance between confessions and silence that writers have to negotiate: the builder Faye employs lives in his van and is looking for someone to listen to his story, while writers are asked to perform a public persona on stage in order to enter the capitalistic system of selling as many copies of their books as possible. This can be analysed as well as placing them in a system of exchange in the symbolic order: here money, elsewhere language. The Woolfian and Lawrentian inspirations are reflected in the agility of the shifts in points of view: some writers reflect on notoriety as a new form of inhibition (T, 101–112), while Faye is conspicuously silent: we are told she reads the speech she has prepared, but we are not presented with what she delivers. Extremes are overtly addressed in this strategic narrative choice when so much of the central scene in *Transit* focuses on the staging of the writers as public characters who may happen to say something deep in the midst of their cacophonous banter (T, 113). 'While I perceive postmodernist rewriting as a deconstructive form of exposing the fabric and playing with the source-text's writing and interpretations, the intention and force of neo-modernist rewriting is primarily constructive' (Latham 2016: 7–8). This is how Latham justifies the classification of Cusk amongst neo-modernists, something which I will follow here, and which manifests already in her decision to show silence as a response to, rather than a lack of, communication. Cusk embarks upon a new form not to play with pre-existing texts but to seek new ways of delving into the psyche of contemporary characters.

The confessional aspect of Cusk's novels does not translate in the unity of a single place or in the development of close bonds between the characters. On the contrary, in order to enhance the ceaseless circulation of words, the characters are always in 'transit', in between planes and houses, as if suspended in mid-air, waiting to be anchored back to life, if mooring is still possible outside the safety measures of a travelling company. Their experience illustrates what Lacan says about the subject being a fleeting presence emerging in discourse, in between travelling signifiers in the metonymic chain of language. Faye seems to be in exile from everywhere, having returned to London after the end of her marriage, to a house that might become a home but is as of now inhospitable and where she knows nobody except her raging neighbours, angry that such a middle-class, single mother should have appropriated their space and put down walls. This symbolic exploration of the house is a recurrent Cuskian aspect (K, 94): she enjoys setting people that seem to be stuck in their homeless houses where they face silence and slow death. *The Country Life* was focused on the maze-like, haunting nature of a country mansion that was both the perfect setting for an escape and the eerie, threatening décor of a possible alienation (Boileau 2013a, 2013b); in *Arlington Park*, the houses of each of the protagonists are approached as an extension, if not a metonymic exploration, of their subjectivity, with a special focus on how space is in fact empty, like speech is silent: Ex-manager Amanda Clapp thus thinks she is pleased with her newly done house with its immense kitchen (the pronoun 'her' is used in the text) in the posh Western Gardens until she realises that 'they had created not space but emptiness' (AP, 64; see Boileau 2022).

The role played by houses in the trilogy is analysed by Valihora as partaking of the way marriage and home are understood as 'a primarily material thing' marked by 'almost compulsive acts of destruction and rebuilding' (Valihora 2019: 31). However, the home is also a metaphor for literature: 'people liked to live in old houses that had been thoroughly refurbished with modern conveniences, and I wondered whether the same principle might be applied to novels' (K, 37). Faye says that she likes to remind people that 'each reader came to your book a stranger who had to be persuaded to stay' (T, 114). The domestic situation of these women is not understood as an alienation to a stereotypical vision of womanhood, but as the site of constant renegotiations of the self. Here is what a student of her creative course explains when she is unable to produce any writing:

> I went to the kitchen and thought about trying to write a story. But all I could think of was a line describing the exact moment I was living in: *a woman stood in the kitchen and thought about trying to write a story.* The problem was that the line didn't connect to any other line. It hadn't come from anywhere and it wasn't going anywhere either, anymore than I was going anywhere by just standing in my kitchen. So I went to the other room... (O, 209)

It would be extremely tempting to read this as metaphorically emphasising the workings of the mind, the absolute aporia of storytelling, exemplified here in the absurd paraphrasis of life that the character who has signed up for a creative writing course is only capable of offering, and the importance of 'connection', which always defies Forster's well-known phrase. Some may even be tempted to use one of the old arguments (Lodge 1992) against Woolf and others that this speech does not sound like 'real speech' (Prose 2018). However, it connects the symbolic to the material, words to the body: 'the building was digesting me' (K, 43).

The literal aspect of this student's account of the writer's block cannot but evoke something more essential about the failure of language to connect with a more metaphorical level of meaning. Here language is used metonymically, as seen in the decision to change rooms in a logic of contiguity rather than association. In Forsterian fashion, Cusk can only envisage connection as sham—as when she opens an unsolicited email from an astrologer who tells her she 'feels a strong personal connection' with her (T, 2)—but it is also the aim of her writing to endlessly strive to achieve a connection of a different nature: this is a leitmotiv obsessively taken on by most of the people she comes across: 'In a way I don't care what I write – I just want that feeling of being in sync again, body and mind, do you know what I mean?' (O, 48). In the second volume, the same idea is taken on by someone else: 'Most marriages worked in the same way that stories are said to do through the suspension of disbelief' (T, 29) This is in part due to the incredible number of people she meets who are writers: the number is disproportionate to any realistic assumption of how many people in real life would devote their lives to writing.

CONFESSIONS, SILENCE AND HOW TALKING CURES, OR HOW MUCH SHE CARES

The characters' temptation for silence and Cusk's work on voices heard and unheard renew the exploration of psychic disorder and, I would argue, constitute the paradoxical, new mode of representation of delirium. Although the likening of Cusk's work with psychoanalysis is not pregnant in the first part of her works, in *Aftermath*, a shrink is mentioned as she tries to find ways of coping with her new celibacy. Jung is being read in *Transit* (T, 210) and psychoanalysis in general is at times referred to in the *Trilogy*: 'If, that is, psychoanalysts are to be believed when they say we are unconsciously drawn to the repetition of painful experiences' (K, 40). Most ironic of all, her direct references to the caring of the mind is the superimposition of psychoanalysis with an estate agent at the very beginning of the second volume: when she describes the estate agent who sold her the flat she is refurbishing, Faye clearly describes him in terms that are comparable to what she would have used for the work of an analyst: people talk to him of their intimacies, they evoke the 'throes of desire' (T, 5) leading him to describe himself as: 'a figure conjured out of the red mist of their desire, an object, so to speak, of transference' (T, 6). Here again, the analogy is more likely to be Cusk's than the estate agent's, especially because of the fairly technical reference to transference, showing that verisimilitude matters less than the flow of conversation and language. Besides, it furthers the association in Cusk's fiction of the house and the mind, as if the domestic sphere was a valid site of cognition. The whole structure of the novel in hindsight of such subtle references evokes the talking cure since the characters babble and associate ideas with only a very few prompts given by Faye, when there are any prompts.

At one point, Faye evokes the 'final surrender of personal consciousness into the public domain' (K, 12), reflecting on the uneasiness she feels at the public exposure of intimate questions that seem to guide contemporary life. This attitude evokes another technical or industrial revolution, of a magnitude comparable to that witnessed during Modernism, that is, the advent of voyeuristic social medias whose injunction is to show the world a life of leisure and luxury desirable and exclusive.

> [M]odernism weaves together the pleasure of the text and the unreadable, a term we understand to designate all that which falls from the process of signification, the literal residuum whose proliferation both threatens the

integrity of the message and confronts the reader with that element of unde-cipherability at the core of his/her own desire. (Alfandary and Nesme 2011:9)

The conflict between silence and excessive talk in Cusk's novels circum-vents the residuum caused by a symbolic order that has failed to be struc-turing. It can be identified as a symptom formation regarding some social or subjective disorder the characters are trying to cope with. She shows them how the written word can be a way of coming to terms with lan-guage that fails to be a choice against, if not a protection from, the mean-inglessness of a disconnected world, as seen in the overall presence of anxiety or depression in her work (O, ch. 4; *The Country Life*; *Arlington Park*).

Central to *Transit* is the staged confession of Julian and Louis, two suc-cessful writers who are given the floor at a book festival. It is unclear whether the confessions of the two writers are well-rehearsed or spontane-ous, but they are clearly based on 'the babbling, the telling... the messiest thing of all' which constitutes the material of the writer's labour because 'it was hard, hard to turn it around, to take the mess of experience and make something coherent out of it' (T, 100). Resounding with the mod-ernist aesthetics and psychoanalytic cure, this expression is soon linked to the word 'inhibition' (T, 101) and the question of defining subjective truth(s), which Louis translates as what he 'assiduously hid from others' (T, 102), except in the one novel he could write before he was known. This explanation leads to a reflection on writing as not dependent on facts, for Louis, unlike for Julian, but on the possibility of allowing oneself to say something and therefore to make it fit into the structure of language: 'A lot of writers seemed to think that the higher a truth—or to be more accu-rate, since truth was something altogether different, a fact—was pitched from the earth the less of a supporting structure it required' (T, 107). The distinction between fact (which concerns shared reality) and truth (which Freud, Lacan and Miller have consistently elaborated as a fleeting pres-ence, which appears like a revelation and escapes any form of psychological and rational scaffolding)[5] is a leitmotiv of the characters in general, who often seem to regard reality as fake, the real as something which surfaces unexpectedly and language as an instrument of dissimulation.

---

[5] I refer readers to Miller's reading of Lacan's interpretation of Freud's conception (Miller 2016).

'Where hair is concerned, Dale said, the fake generally seemed to be more real than the real' (T, 60). The hair salon is not the only place where such unexpected deep reflections are revealed. Another character says she has a 'feeling of unreality' (T, 227) and Gerard, her former lover whom Faye bumps into unexpectedly, thinks 'there's too much irony. You can't be a poseur here. Everything is already an imitation of itself' (T, 26). On board the plane, the man sitting next to her muses that his wife's profession is 'an escape from reality' (K, 34). The associative, metonymic narratives offered by the characters are like the patients in a therapeutic session, they resound and rebound loaded with more meaning than they had to start with, but that meaning is never stopped or fixed until someone like Faye interrupts the meaningful formations by asking a question. Like in such a session, Faye or the characters stop their linguistic meandering according to a subjective logic that is to be interpreted. One of Faye's many recently divorced friends explains: 'There has been a great harvest, he said, of language and information from life, and it may have become the case that the faux-human was growing more substantial than the original, that there was more tenderness to be had from a machine than from one's fellow man' (T, 3). The irony of her reported speech verbs 'He believed' when she is dealing with esoteric beliefs resonates with the emptied-out presence of God and it does even more so as Faye remains silent, allowing the chamber of meaningful echoes to expand.[6]

Less anecdotal is the recurrent but discreet concerns of Faye's acquaintances for psychic instability and their difficulty to cope with it. In the beginning of *Kudos*, which replays the beginning of *Outline*, with a character's confession on the plane, the man starts evoking his daughter's 'depression' (K, 13), thanks to his dog, Pilot, endowed with the capacity to sense disorder and dysfunction well before things get wrong. Faye clearly takes the stance of the analyst, or the interviewer (see metatextual interview K, 144), this time round questioning the man as to why he had not paid attention to his daughter's practising the oboe and why, when he saw her perform well on stage, he had cried, offering an interpretation about his fear that there might have been something wrong with her: 'I said it seemed to me people often found it easier to entertain that idea about their children than about themselves, and he looked at me as though he were momentarily considering that theory before firmly shaking his

---

[6] I laughed enthusiastically at this and was mortified to hear my laughter make its solo flight across the table (Cusk 1997: 122).

head' (K, 17). Unaware that Betsy seems to use the dog as a way of relating to her father, or replacing him during his long absences, and ready to imagine that she likes the dog because 'he couldn't speak and therefore lie' (K, 19), the father explains how behavioural symptoms with no evident causality led him to construct his daughter as an enigma:

> From earliest childhood, he said, Betsy had been unlike other children—and not in a good way. She was unbelievably neurotic… As she grew older the most serious problem of all became her extraordinary sensitivity to what she called lying, but what was actually as far as he could see the normal conventions and speech patterns of adult conversation. She claimed that most of what people said was fake and insincere, and when he'd asked her how she could possibly know that, she replied that she could tell by the sound…he had noticed that his wife was growing increasingly silent, which he believed to be Betsy's doing, by creating such a minefield around communication that it was easier to say nothing at all. (K, 17–19)

Parents are left perplexed by their children's new symptoms because these manifestations often fail to be analysed outside behavioural aspects, and instead come to constitute that which needs getting rid of because they are antisocial. Betsy's concern for the semblance of everyday speech does not lead her to speak the truth, but to stop speaking, as if language itself contained this inescapable semblance of which she would partake—this is suggested by the sounds of language and the voices which one could interpret also from the logic of hallucinations. This is something I can only venture since this 'discreet' symptom is not developed to the full, especially since the series of characters whose dysfunctional relation with language and others is labelled after a psychiatric nosography that obscures the subject's suffering instead of 'explaining' it.

These symptoms of mental disorders are often evoked in conjunction with the question of the couple, which Cusk does not explore solely through lovers but also in the relationship between parents and children. Faye's children incidentally are ghost-like presences that surface in the form of phone calls but from whom she is as distant as she is with other people: she seems to allow them to live off their wits' ends, travelling the world without them. At the very end of the trilogy, her son phones her to express in a very blunt way: 'I feel so lonely, he said, and yet I have no privacy' and he ponders that even slitting one's wrists cannot attract other people's attention (K, 229). He thus underlines what had been outlined before, this tension between the inside and outside that has now become reversed, the tension between urgency and calm, loneliness and solitude. In *Outline*, there is a son labelled as a schizophrenic for symptoms that seem to consist of drug addiction, phone obsession and lack of communication. This is so unbearable in Cusk's world of fiction in which subjectivity verges on an autistic rejection of otherness that the father is led to 'incarcerate' his son and reject his calls because he fears an excess of talk that he himself cannot stomach, no more than his previous wife or the helper they have hired, despite his own endless rants to Faye:

> I asked what was wrong with his son and his birdlike face grew sombre. Was I familiar with the condition called schizophrenia? Well, that was what his son suffered from. He had developed it in his twenties after leaving university, and had been hospitalised several times over the past decade, but for a number of reasons too complicated to explain he was currently in his father's care. My neighbour had judged that he was safe enough on the island, so long as he didn't get his hands on any money. (O, 62)

Schizophrenia is said to be a 'condition' which functions according to different modes of relation and/or connection: if the father knows when the condition emerged and is articulate about ways in which this condition might be managed, he seems to be reluctant to or ignorant of its mode of transmission or infection. His way of handling the child is based on his intention to control him and to keep him safely away from human exchange and connection.

There is therefore a tendency to reflect a world in which disconnection and silence, even when not seen as pathological, are concomitantly perceived as therapeutic. What is also striking in this passage is how slippery the narrative voice becomes, moving from free indirect speech to a return to the narrator as focaliser, as if the narrator and the characters' voices were disembodied echoes that communally signalled the defeat of narration: 'The tone and cadences of Paula's voice seemed almost to be coming from inside me' (T, 178). As the novels unfold, it becomes clear that these subtly detailed yet slightly marginal symptoms of disorders are also a way of reflecting upon the absence of clear-cut boundaries between people, voices and identities and thus no longer any absolute limit to the possibility that 'the world itself is without meaning', to quote *Mrs Dalloway* again (D, 75). Faye dines with two Greek women, one of whom has just returned from a poetry reading where there were only six attendees. Among them was a man who always comes to the events she does and makes faces at her without ever speaking to her: '"I prefer to call it madness," she said, "whether his or my own, and so instead I have tried to become fond of him. I look up and there he always is, waggling his fingers and sticking out his tongue. He is in fact entirely dependable, and more faithful to me than any lover I've ever had. I try to love him back"' (O, 188). The transitivist aspect of this madness subtly and discreetly indicates that everyone is indeed on the verge of a nervous breakdown. The comparison with a lover at this moment obviously points to a connection that needs delving into.

This example points to a connection to be made between the subjective vagrancy noted before and the gradual change from a social order ensured in the middle-class marriage ('it had occurred to her that by calling her husband and putting an end to the feeling of being unmoored and adrift, she may have missed the opportunity to miss something' (K, 56)), and a lack of human stability propelled by the gradual progress of personal devices and autistic forms of enjoyment, the collapse of family ties of which divorce and its 'aftermath' only highlight the warfare individuals have to come to terms with. Faye's son, when anxious that the police may come after him, says: 'Sometimes I feel as if I'm about to fall over the edge of something, and that there'll be nothing and no one to catch me' (K, 229). Needless to say, Cusk is not advocating a return to a sort of glorious, idealised past of white, middle-class stability, but she is dissecting the subjective aftermath of new modes of relationships which dislocate lives, that is, language, bodies and representation. Men and women are thus presented in violent exchanges, their relationship is, when not conflictual, marked by the violence of enigmatic responses and attitudes that are impossible to decipher, as when Faye is violently kissed by a man who up to now had made no move to seduce her and about whom the reader has had no inkling that she could be wanting this kiss. This man has just confessed that he was embarrassed by his father in ways that caused him to feel anxiety. When asked by Faye what exactly his father did, the man confesses that he couldn't articulate it and starts feeling more defiant: 'He didn't know why he had told me that, he added after a while. It was something he didn't usually talk about' (T, 125). The breach of his silence, which is consistent with most of the characters in the novel, although most is done with 'abashed and easy confidentiality' (K, 10), is marked on his body which now acts on an impulse, as if the unleashing of the confession had imposed its violent mark on his behaviour:

When I turned around again, he took two rapid strides towards me. He seemed to be crossing some unfathomable element or chasm-like space, where things fell and broke far down in the darkness against its deeps. His body reached mine and he pushed me back against the door and kissed me. He put his warm, thick tongue in my mouth; he thrust his hands inside my coat. His lean, hard body was more insistent than forceful. I felt the soft, expensive clothes he was dressed in and the hot skin beneath them. He moved his face away from mine for a moment in order to speak...

He kissed me for a long time. Other than that remark, no one said anything. There were no explanations or endearments.... When our bodies eventually came apart, I moved away and twisted the door handle and opened the door a few inches. He stepped back; he seemed to be grinning...

Good night, I said. (T, 126–7)

Perhaps playing with the well-known comedy trope, 'Speak, cousin; or, if thou cannot, stop his mouth with a kiss, and let not him speak neither' (Sharkespeare 1613: II, 1, 286–87), this scene is clearly defined by its enigmatic nature, its verging on abuse. This is how the structure of the novel presents it as a response to a situation in which communication failed in the transmission of meaning but still operates at the level of desire. The abyss between the two characters is evocative of Lacan's assertion that there is no sexual relationship, which translates as meaning that between men and women there is an impassable gulf that is here broken down (Lacan 1975). Faye becomes therefore not so much the voyeur but the object of desire, circulating between people, and fascinating the readers. The failure of spoken words is translated into a bodily encounter that breaks through the rules of propriety like the irruption of something unwelcome, perceived in the description of the sexual act visible on the body. Faye's return to the most hackneyed phrase, 'good-bye', unveils the preceding breach of decency which enacts the subtext of the novels.

DESIRE, THE BODY AND THE COUPLE AS CONTEMPORARY SYMPTOMS

The novels delve into a question nowadays perhaps regarded as conservative, the heterosexual couple that has inherently been perceived as the epitome of a way of thinking about gender as fixed and normative. '[T]he cynicism of our gender politics' (O, 107) results in the following reflection: 'this notion, of the unitary self being broken down, of consciousness not as an imprisonment in one's own perceptions but rather as something more intimate and less divided' (T, 198). The impassable fracture between men and women, in the context of the collapse of patriarchal ideals, discourses and norms and the new wave of feminist and post-feminist thinking is acknowledged in the text: '"talking to this journalist," she continued, "whose name was I have mentioned Olga, I wondered whether my whole existence—even my feminism—had been a compromise. I felt it had lacked seriousness. Even my writing had been treated as a kind of hobby"' (O, 107–108). It is true that almost all the characters have something to say about the patriarchal, outdated model of marriage and the possibility of union forming which seems to have guided their action and behaviour while it is language itself that is affected by this impossible union that silences, makes invisible, and ultimately pushes people to revert to a state of inhibition. The myth of the androgyn with which Lacan starts his exploration of love in *Encore* (Lacan 1975) is here again envisaged, but contrary to when psychoanalysis emerged, it has now become clear romance cannot be successful: 'Each of them saw things solely from his own perspective: there was only one point of view' (O, 83), which is different from a 'shared vision' in which two humans collide. 'He's me, she said…. I'm him, she said, then added, slightly impatiently: we're the same' (K, 134).

A friend of Faye's tells her how he realised that the end of his marriage was about to happen when up on a mountain with his children, he called his wife to let her know that he was panicking and wondered if he might not collapse; his wife responded with a long silence:

> Most of all [our life-long engagement] wanted silence: and this, I realised, was what my conversations with Chrysta were all leading towards, a silence that would in the end remain unbroken, though on this occasion she did break it. I'm sure you'll manage somehow, was what she said. And shortly after, the conversation concluded. (O, 121)

Since silence is a suspicious sign of disconnection, it is often filled in with internal contradictions and interruptions conjured up by the characters in what is clearly a form of storytelling that gives pride of place to gaps, silence and innuendos. '"… an island you certainly would not have heard of, despite its prolixity to some well known tourist destination." Proximity, I said, I think you mean proximity' (O, 8). The slip of tongue becomes a pun enabling Cusk, on the threshold of her fictional space, to infer that proximity may be achieved through prolixity, a programmatic notion of what the author is trying to achieve by exploring voices and silence, chatter and confessions, and so forth.

When Faye discusses couples with her cousin Lawrence, the conservative nature of such essentialising talk is first pointed out when Eloise bursts 'into loud laughter', adding 'what a ridiculous thing to say'. She is responding to her husband's explanation of Faye's distress after her separation: "'That wasn't fate," Lawrence said. "It was because you're a woman"' (T, 241). Lawrence voices a certain idea of women's disadvantage. The scene once again refers to the esoteric, bringing us back to the beginning of the novel, when Faye reads the emails she has received from an unsolicited astrologer. This evokes Lacan's remark that truth has a surreal dimension:

> A truth, if it must be said, is not easy to recognize once it has become received. Not that there aren't any established truths, but they are so easily confused with the reality that surrounds them that no other artifice was for a long time found to distinguish them from it than to mark them with the sign of the spirit/the wit and, in order to pay them homage, to regard them as having come from another world. (Lacan 1966, 405)

Throughout the trilogy, sexist remarks and misogynistic comments surface and indicate one of the modalities of disconnection between contemporary subjects. When she meets a man on the plane to whom she explains that she is a writer going to a literary festival, the answer she gets is: "'My wife's a big reader," he said. "She belongs to one of those book clubs"' (K, 5). The ordinariness of the remark's tone does not preclude its deep misogyny, discreetly announced by the use of 'those' rather than 'one of these' or even more neutral 'a'.

This is the underlying subtext of all the novels, that Faye is indeed intent on getting confessions about how others find a way of coping with solitude and the persistence of other people's silences and meaningless voices, even if this means unveiling a core element of unwelcome violence and dispossession often illustrated by the conflict between men and women. 'Something that looked good on the outside turned out to be full of violence and hatred. And in that scenario, he said, to be female was to be inherently at a disadvantage, just as it would have been in a physical fight' (T, 242). Central to Cusk's writing emerges a silent conflict between the sexes which gives rise to many symptoms, in conjunction with contemporary psychoanalytic diagnoses of pathological use of language—pathologic to be understood here as making the subject suffer and not as inherently pathological. Towards the end of the first volume, a man confesses:

> I realised, he said, that my whole understanding of life had been, in some sense, profoundly adversarial: the story of men and women, for me, was ultimately a story of war, to the extent that I wondered sometimes whether I had an actual horror of peace, whether I thought to stir things up out of a fear of boredom that was also, you might say, a fear of death itself. I said to you, when we first met, that I regard love—the love between man and woman—as the great regenerator of happiness, but it is also the regenerator of interest. It is what you would call the storyline. (O, 166–67)

Storytelling is ultimately the objective of Cusk's reform. True, she is not considering the other of the heterosexual relation, and for that, her vision of love will not appeal to many who are involved in the visibilisation of minorities. Yet what she works on is also, and more importantly, the fragile relation that can be made between subjects, even in heterosexual relationships: 'It was impossible, I said in response to his question, to give the reasons why the marriage had ended. Among other things a marriage is a system of belief, a story, and though it manifests itself in things that are real enough, the impulse that drives it is ultimately mysterious' (O, 12). It is clear that if Faye listens so painstakingly to the stories of others, it is because she is intent on finding out something about a reality that baffles her, but her interest is not to solve the mystery, but to be filled in with partial stories: 'Most marriages worked in the same way that stories are said to do, through the suspension of disbelief' (T, 29).

It is interesting that structurally she returns to the question of the couple at the end of the second novel. Faye is portrayed exiting the house of fiction she has created without saying anything to her hosts, and the only thing that the reader may be able to construe at this stage is that her exit may be related to the fact that she has just been forced to expose and discuss her own divorce: as pointed out at the beginning of this chapter, it is divorce that Cusk places as the tipping-point of silence. She restores the semblance of small talk after the man kisses her during the novel's unfolding, but even that dimension of language collapses once it is her own adversarial relationship with men that is evoked: after a dinner with her cousin, appropriately called Lawrence, his new wife and his/their kids, during which dinner Faye was forced into a confession about having met a new lover, Faye tries to trace the source of the collapse of her marriage. Interestingly, as an echo to the story of Betsy or the schizophrenic son, it is the show of her sons fighting and of the older one banging her younger son's head against the countertop that reveals to her the fracture of her marriage, as if her 'children had merely acted in the service of this knowledge' (T, 234). The violence of the scene is not followed by a conversation discussing its cause, but by a revelation of the truth of this outburst. As if this underlying violence, this rest of the conversation, continued to circulate, she wakes up in the morning and leaves without saying good-bye or meeting her hosts again: 'I felt change far beneath me, moving deep beneath the surface of things, like the plates of the earth blindly moving in their black traces. I found my bag and my car keys and I let myself silently out of the house' (T, 260). Such an ending interrogates the boundaries between illusion and reality, fiction and fact, autofiction and autobiography, narrator and narrative, and enables the 'reader to find, in idealizations, bids for freedom, and dreams of exaltation, something better' (Valihora 2019: 35). The scene also reflects back upon the transient presence of others in one's life, how their exit forces us into strange combinations and uncanny relationships, silence here being echoed with violence, rudeness, impoliteness and the impulsive nature of a body that literally seeks to be off stage, despite the omnipresence of sex.

The body, like the relationships in marriage or families, is the site of a necessary process of connection that fails, as pointed out in the very first pages: 'In a way, I don't care what I write—I just want that feeling of being sync again, body and mind, do you know what I mean?' (O, 48). The body needs more careful scrutiny because it is situated at a place that is normally made invisible by writing: 'But it always surprised me, I said, that writers didn't feel more fear of the physical exposure such events entailed, given that writing and reading were non-physical transactions, and might be said to represent a mutual escape from the actual body' (T, 115). The body emerges from these reflections as inherently different or disconnected from the subject, having a life of its own and it seems that the subject needs to be anchored back to it somehow. Writing therefore constitutes a sort of substitute for this re-connection because it consists in trying to at least fathom the cause of this discomfort.

> As for the weight, he said, you rarely saw yourself with your clothes off, or anyone else without theirs for that matter. He remembered the feeling of estrangement from his own body, as it laboured in the damp, spore-ridden climate of the house; his clogged lungs and itchy skin, his veins full of sugar and fat, his wobbling flesh shrouded in uncomfortable clothing. As a teenager, he was self-conscious and sedentary and avoided any physical exposure of himself. (O, 38)

The last scene of the trilogy offers itself as an enigmatic conclusion that ties all these elements back together without necessarily offering a conclusive meaning: Faye, who has just been on the phone to her son who wants her to come home, prolongs her stay abroad by going to the beach which 'was wild and strewn with litter' (K, 230). There she comes to a beach that is a nudist, if not a cruising, male gay area, described first in a sort of apocalyptic vision (wind and waves unleashed, no visibility, human presence in shadow or 'low sound of conversation') where she clearly is unwelcome: there is a group who 'turned to look at me like animals surprised in a grove' (K, 231). After going into the sea for a swim, she comes back out of the water to witness a man coming in the other direction, resolutely flashing his manhood at her:

> He came to a halt just where the waves broke and he stood there in his nakedness like a deity, resplendent and grinning. Then he grasped his thick penis and began to urinate into the water…. He looked at me with black eyes full of malevolent delight while the golden jet poured unceasingly forth from him until it seemed impossible that he could contain any more. The water bore me up, heaving, as if I lay on the breast of some sighing creature while the man emptied himself into its depths. I looked into his cruel, merry eyes, and I waited for him to stop. (K, 232)

The mythical creature of the sea shows Cusk recalling some of the most persistent images to evoke *jouissance* in a mixture of pleasure and pain, sex and primitive needs, malevolence and connection which she here knots back together in a scene that is threatening and menacing, but which also enables her to make him stop, to become stronger as a result, where she was first thought to be so frail, hidden in her silence.

If Cusk's silence in the form of her narrator, Faye, has strained some critics' nerves, it may well be because, like the delirium of Septimus, this silence is mysterious, impossible to interpret and forces us (as well as the characters) to face the aporia of contemporary relationships in which Cusk only sees confrontation or tragic break-ups. 'I read aloud what I had written. When I had finished I folded the papers and put them in my bag' (T, 113). Time and again, the narrator–writer is portrayed in her absence, her capacity to listen but not speak, her elusiveness. It is as if she was either entirely constrained by her own fear of exposure or entirely dependent upon the words of others which are the only way for her to circumscribe a meaningful experience. The last volume, *Kudos*, starts with an epigraph of a poem by Stevie Smith, only published for the first time in 2015 by Faber and Faber, but initially written in the 1960s: 'She got up and went away/ Should she not have? Not have what? Got up and gone away'. The poem's iterative style, using childish phrasing, borders on emptiness and enables Cusk to comment on the ending of the previous novel in which she got up and went away, tracing the trajectory of her own character back to other authors but also perhaps as far back as *Genesis* where the phrase is borrowed from. Cusk is implying both a lineage with other such women whose resistance could be comprehended in their opposition to the discourse of truthfulness and confession in which we now live, as well as suggesting that what was once described in the refrain of Stevie Smith now needs a new mundane form of expression. At the beginning of *Transit*, Cusk devotes a fair amount of her narrative to the refurbishing of the place Faye has just bought, placing great emphasis on the builder's sorry feelings for her bad choice. His unexpected confession to her signifies the tension she explores between the outward exposure of everyone's intimate feelings and thoughts and the solitude of someone who is ready to connect with a client. The builder's attention to being requested for the most belittling tasks ('He hadn't literally been asked—if I would excuse his language—to wipe someone's arse for them' (T, 53)) together with his insistence on the debasing effects of his divorce are put an end to when Faye attentively observes the insides of his van, where all she can see is the litter of a solitary quotidian:

> I saw the cab was full of empty carboard coffee cups and discarded food packaging and scraps of paper. Like I said, the builder said ruefully, the job involves a lot of driving. Sometimes he was in his van the whole day and ate all three meals there. You end up sitting in your own leavings, he said, shaking his head. (T, 58)

This rest, the litter of life, which is here materialised, is what literature has to deal with and all the subjects in Cusk's fiction have to expose this rest, which is no longer carefully hidden by any process of repression. They thus show her with affected, if not humorous, regret, rather than shame, what it is their lives are filled with and her fiction is indeed based on the delicate equilibrium she seeks to achieve, a form of transient order that she writes about, lest we become obsessed with the mess.

BIBLIOGRAPHY

PRIMARY SOURCES

Cusk, Rachel (1997). *The Country Life*. London: Picador.
Cusk, Rachel (2009). "Shakespeare's Daughters", *The Guardian*. 12 December 2009. http://www.guardian.co.uk/books/2009/dec/12/rachel-cusk-women-writing-review
Cusk, Rachel (2018). Kudos Trilogy. Outline. 2014; Transit. 2016; Kudos. 2018. London: Faber and Faber.
Shakespeare, William (1613). *Much Ado About Nothing*. London: Penguin, 1996.

SECONDARY SOURCES

Alfandary, Isabelle and Nesme, Axel (eds.) (2011). *Modernism and Unreadability*. Montpellier: Presses Universitaires de la Méditerranée.
Biggs, Joanna (2012). "Clytemnestra in Brighton." *London Review of Books*, 34: 6, March 22, 2012.
Boileau, Nicolas Pierre, Hanson, Clare & Tang, Maria (eds.) (2013). "Kay Boyle/Rachel Cusk: (Neo) Modernist Voices." *E-Rea*, 10.2, 2013 https://journals.openedition.org/erea/2966
Boileau, Nicolas Pierre (2013a). "A Novelist in Changing Rooms: Motherhood and Auto/biography." N. Boileau et al. (eds.) (2013) https://journals.openedition.org/erea/3243
Boileau, Nicolas Pierre (2013b). "Not feminine enough? Rachel Cusk's highly-feminised world and unfeminine characters in *Saving Agnes* and *The Country Life.*" *Anglistik*, "Focus on the Feminisation of Writing", Barbara Puschmann-Nalenz (ed.), Spring 2013, 39–49.
Boileau, Nicolas Pierre (2015). "'In Some Rare and Sacred Dead Time…, there is a Miracle of Silence.' On Not Lifting the Veil in Mc Gregor's and Cusk's Novels." *L'Atelier*, vol.7, No. 2, 2015, http://ojs.u-paris10.fr/index.php/latelier/article/view/428
Boileau, Nicolas Pierre (2022). "Suburbia, or *Para*-urbia: Rachel Cusk's Gendered Readings of Suburban Spaces and the Role of the Writer in *Arlington Park.*" M. Bouchet, I. Keller-Privat et al. (eds.) (2022). *Suburbs. New Literary Perspectives*. Rowman and Littlefield.

Bradbury, Malcolm & McFarlane, James (eds.) (1976). *Modernism (1890–1930)*. London: Penguin Books, reprinted 1991.

Childs, Peter (2012). *Contemporary Fiction: British Novelists since 1970*. London: Palgrave Macmillan.

Cohn, Dorrit (1978). *Transparent Minds, Narrative Modes for Presenting Consciousness in Fiction*. Princeton. Princeton UP.

Derbyshire, Jonathan (2012). "A Writer with a Splinter of Ice in her Heart". *The New Statesman*, 5 March 2012.

Gallagher, Lucy (2011). *The Contemporary Middlebrow Novel*. Unpublished Ph.D. thesis, Newcastle University, 2011.

Kellaway, Kate (2001). "Mother's ruin." *The Observer*, 9 September 2001.

Kellaway, Kate (2014). Interview of Rachel Cusk, 24 August 2014, last checked May 2022. https://www.theguardian.com/books/2014/aug/24/rachel-cusk-interview-aftermath-outline

Lacan, Jacques (1966). *Écrits* I. Paris: Éditions du Seuil, "Essais Points", 1999.

Lacan, Jacques (1975). *Le Séminaire, Livre XX, Encore* (1972–73). J.-A. Miller (ed.). Paris: Éditions du Seuil.

Latham, Monica (2013). *"Arlington Park:* Variations on Virginia Woolf's *Mrs Dalloway"*. Boileau et al. (eds.) (2013) https://journals.openedition.org/erea/3216

Latham, Monica (2016). *A Poetics of Postmodernism and Neomodernism*. New York: Routledge.

Lockwood, Patricia (2018). "Why do I have to know what MacDonald's is?" *London Review of Books*, vol. 40, No.9, 10 May 2018, https://www.lrb.co.uk/the-paper/v40/n09/patricia-lockwood/why-do-i-have-to-know-what-mcdonald-s-is

Lodge, David (1992). *The Art of Fiction*, London: Vintage, 2011.

Lucey, Michael (2022). *What Proust Heard and the Ethnography of Talk*. Chicago: The University of Chicago Press.

Lyotard, Jean-François (1984). *The Postmodern Condition, A Report on Knowledge*. Minneapolis: University of Minnesota Press.

McAlpin, Heller (2018). "An Epic Conversation Draws to a Close in *Kudos*." https://www.npr.org/2018/06/05/613465563/an-epic-conversation-draws-to-a-close-in-kudos?t=1622381639864 last checked May 2022.

Messud, Claire (2017). "Fierce, She Got Outside the Moment". *The New York Review of Books*, March, 23rd, 2017: https://www.nybooks.com/articles/2017/03/23/rachel-cusk-transit-fierce-outside-moment/ (checked in May 2022)

Prose, Francine (2018). "Real Talk: Rachel Cusk's *Kudos"*. *The Sewanee Review*, 126.3, 520–534.

Rannou, Isabelle (2013). "'Like journeying through a painting': Travel Writing and the Exploration of Textual Boundaries in Rachel Cusk's *The Last Supper"*.

E-rea, 10.2 | 2013, checked on 27 Dec. 2017. URL: http://journals.openedition.org/erea/3235

Ricœur, Paul (1984). "Entre le temps mortel et le temps monumental: *Mrs Dalloway*". *Temps et récit*, vol. 2, *La Configuration du récit de fiction*. Paris: Éditions du seuil, 1984, 192–212.

Tang, Maria (2013). "Bodies at Risk: Ambiguous Subjectivities in *Arlington Park*. A Beauvoirean Perspective". Boileau et al. (eds.), 2013.

Tayler, Christopher (2005). "Imbued... with Exigence". *London Review of Books*, vol. 27, No.18, 22 September 2005, https://www.lrb.co.uk/the-paper/v27/n18/christopher-tayler/imbued-with-exigence

Valihora, Karen (2019). "She Got Up and Went Away: Rachel Cusk on Making an Exit". *English Studies in Canada*, 45.1–2 (March/June 2019): 19–35.

CHAPTER 8

Ali Smith's Voices: Everyone Is Delirious

The examples taken in this book have contributed to identifying voice and silence as core symptomatic formations in response to the enigmatic, opaque and fragmentary experience of contemporary life. Since Septimus Warren Smith in *Mrs Dalloway*, British novelists have expressed the disconnection from direct access to reality through communication that fails, characters that are dialectically pitted against one another and forms of speech that explore the edge of signification, where language may be a mode of enjoyment instead of a way of communicating feelings and meanings. The novels studied so far have circumscribed a hole in knowledge and expression, without seeking to resolve it: the characters are shown to be able to invent temporary solutions, often through singular ways of negotiating their relations with others. I argue that these novels' connection to the modernist aesthetics can be traced at this juncture, where voiced thoughts point to the failure of communication and the necessity to find substitutes that secure connections and bonds with others all the same. In 2016, Ali Smith decided to further this exploration of fragmentation by publishing successively four novels titled after the seasons, one novel published every year (2016–2020). The project was announced before the novels were completed, and the covers designed before the novels had been written, already pointing to a taste for indeterminacy and lack of linearity. The stories are almost independent, even if in *Summer*,

© The Author(s), under exclusive license to Springer Nature Switzerland AG 2023
N. P. Boileau, *Mental Health Symptoms in Literature since Modernism*, Palgrave Studies in Literature, Science and Medicine, https://doi.org/10.1007/978-3-031-37630-6_8

the last volume, some of the characters return and previously unsuspected connections are made apparent. The novels have now become examples of 'Brex-lit' (Shaw 2018: 21), a literature produced as a consequence or explanation of Brexit, a major political event that seems to consecrate the willingness of the British people to be set apart from the rest of Europe. The cycle of Smith's novels seems to have originated in the feelings of ultimate severing of ties and disconnection caused by the vote that the United Kingdom would leave the European Union. Reflecting about the state of the nation now that separation is branded as valid policy, Smith suggests that separation does not preclude a form of community that her novels seek to restore.

Commentators of contemporary fiction have already hailed the quartet as masterpieces, notably emphasising such themes as the link between politics and time (Anderson 2012; Shaw 2018; Rau 2018; Bernard 2015, 2019: par.27; 2022; Mulalić 2020), and the novels' impregnation in its own present: 'Context. It matters', says Sacha's mother to her daughter who is reluctant to find out the source of a quote by Hannah Arendt she would like to use for an essay on forgiveness (SQ4, 10). Some have explored political conflicts (Heynders 2021) or the questions of migration, borders and the present (Masterson 2020). The novels' political nature is undeniable, but I want to argue that it goes far beyond the contextual question of Brexit: Bernard talks about its 'political valence' (Bernard 2022: 15) 'delineat[ing]… a dark collective fate whose inexorability seems the outcome of a systemic necropolitics affecting both the body politic and the planet threatened with ecocide' (Bernard 2022: 21). I follow Wally, who makes a crucial distinction between political strategies and politics in a novel (Wally 2018: 81), a distinction that enables her to study the novels without much heed to the contemporary present of Brexit and to highlight instead Smith's concern for notions of ethics and engagement.

Another important idea that has attracted the critics' attention is the link between this general definition of politics and the question of illness. Thus, the novels are said to 'interrogat[e] the nation's pathology that resulted in the referendum campaign and subsequent fracturing of the populace' (Shaw 2018: 22). The metaphor of a sick body politic is often used, underlined by the concept behind the novels since the seasonal titles evoke the cycle of time as well as the inevitable loss resulting from such time passing. Heynders, for example, quotes Rancière's definition of writing as 'deciphering the symptoms of a state of things' (Heynders 2021: 40). Political divisions are said to have inspired the analogy: Hughes further argues that Brexit is often described in a psychiatric language, as 'madness' (Hughes 111), 'mental disorder', 'national masochism and self-harm' (Hughes 113) (qd in Dobrogoszcz 2021: 141); the Covid pandemic, which is referred to in *Summer*, happened while Smith was writing and publishing the tetralogy, inviting such comparison between the state of the nation and images of sickness too. It could not but consolidate the image of a body politic whose health needed tending to. It has become customary to think of contemporary fiction as exploring crises in terms of disease through the prevalent concept of trauma: 'employing self-conscious and ironic textual devices that question trauma's prominent post-9/11 placement, both as a diagnostic category and as a cultural and political discourse' (Horton 2012: 639). Horton talks about the trauma of fantasy and not just 'event-based' responses of a traumatic nature. This analogy was further developed by Bernard who suggests literature comes to 'crystallize [the full magnitude of the identity crisis of Brexit] in a dizzying conflation of political agency and symptomatology' (Bernard 2019: par.2) before analysing the effect of the four novels along the lines of immunology and Covid (Bernard 2022; Masterson 2020). I want to show that there is another type of illness that is hinted at, madness, but in its generalised form and as a subjective experience. This means that Smith foregrounds the originality of subjective responses to reality, while norms and accepted or shared views of the world collapse. This has resulted in political and sociological turmoil: the author presents us with characters that are faced with the pluralisation/multiplication of master narratives that leaves them all fairly vulnerable in their ways of inhabiting language and in their subjective place.

The novels immediately strike one as situated on the edge between legacy and modernity, replaying some of the tropes of modernist, postmodern and contemporary fiction (Germanà 2017: 99) in such a special way that form at times seems to be conspicuous and overwhelming. Smith has now a reputation for her postmodernist strategies and intertextuality (Bernard et al. 2014: par.14–17). Diane Leblond explains: 'Wordplay reminds us that the main concern in linguistic creativity is to reach out to a listener or a reader' (Bernard et al. 2014: par.24). As with many novelists, critics fail to agree on whether she is or isn't a modernist (Mulalić 2020: 48): 'many reviewers … place *Autumn* in the tradition of high modernism, relating the novel to works such as Marcel Proust…*Autumn* is ultimately a meditation on human identity' (Wally 2018: 77). Opposing this view, Ley calls Smith's style 'a kind of ersatz modernism' (Ley 2020).

Smith's formal experimentations are often compared to D.H. Lawrence's, Mansfield's (with the reference to 'Bliss' (Orosz-Réti 2021: 64)) or Woolf's (Germanà 2017: 99). Like Woolf, Smith is accused of giving a voice only to the middle classes and not being convincing about the subaltern voices of migrants (Mulalić 2020: 47). Perhaps the references to Lawrence and Woolf are the most consistently indexed to her major works, as Ryan-Sautour underlines: 'Virginia Woolf clearly haunts the pages of *Shire*' (Bernard 2015: par.27) or 'It can be considered that Smith, like Woolf in *Mrs. Dalloway*, "creates a common world that includes separation itself"' in the words of Jacques Rancière (Tollance 2020: 83).

Whether successful or not, Smith connects her own work to that of her modernist predecessors, offering a lineage that pays tribute to the Modernist attempts at capturing the loss inherent in subjective experience. In *Spring*, Smith praises Mansfield who 'made them seem suburban, Woolf, Bell, the Bloomsburys…' (SQ3, 39). In *Summer*, the author makes an indirect reference to the literary canon again, when one of the characters reads a novel that she thus describes: 'It's okay, sub-Woolfian, well' (SQ4, 161). More structural perhaps is the example of how intersemiotic references work in *Autumn*: Elisabeth is a specialist of an artist, Boty, who made her name as a collage artist, one of the fragmentary artforms that emerged with modernism (Reynier 2021: 24) and is evoked in the opening scene of *To the Lighthouse*. This goes to show that however slippery the reference, Smith is aligned with Woolf in her quest for a form to accommodate the fragmentary/fragmented nature of experience and account for the infinitesimal, even if she is aiming for the bigger picture too. Like in *Mrs Dalloway*, *Cymbeline* is referred to in the tetralogy (SQ2, 200), but beyond these clues that perhaps say more about the critics' ability to recognise them than about their meaningful function, Smith's connection to Woolf has become public knowledge when she praised the work of her 'foresister' in *Artful*, by underlining what makes them so close stylistically speaking—their shared interest in the way the novel's form shapes and reflects life:

> Even Woolf, who knew the novel form differently, being one of the few people successful in remaking it (interestingly enough via a great deal of initial help from the critical eye and advice of her friend and rival, the short story writer Mansfield), depends on chronology. The wanderings in time of *Mrs. Dalloway* have to be held in the matrix of a single day. (Smith 2012: 30)

An undeniable feature of Smith's Modernism is her interest in voices and bodies, two attributes of singularity that she questions in moments of crises, especially when meaning escapes. Both are shown to be affected by pathological troubles or disorders: one character has willingly stopped speaking in *Summer* while *Autumn* opens with one character in a coma, Mr Gluck, and his lifeless body is observed until he dies in *Summer*. However, at the end of the books, it becomes clear that rather than conceiving crisis as a temporary state of disruption or malfunction, Smith sees the plight of human beings as a perpetual state of crisis that they have to negotiate and create responses to.[1] Just like Cusk's trilogy plunges us again in a world of endless voices and echoes that try to bridge the gap of an experience that fails to be inscribed, Smith's narrative strategy seeks to work on various ways of expressing the hole at the heart of life: elliptical beginnings, her refusal to make the narrator's identity clear, her playful use of punctuation signs between speech and reported speech, all of these stylistic techniques allow her to place readers in a position of mis-reading, or mis-recognition. The meaning of the text is both deferred and lost, slippery at best, because there does not seem to be any structure that holds, while the polyfocal and polyphonic perspectives that Smith forces us to face (Tollance 2020: 75; Dobrogoszcz 2021: 138) can be analysed as the discreet signs of a generalised foreclosure in the contemporary world of disconnectedness.

> The substantial, symbolic Other in which the subject had emerged since the dawn of time now appears as lacking: the disenchantment of the world (Gauchet 1984), the ideologies of suspicion (Marx, Nietzsche, Freud) and the revelations concerning the incompleteness of modern science have challenged the order of this stable Other… The decline of the Ideal, typical of the western world, causes the conditions in which the figures of the law multiply. The modern subject no longer finds their direction according to the notion of an exceptional One, promoting a signifying castration that is the principle of the morals of austerity, abnegation and sacrifice. (Maleval 2019: 9)

Even before the tetralogy, Smith had worked on contemporary forms of disconnection and the lack of a stabilised structure that could ensure the subjects' inscription in the social order. She has long worked on

---

[1] The word plight was used until the nineteenth century as a word designating good or bad health.

cacophonous novels in which voices need to be reconnected to the body and language but are first heard as enigmatic expressions of characters unknown: 'Voices are disembodied', as Ryan-Sautour explains, 'echoing in playful, often distanced spaces within the short story narrative. And puns abound, as Smith's fascination with the play of language is evident in all of her fiction, and increasingly foregrounded as she progresses in her career' (Bernard 2015: par.32). Ryan-Sautour's programmatic vision was proven correct with the tetralogy: the absence of punctuation, or even verbs of reported speech, creates a case of extreme fluidity between speech spoken and/or thought, discourse, voices, and the collapse of the barriers between people that is a political statement (Masterson 2020). Smith, I argue, shows the way subjects try to grapple with the knotting back of the symbolic and the real, that is, the operations by which, faced with examples of dysfunctional relations and relationships—be it medical, social or amorous—their insistence on writing, speaking and thinking with language is the sign that they are trying to reconnect language to their bodies. In that respect, Smith can be said to prolong the stream-of-consciousness narration into the twenty-first century, where statements are heard, echoed and repeated without much heed to their effects, as can be seen in social media practices.

I will therefore look at various symptomatic formations in which paradoxically communication between the characters fails while connection still is established, with a view to unveiling how the subjective logic in Smith's tetralogy consists in repeatedly enacting a desire for commonality and sharing that defies contemporary excesses of individuality and disconnection. If 'identity is a relational category' (Wally 2018: 78) for Smith, it is only because she notes how fraught that characteristic is and how literature as a language must come to support, if not cure, the disconnection inherent in life. I will first look at these examples of disconnection that renew the modernist *topos* of 'only connect', underlining the tremendous paradox that is the basis of contemporary life. Then I will analyse how art is presented as a form of meaning and structure to the real of experience the body is the epitome of, before arguing that where communication fails, human connection is restored, if only fleetingly: 'Well, the project's finished, and nothing is over. The novel's a form of continuance' (Smith 2020a, b).

DISCONNECTION AND 'BARE-INGS' (SA1, 7): LOSS AND GAIN

When comparing the tetralogy to Smith's previous novels, a number of stylistic devices, consistently used, have also been noted: 'Metaphors and images of division and dismemberment create the background against which the story unfolds' (Mulalić 2020: 45). The beginnings of the novels present us with a situation of utterance or communication that is impossible to situate, creating an impression of being on the edge of narration and words, in a state of crisis that the novel then will have to stitch up back into some shape. The facetiousness of a narrative that derives so much of its appeal from the play on words, puns and unidentifiable narrator dramatises even more the darkness of disconnectedness—analysed by Ley as contained in the reference to Shakespeare (Ley 2020) and literalised in the body which, within the first pages, is presented as putrefied, dead: 'His body's still the old body, the ruined knees' (SQ1, 4). This would seem to suggest a point of connection between the body decadent and the body flamboyant, between the body as a whole and the body part that is now 'ruined'. It must be analysed in relation to what follows immediately. The metaphor of the tree and its stability in the environment calls for a similar effort on the part of humans to say in contact with their land: 'I can see the stem connecting that leaf to that tree' (SQ1, 5). Again, for some, the analogy of the body and death is achieved through the vision of a decaying nature (fully explored in Sacha's character in *Summer*) and it is a political one: 'the image of the head, separated from the body in the photograph, invites comparison with the dismemberment of the body politic... through the divisive referendum (Mulalić 2020: 45). However, in this final chapter, I want to argue that in itself, the question of connectedness and subjective relation to the body is political in a larger sense, namely, the ethics of the individual within society, without necessarily including the background of Brexit or rather as a sufficient factor in itself, Brexit becoming only one of its manifestations.

In keeping with the musical metaphor of their final title, the novels of the 'quartet' can be said to be marked by a predominance of a flow of discourse: very few passages can be regarded as part of narrative or description and even when they are, they often are delivered in the form of speech, as if someone was addressing the readers, or as if the readers were active participants in the text, expected to respond to it. Despite this stylistic feature, which lays the emphasis on speech and expression, the experience of the characters' reality is one of disconnectedness. The novels probe the loss of relations between the various protagonists, their absence of physical and social presence in the world that seems to unfold as a backdrop to their lives. None of them are fully integrated in communities: mothers in particular, who might traditionally have been regarded as agents of social connection, are lonely beings. Elisabeth's mother has attracted the ire of her fellow villagers who voted leave; Art's mother is dying alone after falling out with her sister and separating from Art's father; Sacha and Robert's mother is a retired actress with apparently no more work. Sacha and Robert's stepmother, Ashley, has stopped speaking and Robert 'silents himself out of his room and down the loft stairs again. Then silents himself down the staircases. Halfway down the last flight Robert Greenlaw sits, but with his feet well up off the next step because it's the creaker' (SQ4, 66). The verbing of the noun 'silent' is a coinage that enables Smith to suggest a willing state of silence designed to avoid arousing the attention of the people around. It is the opposite of the verb silence, which usually refers to the act of making sure others are or remain silent. Despite the novel's clear inscription within modern-day families, what is shown is the absence of communication, the distancing of beings and the solitude of the contemporary world where connection has been secured by machines—the Internet and phones are instruments of the characters' sickness. This does not suggest a melancholy vision of a bygone era in which families were more stable, but it denotes the end of the Oedipal families and the necessary changes this has caused. Quite characteristically, like in Cusk's trilogy, marriages have broken down and readers are told stories of characters that are isolated, in single families, in relationships that are dysfunctional (Art and Charlotte), based on fantasy (Robert and Charlotte; Richard and Paddy; Mansfield and Rilke), unconventional (Elisabeth and Daniel) or conflictual (Iris and Art's mother), and so on. Families are often without fathers or father figures—Elisabeth's mother's suggestion that Daniel must be gay because otherwise he wouldn't enjoy the company of her daughter is telling of this—and siblings do not get on well, when siblings there are.

During lockdown, while people are trying to avoid the Covid pandemic going through the roof, Art suggests a daily phone conversation to a girlfriend from whom he is separated. He has imagined that during these conversations, they would tell each other stories or what they thought about during the day. Charlotte's answer is: 'Us phoning each other, she says. That's your Eureka?/Calling each other expressly every single day;

he says, just for a few minutes, no pressure. But also, get this. We make it an aesthetic practice' (SQ4, 324). Charlotte seems to think the act of phoning is too random and banal to be elevated to the rank of a solution for the separation and estrangement from her boyfriend in this time of crisis. And yet, Art's idea—the many puns of which are both self-evident and intricate enough to demand a development of their own—is interesting because it uses a device that instead of bringing people together has led to their feeling more and more disconnected, forcing them to constant attachments to objects in lieu of the emotional relations to other beings (Boileau 2015). The idea that the telephone is a device of disconnection and solitude is beautifully expressed in the metonymic suggestion of a fancied lapsus: 'I have a theory that he hears the word *internet* and thinks the word *internment*' (SQ4, 144). Being 104 years old, Gluck's vision of technological devices branded as instruments of freedom and enhanced communication is determined by his long experience of humans' alienation to the wor(l)d, rather than their freedom, being himself a survivor of a detainee camp in Britain. The pessimistic, oppressive view of contemporary modes of relation is underlain in all the novels, either through the obsolete practice of letter writing in *Summer*, even if the character has no guarantee that their letter is received and read, or the facetious but realistic examples of relational paradoxes: 'Don't speak to me, the man says. I'm on Facetime' (SQ2, 289). Contemporary devices of 'connection' turn out to be unsatisfactory if not useless services to human beings whose body is at best inexistent (very few descriptions of bodies are shown; when the characters' bodies are referred to, they are often so as isolated elements), if not ill and dysfunctional.

The novel's fragmentation of style is in keeping with or makes apparent the fragmentation of human relations: 'Smith has made it clear since *Artful* that art does not imitate but fashions' (Ley 2020). I would argue with Ley that Smith's invention of a new mode of stream-of-consciousness shapes our vision of what today's subjects may have to grapple with, in particular their desperate attempts to make connections based on a language that escapes. This ostentatious aesthetic practice—further highlighted by the intertextual structure of the book and the intersemiotic practices (Boty, for example; Hockney in the choice of the covers; Rilke and Mansfield)—echoes the Brexit dis-union both between Britain and Europe and within Britain, between remainers and leavers (Shaw 2018: 21). The opening of *Winter* sees the character getting caught in the buzzing outrage of social media. Art seeks to avert the conflict by shutting his account and getting away to his mother's home in Cornwall with a pretend girlfriend. Ironically, this happens just before Christmas, the family gathering *par excellence* in Europe, but Smith only pays lip service to comedy by turning the family event into an epic failure: the host is ill, her son introduces her to a false girlfriend and has invited his mother's estranged sister for what promises to turn out to be the antithesis of the stereotypical Christmas, which is not celebrated. Art's mother, as it happens, lives secluded and is well aware of the potential dangers of human contact:

> And in a strange way it was a relief to because having a talk with someone, even the smallest, casual of talks, was sometimes quite hard because you always felt they judged you or you always felt shy or that you were saying a stupid or wrong thing. The pitfalls of human exchange, Sophia said. (SQ2, 36)

Such reflection takes us back to Clarissa and Septimus's response to small talk which, to a certain extent, threatens them in ways that are baffling because the insignificance of the speech content is disproportionate to the effect it bears on the subjects.

It is evident that language does not pose a risk because of the content or meaning of the talk, which is almost inexistent here. What language does is threaten the secure place of the subject by displacing them or potentially inscribing them elsewhere, in a flux of conversation where the subject is bare and loses their 'bare-ings'. Thus, Art's mother thinks it is safer to stay away from the trouble of social contact, a discreet sign of a mode of enjoyment that is self-harming: 'the *jouissance* of the body in the Speaking being implies that the body be marked or hit by the signifier. Enjoying a body for the species known as Speaking beings always means that it is going to be beaten, abused in a way, hit or even destroyed' (Miller 2018: 68). This has been exemplified before in a scene of social awkwardness during which Sophia's interaction with an optician is filled with misunderstandings: Sophia, apparently unaware of it, constantly mixes the common, phatic usage of 'see' as 'think' and her recent seeing impairment which she has come to have checked. Sophia is perplexed by the acknowledgement of the puns she is apparently making in total lack of awareness, while the optician does not know how to respond to her lack of realisation of what her words implicate. Sophia's body clearly escapes her, but her fascination for the floating body in her eye which she interprets as a head, as the presence of an Other, also signifies that she is trying to knot together language (in the puns), the image of her body and the real experience of this body that she cannot control. This could be seen as a sign of the pathological suffering she testifies to, well beyond the physical symptom of her eye that causes a subjective imprint. Each character has to make do with a world that does not provide a method or structure that you simply can conform to. Illness, whether physical or psychological, forces the subject to redefine their relations to others and the language they use for it.

All the characters in the tetralogy are shown to struggle with human contact and communication: a significant aspect of the appeal of the texts lies in the way dialogues are based on an absence of direct responses to the questions posed, a constant deferral of meaning and an apparent disregard for the most basic rules of phatic communication. The overall impression is one of disconnection and separation which goes hand in glove with the Brexit-inspired tale.

Yet, towards the end of the tetralogy, a counter-discourse is made possible, according to which this fragmentation is not only posited, shown or lamented but becomes the instrument of an attempt at raising the issue of how to fix it to ensure the preservation of society. Thus, individual solitude is paired with the question of commonality. Connection is re-affirmed as a virtue which the characters envisage not so much as actual but as a promising potentiality: 'On the contrary, time and space are what lace us all up together, Hannah says. What makes us part of the larger picture. Universally speaking. The problem is, we tend to think we're separate. But it's a delusion' (SQ4, 196). This passage is concluded by: 'It makes you and I more than just you or I, Hannah says. It makes us us' (SQ4, 197). The union is primary, despite the feeling of separateness, and the question Hannah seems to raise is how to find ways of achieving what, in everyday life, is veiled, hidden or undiscovered. The tautological sounding response is also a way of making the connection happen in language, of placing it logically in the conversation, perhaps to ensure that it exists and make sure it is not made equivocal by the sophistication of language. The relentless solution found by most characters is the contemplation or analysis of art: Elisabeth is an art specialist of Boty; Art has set up an online project with artful pictures of nature and has erased his name, Arthur, in the short but evocative nickname; Sophia imagines she is on the radio: 'it touches us deeply because it is insistent about both loneliness and communality, she told the millions of listeners not listening' (SQ2, 39). When they speak or write or become creative, the characters seek to find temporary solace to the hardships of simply living, recalling what Woolf wrote of Clarissa: 'She had a perpetual sense, as she watched the taxicabs, of being out, out, far out to sea and alone; she always had the feeling that it was very, very dangerous to live even one day' (D, 7).

Besides, the characters raise an even more crucial question of how to share the experience with an Other that is almost never a guarantee: parents are unreliable, the State has only created inefficient and humiliating bureaucracy, and so forth. In a very romantic, if not traditional approach, art, even the art of collage that shows the divisions and cuts, seems to have the function of stitching up together the dislocated relations that characters experience, witness or cause:

> If this writer from this place can make this mad and bitter mess into this graceful thing it is at the end, where the balance comes back and all the lies are revealed and all the losses… It's like the people in the play are living in the same world but separately from each other, like their worlds have somehow become disjointed or broken off each other's worlds. (SQ2, 200–201)

In psychoanalytic terms, one could say that the 'ready-made' response to the world that the Oedipus complex used to stand for as a familial structure that was common ground is shown to be inoperative. Fragmentation, dislocation, dismemberment infuse the texts with many images and cannot but be related to the many examples of disjointed bodies which people the tetralogy, evoking Jacques-Alain Miller's notion that the body is first and foremost experienced as a mass of disjointed pieces (Miller 2004).

ILLNESS AND THE BODY

Many episodes in the novels show this experience of dislocation and disconnection through fragmented bodies and the experience of disease. In *Autumn*, the passport scene uses the comic tone to suggest something of greater programmatic relevance for the tetralogy. After waiting for a long time with absolutely no human contact in the waiting room of a local post office, Elisabeth is frustrated that she hasn't been able to complete the administrative formality of renewing her passport. The clerk meant to receive her passport application is intent on closing his desk and in a parody of bureaucracy, her application is rejected because her head in the photograph came out the wrong size, which the clerk insists on writing on a piece of paper to (a) testify that he has been meticulous in the handling of this issue and (b) make sure he remembers why the application was not accepted: 'hope you won't take it the wrong way if I write in this box that you're wrong in the head, the man says' (SQ1, 5). The humorous nature of this 'resides essentially in a kind of inadequacy or impropriety' (Pollock 2001: 85). The clerk's aporetic formulation with the repetition of 'wrong' disjoints Elisabeth's body, replaying the Western tradition of separating mind and body and announcing one of the recurring motifs of the tetralogy, the head detached from a body that needs reconnection. In addition, Smith also suggests that there is something wrong with some clerk not being able to appreciate the wrongness of his declaration, proving that if not everyone is mad, then everyone does seem delirious in their use of language. Elisabeth notes the awkwardness of the phrase but makes nothing of it, as if there was no point in trying to correct or fix something that was not going to work. The clerk's absence of affect and humour whenever she tries to make contact with him further establishes that the world itself is askew.

Autumn clearly sets the tone of the novels by showing characters that have to make do with illness, related to old age in particular. The last novel takes place during the ongoing Covid-19 pandemic, so the question of the suffering body is metaphorically and structurally used to reflect back upon the identified feelings of disconnection and estrangement the novels highlight. Elisabeth wonders what has happened to all the care assistants (SQ1, 111), reminding us of an obsession of British literature and artistic creations, but also of one of the current critical interests in stories of migration and foreign-ness (Masterson 2020). Instead of providing care, the health staff manages patients, and their aim is to ensure the stability of an institution that does not function—perhaps a metaphor of British society's malfunctioning: 'The receptionist smiles a patient smile. (A smile especially for patients)' (SQ1, 104). In *Winter*, Sophia experiences an eye phenomenon that the reader is first made aware of through her hallucination that she sees a head. It becomes gradually clear Sophia is attached to this disorder as if it enabled her to cling back to life and this gives rise to a reflection that recalls Woolf's 'On Being Ill': 'Though it might be worth it, to re-experience what it's like to be sick, because from what she remembered there was a certain pleasure in it, anarchic force of clearance, one of those powerful liminal times in a life when death isn't just preferable to being alive' (SQ2, 109). The state of illness is far from being, perhaps like a crisis, lamented because it makes one more attuned to life and the materiality of the body.

This view might derive from Smith's own experience of illness (Germanà & Horton 2013), but it still connects body and subject in a very specific fashion that brings it back to life: hence perhaps the fact that in the floater in her eye, Sophia cherishes the presence of a child's head that accompanies her, making up for the absence of her own son. In truth, Sophia is less alone or lonely with her illness than she was before: 'The head on the table raised its eyebrows at her. As if it could read her mind, it gave her a little Mona Lisa smirk. Very funny. Very smart' (SQ2, 12). Throughout the tetralogy, the enjoyable nature of the state of being sick resounds with new possibilities for the contemporary subjects; it gives them access to their past: 'The summer when I was thirteen, I remember, was a summer of migraines. The migraines were partly enjoyable, like a private light show on' (SQ4, 205). The state of physical or mental suffering is paradoxically hailed as a way into well-being, forcing us to reconsider what we hold as a natural distribution between healthy and non-healthy: 'And also. I'm somatizing. This project's making me feel, all right. It's making me feel very all right…' (SQ3, 287). Richard, throughout the third volume, hesitates between the anxiety caused by the possibility of having an incurable illness and the paradoxical excitement that the illness reveals his body is still alive. When he feels nauseous, he hopes this connects him to the life of Rilke, whose poetry he is inspired by: 'He might well *be* sick./(Is that a symptom of leukemia?)' (SQ3; 49).

Daniel Gluck's body, which was taken for dead in the first novel, is now described with a particular emphasis on his wounds: these form curlicues and traces that evoke writing and enable him to reconnect with the losses of his life and experience: 'But he can still feel the place the doctor took it off and left a line of stitches. He can still feel the line where something was that's gone, where the gone thing healed' (SQ4, 174). The persistence of the line also evokes the persistence of the text and language in art. Gluck's body is like Boty's art, a collage that patches up the past back together, just like a text tries to account for an experience of loss by bringing together the fragmented pieces in the hope that it transforms it into a whole: 'I don't really know, Art says. There's a sort of hole in my life, where the word father is. He played a gay person on TV and in panto(mime)' (SQ2, 179).

The rewriting of this dichotomy between the mind and the body, in keeping with contemporary trust in the brain as the sole location of subjectivity, is central to the opening of the second novel: 'She was speaking to the disembodied head./It was the head of a child, just a head, no body attached, floating by itself in midair' (SQ2, 7). It turns out the head is a floater she sees due to sight problems, but the effect remains that Sophia does not seem as bothered as she should be that there is a head in the air. It seems that Sophia perceives the body as detached; that the floaters in her eye are articulated to her sense of being disturbed in her solitude and the threat of the other within. She happens to live in the house whose Cornish name, when finally deciphered after much speculation, underlines that trait again: 'The name of the house... House of the mind, of the head, of the psyche. Psyche's house' (SQ2, 270). Again the comedy should not blind us, as it were, to the function played by Smith's use of this hackneyed metaphor because it points to the pathologisation of behaviour and bodies and the resistance of subjective experience to the planned obsolescence of the subject. Just like the house's name, the psyche needs decoding, but Smith employs another strategy than the disclosing of the thing repressed, since in her fictional world, the logic is one of excessive information.

The text does not show any therapeutic scene, just as Cusk's trilogy, but the presence of therapy, whether physical or mental, is referred to at times. This culminates in the last novel. Although the text itself is not concerned with mental health as such, there is a growing concern for health indeed: the characters are often forced to associate their dislocated thoughts with the one theory that has made these no longer pathological, namely, psychoanalysis, although Smith presents it as a theory that is outdated and possibly unknown to most other than as a cultural reference: 'Your songs came over me like a lullaby, he says. Like the unconscious has a language it can speak in. The unconscious, the subconscious. I've never known the difference. What I mean is, it sounded like one of them was singing' (SQ3, 253). The vagueness of the terms and definitions does not stop the subconscious from being a point of reference for the characters and the interpretative, associative process that has been so central to the progress of the narrative since the beginning is given here some theoretical structure: '[The bleeding ghosts]'d been in my unconscious for too long' (SQ4, 269).

In the novel, the surprising persistence of psychoanalytic discourse is presented as carrying a potential for disruption. The reference to psychoanalysis is treated lightly only to convince readers even more of its influence upon ways of telling stories: 'Funny you should mention Freud, Art says (though nobody has mentioned Freud). The dream I had last night, this morning, I woke up from it actually saying out loud the word Freud' (SQ2, 210). The enigmatic character Danie Gluck, who has a fondness for art, stories and literature, tells Elisabeth straightaway that his name is a reminder of the importance of dream interpretation in connection with myth: 'And if you ever have a dream and you don't know what it means you can ask me. My first name also designates an ability to interpret dreams' (SQ1, 51). It is as if psychoanalysis had to do with the interpretation of esoteric phenomena that account for strange, enigmatic connections. One of these phenomena, which no scientific discourse can measure, describe or explain, is silence: 'The pauses are a special language, more a language than actual language is, Elisabeth thinks' (SQ1, 41). It is therefore no wonder the whole tetralogy should be interested in writing as an art form, writing as an art of making sense of what does not have any. In keeping with the choice of David Hockney's paintings to illustrate the novels' covers, Smith deploys a world in which art is everyone's solution against the angst of the times: painting, criticism, film making and essay writing, among others. Like Cusk, her appreciation of the overwhelming difficulty there is in naming one's cause(s) of discomfort results in either insignificant chitchat or endless silence, two kinds of response to the same danger: 'The thing is, it's very much about not talking. About two men who are friends and both deaf mutes who can't talk like everyone else does, so…' (SQ4, 110). Art provokes changes, quite literally in the second volume since this is the name of one of the main characters. The role of Art is to bring back together his mother and aunt and it is concomitant with his separation from his girlfriend—it is as if the equivocation of his name placed him in a strategic site of negotiations in order to solve tense connections between beings, which can be made or come undone.

If Freud is quoted as an authority in the interpretation of dreams mostly, the interpretative model followed by the characters is influenced by a sort of pop-Freudianism which serves as an underlying narrative to make sense of the characters' dismay: 'I don't have a father fixation, Elisabeth says. And Daniel is not gay. He's European' (SQ1, 77). The characters can at times use the reference to psychoanalysis as an instrument of conservatism for the gender divide and hierarchy, not without suggesting the playfulness of unqualified statements: 'It is driven by a Freudian envy of young people, especially her daughter… because being a man is all about spreading our seed./Robert! (chorus of voices)/And basically everybody, including quite a lot of women, think that women should shut up, he said' (SQ4, 34). Elsewhere psychoanalysis is portrayed as an authoritative discourse, the implications of which must be dreaded for what they reveal of the person: 'That'll be where the flower dream came from. What Freud would say. God almighty. It is the dregs really, to be living in a time when even your dreams have to be post-postmodern consciouser-than-thou' (SQ2, 158). The comedy of these references should not make us overlook the fact that the language of Smith's prose is indeed connected to the unconscious in its repetitive fragmentation and dislocation, its reduction to dense puns, play on words and misunderstandings, all of which being treated as possibly meaningful: 'She remembers the dream (of her father) for a fraction of a second, then she remembers where she is and she forgets the dream' (SQ1, 205). The paratactic style seems to preclude any interpretation based on a dialectic of cause and consequence: and yet, the random aspect of the dream resurfacing in her mind is signified in its disappearance, almost as random as its apparition. It seems to show a split in the character's psyche between the here and now of the experience and another, subconscious scene which is not just a repository of past events but which, in itself, produces meaning and memories.

The signifiers of psychiatry and mental health are used equally for medicated cases and metaphorical ones. People search for an explanation that there does not seem to be a reality that holds for everyone, a reality everyone can rely on:

> *deranged*. Nobody who isn't deranged can live like she does. Psychotic. Psychotic people see the world in terms of their illusions and delusions, Arthur. You can't accommodate you on your own terms like she does. You can't expect to live in the world like the world's your private myth. (SQ2, 156)

Arthur's mother thinks 'psychosis' is a subjective mode of apprehension of the world and as Lacan says in the beginning of his seminar on psychosis (Lacan 1981), she does not think you can choose to be psychotic. Through this character, Smith re-instates the mystical, this presence that religion feeds on and that has been excluded from a world defined by its scientific methods and causality. 'Visitor/Visitation/There seems to be a force which bodies, by their very presence, exert upon each other' (SQ4, 76–77). She reclaims the metaphorical meaning of mental illness too: 'My sister was psychotic about banning the bomb, Charlotte, at the time, his mother says. We all have our visions' (SQ2, 209). Madness becomes a shared experience of visions and Smith defies the ciphering of the world that neurology and science force us into thinking as the only object worth of worship: 'the whole town danced and danced, because of madness and poverty. Driven to joy' (SQ4, 174).

The first novel germinates a number of recurring motifs in relation to the idea of fragmentation and incoherent language as signs of a disorder that needs fixing. In the middle of the novel, as Elisabeth and her mother fight over the role of art and Mr Gluck's idea of its function, Elisabeth is said to only remember these dribs and drabs of a conversation with her mother:

> Unnatural.
> Unhealthy.
> You're not to.
> I forbid it.
> That's enough. (SQ1, 83)

These isolated words are repeated 'verbatim' (SQ1, 83) at the end of the novel, interspersed with passages in which Elisabeth's mother reflects upon her relationship with her new lover, Zoe (SQ1, 238). These fragments are pronounced like interjections, injunctions, orders coming from an other. Above all, they evoke the reduction of language to its 'litter' as Smith describes in *Artful*: 'Litter-ature! Litter is even brighter than, more powerful than, more enduring than art', she says when she describes a 1987 poem by Edwin Morgan (Smith 2012, 70).[2] The association of language and litter is a recurring motif since she opens *Spring* with a similar image of waste: 'rubbish depot. Landfill' (SQ3, 12). I am far more interested in the logic this suggests than in the content or meaningful associations which careful analysis of the expressions could reveal about the plot dynamics. In the quote recalling Elisabeth's argument with her mother, Smith constructs true love (outside patriarchal norms) as expressed in incoherent language, pathologising a relationship that cannot be made sense of, but the iteration of the words is interesting because it shows that the body is marked by the signifier which, beyond the meaning of it, fixes/

---

[2] I cannot affirm that she knows she is not the first author to suggest this interpretation but in *Artful*, she does not mention that she does. However, Lacan notes this pun in Joyce between letter and litter and writes an essay entitled 'Litturaterre', in which he explores the ramifications of this pun (Lacan 1971, 11). The metaphor connects the works studied in the present book, since waste and litter have been quoted about Lessing, Cusk, Woolf and now Smith.

mortifies the relationship while literature re-ignites it by reincorporating elements in between that dislocate the memory fixed. The words, ordered like the lines of a poem, all seek to circumscribe a form of excess, or *disorder*. They infer the idea that Elisabeth's mother castigates and seeks to police her daughter, but it is her own language that deteriorates.

When they discuss Boty, Zoe, Elisabeth's mother's new girlfriend, and Elisabeth have a conversation which, underneath the veneer of clichés, tries to connect language to the body and to subjective experience. Zoe starts by manipulating stereotypical visions of the 'mad' (SQ2, 213) artist.

> Victim of abuse, I expect, Zoe says.
> She winks at Elisabeth. Elisabeth laughs.
> Just the usual humdrum contemporary misogynies, she says.
> Committed suicide, Zoe says.
> Nope. Just the usual humdrum completely sane occasional depressions, Elisabeth says.
> Ah. Died tragically, then, Zoe says.
> Well, that's one reading of it, Elisabeth says. My own preferred reading is free spirit arrives on earth equipped with the skill and the vision capable of blasting the tragic stuff that happens to us all into space, where it dissolves away to nothing whenever you pay any attention to the lifeforce in her pictures.
> Oh, that's good, Zoe says. That's very good. All the same. I bet she was ignored.
> She was after she died, Elisabeth says.
> I bet it goes like this, Zoe says. Ignored. Lost. Rediscovered years later. Then ignored. Lost. Rediscovered years later. Then ignored. Lost. Rediscovered ad infinitum. Am I right?
> … What's her story, then this girl?….
> Her story? Elisabeth says. Got ten minutes?' (SQ1, 239–40)

This extract enables me to underline how, straight from *Autumn*, Ali Smith knots together the various aspects of her narrative via this seemingly insignificant small talk. In truth, the passage resonates with the therapeutic scene of the talking cure since the association of ideas is conducive to the expression of some truth about the function this artist has in the life of Elisabeth. Exchange is the site of a construction of a reality that defies expectations and preconceived ideas about creativity, art and mental health. Zoe's resorting to a traditional view of the mad artist is likely to come across as a piece of comedy but I think it serves the purpose of suggesting that madness, despite its biomedical treatment in recent years, hasn't been solved and its manifestations resurface in the most banal of talks, becoming particularly relevant in its potential for stories—the next ten minutes will prompt an articulation of this reality that would otherwise be forgotten and continue to unconsciously influence the narrative of society.

ART-FULL: SATURATION OF ART AS A MEANS OF CONNECTION

The interpretative process stemming from the enigmatic nature of life lived is problematised in the novels by a narrative that juxtaposes, entangles and unwinds various voices and visions that have been accepted as truthful because deemed rational and reasonable, and yet which are contradicted by people's experience of truth, which remains disconnected from facts. Art, and especially the writing of visions, becomes a means to oppose the sickness of the times and the humdrum depression of the modern day. Storytelling, its margins and its edges are the founding principles of the novel because nobody seems to be intent on hearing, comprehending or even connecting stories back to the singularity of the subject experiencing them: in the quote above, Zoe thinks Boty can only be one in a million such cases. It is no wonder talk should come to epitomise this disconnection between symptoms of unease or suffering and the subjective articulation of someone to their bodies because often, it is the sound of a voice that is rejected or regarded as unbearable: 'the sound of his own voice in his ears saying stuff disgusts him …/Oh nothing nothing nothing' (SQ3, 56). The nothingness of the thing said hides the everything of the voice's role in carrying some truth about the subject that once again interlaces language with litter, makes of literature a place where the rest, the leftovers of language are replayed and resituated within the subjective presence of the characters. Storytelling is therefore restored in all its therapeutic function of not just recounting events but accounting for the subject's ethical presence in them and their function. As argued by Butler, it is precisely in virtue of its opacity that the subject needs to be ethically held responsible for its connection to others (Butler 2005).

In that respect, the novels' interest in everyone's capacity for storytelling and for interpreting through reflections of their own about the 'state of the union', to use a phrase that returned with more force after Brexit,[3] is most visible in *Spring*, in which Richard tries to find the best strategy to tell his story. This director is dispossessed of his ability to find a way of structuring his account of reality and this is densified in the simplest of terms: 'there's no story. He's had it with story' (SQ3, 11). Set in the post-truth, obsessional fact-checking practices of the Trump era, Ali Smith's novels also show how the collapse of grand narratives affect the contemporary subject's view of the world as unbearably ungraspable, and how the lack in the Other, which used to be veiled by the substitute offered by the Name-of-the-Father (Maleval 1997), is here exhibited, out in the open, for everyone to see. One could almost construe that *Spring* is the pivotal novel about the function of storytelling and interpretation because the two running, parallel stories pit against one another Richard's barrenness and the girl's multiplication of invented stories (or lies?) which she uses because she has been bereft of her own story: She gets away with everything, including boarding a train to Scotland without a ticket by talking the conductor into allowing her to, thereby achieving to be as clandestine in language as she is forced to become in reality because of British politics. Were it not for Brittany, nobody would be interested in hearing her story and Brittany learns more by listening to the little girl's imagined or unwilling creations than by the truthful account she could give, if she was to be interviewed by the authorities. This links the two stories together, as it offers two accounts to make sense of what Richard's friend had told her, and which has somehow guided his search: 'There's a difference between narrative strategy and reality but they're symbiotic, she said to him one day in the 1970s' (SQ3, 63).

Spring is presented by the editors as 'the great connective', 'the impossible tale of an impossible time' (SQ3, back cover), but what is at stake indeed is the difficulty of the connection. After she has just boarded the train taking them to Scotland, Brittany tries to know more about this girl she's accompanying. The girl's response to all of Brit's questions is 'private private private, the girl says. Private private. Private. Private. You?' (SQ3, 188), leading Brit to reflect: 'But how do we get to be friends, or even know each other at all, without you telling me a bit about what your life's

---

[3] This figurative approach to Brexit was prompted by the BBC series written by Nick Hornby and directed by Stephen Frears, entitled *State of the Union* and broadcast in 2019 for the first series. The series looks into the intimacy of a couple who meets up in a pub before their weekly, joint therapy session.

like and me swapping with you what mine is like?'/'Making friends with a machine, the girl says. No way. It's quicksand' (SQ3, 189). The dangers of human contact are reiterated here but *Spring* brings about some hope that it can be restored because Brit's insistence on exchanging, even fictional stories, gradually wins over the girl, now named Florence (hence perhaps the reference here to the machine, which connects to the joke of the indie UK singer Florence and the machines). The symbolic order therefore is not 'dead' to parody the beginning of *Winter* and literature seeks to make it work again, despite its failings.

This is in keeping with what Smith says in interviews: 'fiction tells you by the making up of truth, what really is true' (qd in Ley 2020). This recalls Woolf's definition of truth in *A Room of One's Own:* 'Fiction here is likely to contain more truth than fact' (Woolf 1929: 4). F. Regard has analysed this as the feminine, not in its opposition to the masculine, but in its insistence to get out of the binary system of gender politics: 'the feminine will have been the operation of othering, othering not as based on polar opposites but one that admits contraries, laughs at its contradictions and lives a difference that is split and made dynamic' (Regard 2002: 7). And Warner tells us that since Woolf began *A Room* with 'But...' 'there has not been another writer who can make a little do so much' (Germanà and Horton 2013: ix). Because of this and her interests in gender fluidity, Smith has sometimes been regarded as creating characters that are more archetypal than individuated, like Woolf feared she lacked the knack of making characters. Each novel in the tetralogy starts with a litany-like, myth sounding opening which forces the readers to interpret, imagine, think about the ramifications and exploitations such parts constitute: 'God was dead: to begin with./And romance was dead' (SQ2, 1–2). We'll learn later that this is Art playing with the search bar of his computer to try and find a word which is not statistically combined with dead. However, without this element of context, the text seems to mock the language of the grand narratives as well as to mock the epitome of said authority. Interestingly, God, who is not a story but about whom stories circulate, sometimes incompatible ones, is followed by the word 'romance' whose meanings are multifarious, but which suggests a story of an extraordinary or outstanding nature, not unrelated to myths and legends. In other words, the story starts with the idea that the paragon of heroes and the means by which their story is recounted are dead, calling for a new form to account for new myths while also suggesting that Smith's novels are an attempt to contradict this interpretation. It so happens that throughout the novel Sophia calls her sister Iris 'mythologiser' when she refuses to deliver to Lux, her son's pretend lover, a story she thinks is too private (SQ2, 255). Romance is both the literary tradition of the epic, medieval genre and the literary tradition of codified love stories. In Smith, this language is not the proper story of love and her characters intend to make it known or heard in a slightly different way: 'And I like a good fuck as much as the next person, and that was a very good fuck. Thanks' (SQ3, 246). The relationship is here reduced to the sexual act because there is no story to be told from there, suggesting thereby that the story of love is one that is much more complex than facts. This does not mean that we should return to a literature of the flight of fancy or the substitution of the amorous act by words of propriety. On the contrary, the solution is to see the act as it is, without the barrier of the repressed, while understanding that in itself it does not strive to connect people: in-yer-face sex is just a physical approach that bears no relation to the subjective function of the symbolic exchange that the act leads to: 'He understands now why porn isn't all the same thing as love' (SQ4, 86).

In that context, one may as well return to the beginning of the last novel and hear the time-honoured, hackeneyed swearing as a reinterpretation of the function of coupling, mating, sex in contemporary forms of relations: 'yep, there, see,/Nobody gave a fuck,/Sign of the times,/Nobody even saw, or if they did, cared' (SQ4, 57). For Smith connects language and sex in the bluntest fashion: 'Everybody said: so?/Okay, not everybody said it. I'm speaking colloquially, like in that phrase *everybody's doing it*' (SQ4, 3). The novel *Summer* starts with the conundrum of the clichés of language, the way they distort reality and the way they are connected to a form of *jouissance*, the sexual nature of which is only made evident here, despite the fact that the narrative focuses on the indifference suggested by the phrase, 'so?' Yet, in *Summer*, the author also shows us the way by resorting to an ek-phrasis within the first chapter, one that is declared impossible because it deals with a movie: 'There'd be no point in showing you a still or a photo of this. It's very much a moving image' (SQ4, 6). Smith has just provided what she says has no point and concludes with 'so:', without the question mark. She is about to demonstrate to us that what is impossible does not preclude that we try because we may at least temporarily succeed in being ethically placed as subjects, that is agents, in language. Smith restores the symbolic function of language (all of her books are about writing, says the author (Germanà and Horton 2013: 41)) to render the truth of another work of art, the reinstation of mediation. This is why symbolic articulation is central to understanding the way these four novels interconnect in their semblance of fragmentation and disconnection: 'Now what we don't want is facts. What we want is bewilderment. What we want is repetition' (SQ3, 3).

The novels explore this relentless hesitation between facts, reality and truth, in an age that has been designated as 'post-truth', but which is not exactly the kind of post-truth Smith advocates: 'Here's an old story so new that it's still in the middle of happening, writing itself right now with no knowledge of where or how it'll end' (SQ1, 181). She offers a panoramic vision of a subject's development in relation to this question via Elisabeth as a child whose clear-cut definitions are indicative of a wish to classify rather than a sign of her lack of complexity: 'You mean there's truth, and there's the make-up version of it that we get told about the world, Daniel said. No. The world *exists. Stories* are made up, Elisabeth said' (SQ1, 119). Her reaction to Daniel's suggestion is the certitude of madness (cf. Trollope's *He Knew He Was Right*): to the possibility of contradictions, Elisabeth as a child opposes the notion of a binary system that has been proven wrong and inoperative during her lifetime.

For it is indeed language altogether that is now perceived as inoperative and whose function for the subjects is no longer connectible to meaning: 'He tells her the artist said that she was tired of faces and of dramas and that she wanted a universal language./One where the world itself speaks, he says, not just us' (SQ2, 273). As we can see here, Ali Smith does investigate the function of language at the subjective level, but she does not suppress the ethical question of how to share and find common ground for this subjective knowledge to enable some form of connection, which is one of the determining factors for making her fit into the Modernist aesthetics. As could be seen here, Ali Smith produces novels in which disembodied voices, actual floating words and signifiers, seem to point to a world of crisis, fragmentation and broken pieces. Yet, this pathological language is only exposed as a way of taking stock of contemporary forms of enjoyment in which subjects are reduced to their bafflement with a language that no longer operates, whose function is thought to have been erased, if not altogether made redundant. Yet, Smith's insistence on art, literary language, the function of articulation and expression, even if it be only a school assignment, tends to point to the most mundane effects of language in offering a kind of structure for what is left over by the operation of language, the waste of meaning that she expresses thus: 'It was the demonstration that everything symbolic will be revealed as a lie, everything you revere nothing but burnt matter, broken stone, as soon as it meets whatever shape time's contemporary cudgel takes' (SQ2, 110). One of the most blatant examples of this destruction and mortifying power of language is found in the commonest mistake: 'Brittany Hall. I'm a DCO at an IRC./The female assistant wrote it down without asking what it was. She wrote it down like the Britney in Britney Spears. People are often careless like that. She wrote it all down. Britney Hall DC RC/So it didn't really matter, then, what or who Brit was' (SQ3, 164). The humour does not repress or hide the tragic aspect of this mistake which, by denying Brittany her place in the symbolic order, denies her very existence and symbolic value. The absurd identity check is made fun of to signify that the wor(l)d has become dangerously slippery and the hailed fluidity of identity must be reconsidered, lest it jeopardises the life of the subjects:

> I certainly have a proper name through which I am recognized but this name never reaches to the core of my singularity which is my self… Is the self impossible to say? It is always betrayed by language, which Bergson has rightfully reminded us that it was mechanical, impersonal and static, and for all these reasons, language is far from being able to express the fragile threads of interior life. (Auregan 1998, 5)

BIBLIOGRAPHY

PRIMARY SOURCES

Smith, Ali (2012). *Artful*. London: Penguin, 2013.
Smith, Ali (2020a). *Seasonal Quartet*. London: Penguin Books (2016–2021), with *Autumn* (2016), *Winter* (2017), *Spring* (2019) and *Summer* (2020b).
Woolf, Virginia (1929). *A Room of One's Own*. London: Penguin Books, "Great Ideas", 2004.

SECONDARY SOURCES

Anderson, Sarah Wood (2012). *Readings of Trauma, Madness and the Body*. New York: Palgrave Macmillan.
Auregan, Pierre (1998). *Les Figures du moi et la question du sujet depuis la Renaissance*. Paris: Ellipses, "Culture et Histoire", 1998.

Bernard, Catherine et ali. (2015). "Recent British Fiction (Part 3)". *Études britanniques contemporaines*, 49/2015. https://doi.org/10.4000/ebc.2753

Bernard, Catherine (2019). "'It was the worst of times. It was the worst of times. Again.' Representing the Body Politic after Brexit." *Études britanniques contemporaines*, 57, 2019. https://doi.org/10.4000/ebc.7401

Bernard, Catherine (2022). "Vibrant Allegories: Questioning Immunity with Ali Smith's Seasonal Quartet." *Études anglaises*, 2022/1, vol. 75, 13–29. https://doi.org/10.3917/etan.751.0013

Bernard, Catherine et ali. (2014). "Recent British Fiction". *Études britanniques contemporaines*, 47/2014. https://doi.org/10.4000/ebc.1992

Boileau, Nicolas Pierre (2015). "'In Some Rare and Sacred Dead Time…, there is a Miracle of Silence.' On Not Lifting the Veil in Mc Gregor's and Cusk's Novels." *L'Atelier*, vol.7, No. 2, 2015, http://ojs.u-paris10.fr/index.php/latelier/article/view/428

Butler, Judith (2005). *Giving an Account of Oneself.* New York: Fordham University Press.

Dobrogoszcz, Tomasz (2021). "Are We In This Together?: The Polarisation of the British Society and the Marginalisation of Otherness in Ali Smith's *Seasonal Quartet*." *Porównania*, vol. 3 (30), 2021 DOI: https://doi.org/10.14746/por.2021.3.9

Germanà, Monica (2017). "Ali Smith: Strangers and Intrusions". J. Acheson. *The Contemporary British Novel Since 2000.* Edinburgh: Edinburgh University Press.

Germanà, Monica & Horton, Emily (eds.) (2013), *Ali Smith: Contemporary Critical Perspectives*, London: Bloomsbury Academic.

Heynders, Odile (2021). "Dissensus in Ali Smith's *Seasonal Quartet*". *Frame, Journal of Literary Studies*, No. 34.1, May 2021, 35–51.

Horton, Emily (2012). "'Everything You've Ever Dreamed': Post-9/11 Trauma and Fantasy in Ali Smith's *The Accidental*". *Modern Fiction Studies*. Fall 2012, Vol. 58, No. 3, 637–654.

Lacan, Jacques (1971). "Lituraterre". *Autres écrits*, Paris: Éditions du seuil, 11–20.

Lacan, Jacques (1981). *Le Séminaire*, Livre III, *Les Psychoses* (1955–56). J.-A. Miller (ed.). Paris: Éditions du Seuil.

Ley, James (2020). "Brexit, Pursued by a Bard". *The Sydney Review of Books.* December 4, 2020. https://sydneyreviewofbooks.com/review/smith-autumn-winter-spring-summer/

Maleval, Jean-Claude (1997). *Logique du délire*. Paris: Masson, "Ouvertures Psy", 2000.

Maleval, Jean-Claude (2019). *Repères pour la psychose ordinaire*. Paris: Navarin Éditeurs, 2019.

Masterson, John. "'Don't tell me this isn't relevant all over again in its brand new same old way': Imagination, Agitation, and Raging against the Machine in Ali Smith's *Spring.*" Safundi 21.3 (2020): 355–372. https://doi.org/10.1080/17533171.2020.1776961

Miller, Jacques-Alain (2004). "Pièces détachées", *L'Orientation lacanienne,* lesson of 17 November 2004, unpublished.

Miller, Jacques-Alain (2018). *L'os d'une cure.* Paris: Navarin éditeur.

Mulalić, Lejla (2020). "Politics and the Novel in a Post-Brexit World: Ali Smith's *Autumn*". *Journal of Education and Humanities.* Volume 3, No.1, 43–52.

Orosz-Réti, Zsófia (2021). "Covidian Metamorphoses: Art and the Poetics of Transformation in Ali Smith's *Seasonal Quartet*". *Acta Universitatis Sapientiae, Philologica.* Vol. 13, No.1, 60–72.

Pollock, Jonathan (2001). *Qu'est-ce que l'humour?* Paris: Klicksieck.

Rau, Petra (2018). "*Autumn* After the Referendum". R. Eaglestone (ed.) (2018). 31–43.

Regard, Frédéric (2002). *La Force du féminin, Sur trois essais de Virginia Woolf.* Paris: La Fabrique Éditions.

Reynier, Christine (2021). "Virginia Woolf's Radical Vision of Recycling". In Latham, Monica, Marie, Caroline & Rigeade, Anne-Laure (eds.). *Recycling Virginia Woolf in Contemporary Art and Literature.* Londres: Routledge.

Shaw, Kristian (2018), "Brexlit". R. Eaglestone (ed.) (2018). 15–30.

Smith, Ali (2020b). "Before Brexit, Grenfell, Covid-19... Ali Smith on writing four novels in four years". *The Guardian*, August 1st, 2020, https://www.theguardian.com/books/2020/aug/01/before-brexit-grenfell-covid-19-ali-smith-on-writing-four-novels-in-four-years

Tollance, Pascale. "Penser l'être-avec: hôtes et parasites dans la fiction d'Ali Smith". *L'Atelier*, 12.2, 2020, 75–91.

Wally, Johannes. "The Return of Political Fiction? An Analysis of Howard Jacobson's *Pussy* (2017) and Ali Smith's *Autumn* (2016) as First Reactions to the Phenomena 'Donald Trump' and 'Brexit' in Contemporary British Literature", *AAA – Arbeiten aus Anglistik und Amerikanistik*, Issue 43 (2018), online.

BIBLIOGRAPHY

BIBLIOGRAPHY SYMPTOM

PRIMARY SOURCES

Barker, Pat (1991). *Regeneration*. London: Penguin Books, 2008.
Barker, Pat (1993). *The Eye in the Door*. London: Penguin Books, 2008.
Barker, Pat (1995). *The Ghost Road*. London: Penguin Books, 2008.
Collins, Wilkie (1883). *Heart and Science*. Stroud: Alan Sutton, 1994.
Cusk, Rachel (1993). *Saving Agnes*. London: Macmillan.
Cusk, Rachel (1997). *The Country Life*. London: Picador.
Cusk, Rachel (2001). *A Life's Work*. London: Faber and Faber, 2008.
Cusk, Rachel (2005). *Arlington Park*. London: Faber and Faber.
Cusk, Rachel (2006). *The Last Supper*. London: Faber and Faber.
Cusk, Rachel (2009a). *The Bradshaw Variations*. London: Faber and Faber.
Cusk, Rachel (2009b). "Shakespeare's Daughters", *The Guardian*. 12 December 2009. http://www.guardian.co.uk/books/2009/dec/12/rachel-cusk-women-writing-review
Cusk, Rachel (2012). *Aftermath: On Marriage and Separation*. London: Faber and Faber (Kindle version).
Cusk, Rachel (2018). *Kudos Trilogy. Outline*. 2014; *Transit*. 2016; *Kudos*. 2018. London: Faber and Faber.
Dawson, Jennifer (1961). *The Ha-Ha*. London: Panther Books, 1966.

© The Author(s), under exclusive licence to Springer Nature   259
Switzerland AG 2023
N. P. Boileau, *Mental Health Symptoms in Literature since
Modernism*, Palgrave Studies in Literature, Science and Medicine,
https://doi.org/10.1007/978-3-031-37630-6

Forster, Edward M. (1927). *Aspects of the Novel*. Orlando, Florida: Harvest Book, 1955.

Frame, Janet (1961). *Faces in the water*. London: The Women's Press, 1980.

Frame, Janet (1982–85). *An Autobiography*. London: The Women's Press, 1990. (*To the Is-Land*. 1982; *An Angel at my Table*. 1984; *The Envoy from Mirror City*. New York: George Braziller, 1985)

Hollinghurst, Alan (1998). *The Spell*. London: Vintage, 1999.

Hollinghurst, Alan (2004a). *The Line of Beauty*. London: Picador, 2005.

Hollinghurst, Alan (2011). *The Stranger's Child*. London: Picador, 2012.

Kaysen, Susanna (1995). *Girl, Interrupted*. London: Virago Press, 1995.

Lessing, Doris (1950). *The Grass is singing*. London: Flamingo, 1994.

Lessing, Doris (1952). Martha's Quest. New York: HarperPerennial, 2001. Part of the *Children of Violence* series (1952–1969).

Lessing, Doris (1962). *The Golden Notebook*. London: HarperPerennial, 2008.

Lessing, Doris (1973). *The Summer Before the Dark*. New York: Vintage, 2009.

Lessing, Doris (1985). *The Good Terrorist*. London: HarperPerennial, 2007.

Lessing, Doris (2002). *Briefing for a Descent into Hell*. London: Flamingo.

Lessing, Doris (1988). *The Fifth Child*. London: Random House.

Lessing, Doris (2000). *Ben, in the World*. London: Fourth Estate, 2012.

McGrath, Patrick (1993). *Dr. Haggard's Disease*. London: Viking.

McGrath, Patrick (1996). *Asylum*. London: Penguin Books, 2015.

McGrath, Patrick (2005). *Ghost Town, Tales of Manhattan Then and Now*. London: Bloomsbury, 2006.

McGrath, Patrick (2008). *Trauma*. New York: A. A. Knopf.

Plath, Sylvia (1966). *The Bell Jar*. London: Faber and Faber.

Shakespeare, William (1607). *Anthony and Cleopatra*. London: Penguin.

Shakespeare, William (1613). *Much Ado About Nothing*. London: Penguin, 1996.

Smith, Ali (2012). *Artful*. London: Penguin, 2013.

Smith, Ali (2020a). *Seasonal Quartet*. London: Penguin Books (2016–2021), with *Autumn* (2016), *Winter* (2017), *Spring* (2019) and *Summer* (2020b).

Woolf, Leonard (1964), *Beginning Again, The Autobiography of the years 1911–1918*. London: The Hogarth Press.

Woolf, Virginia (1919). *Night and Day*. London: Penguin Modern Classics, 1976.

Woolf, Virginia (1922). *Jacob's Room*. Oxford: Oxford World's Classics, 1992.

Woolf, Virginia (1925a). *Mrs Dalloway*. Oxford: Oxford World's Classics, 2009. Introduction by David Bradshaw (2000).

Woolf, Virginia (1925b). *The Common Reader, First Series*. New York: Harcourt Inc., with an introduction by Andrew McNeillie, 1984.

Woolf, Virginia (1926). "On Being Ill" (1930) in Woolf 1948, 9–23.

Woolf, Virginia (1927). *To the Lighthouse*. London: Penguin Popular Classics, 1996.

Woolf, Virginia (1928). *Orlando*. London: Penguin Popular Classics, 1996.

Woolf, Virginia (1929). *A Room of One's Own*. London: Penguin Books, "Great Ideas", 2004.

Woolf, Virginia (1948). *The Moment and Other Essays*. London: Harvest Book.
Woolf, Virginia (1978). *The Diary of Virginia Woolf*, volume 2, 1920–24, A. O. Bell (ed.), London: Penguin Books, 1981.
Woolf, Virginia (2002). *Moments of Being, Autobiographical Writings*, Jeanne Schulkind (ed.), intro. by Hermione Lee, London: Pimlico Edition.

SECONDARY SOURCES

DSM-5   https://cdn.website-editor.net/30f11123991548a0af708722d458e476/files/uploaded/DSM%2520V.pdf
Abel, Elizabeth (1989). *Virginia Woolf and the Fictions of Psychoanalysis*. Chicago: The University of Chicago Press, "Women in Culture and Society".
Acheson, James & Ross, Sarah E. (eds.) (2005). *The Contemporary British Novel Since 1980*. Edinburgh: Edinburgh University Press.
Anderson, Sarah Wood (2012). *Readings of Trauma, Madness and the Body*. New York: Palgrave Macmillan.
Alderson, David (2017). "Attachment and Possession: The Romance of Family, Politics and Things in *The Line of Beauty*". M. Mathuray (ed.), 129–149.
Alfandary, Isabelle and Nesme, Axel (eds.) (2011). *Modernism and Unreadability*. Montpellier: Presses Universitaires de la Méditerranée.
Auregan, Pierre (1998). *Les Figures du moi et la question du sujet depuis la Renaissance*. Paris: Ellipses, "Culture et Histoire", 1998.
Baker, Charley, Crawford, Paul et al. (2010). *Madness in Post-1945 British and American Fiction*. London: Routledge.
Barber-Stetson, Claire (2016). "*On Being Ill* in the Twenty-First Century". *Woolf Miscellany*, 48–50.
Barrett, Michèle (2012). "'Regeneration' Trilogy and the Freudianization of Shell Shock". *Contemporary Literature*, Vol. 53, No. 2, 237–260.
Berets, Ralph (1980). "A Jungian Interpretation of the Dream Sequence in Doris Lessing's *The Summer Before Dark*". *Modern Fiction Studies*, vol. 26, No.1, Spring 1980, 117–130.
Bernard, Catherine (2007). "Pat Barker's Critical Work of Mourning: Realism with a Difference." *Études anglaises*, 2007/2, vol. 60, 173–184.
Bernard, Catherine (2018). *Matière à réflexion: du corps politique dans la littérature et les arts visuels contemporains*. Paris: Presses Universitaires de Paris-Sorbonne.
Bernard, Catherine (2019). "'It was the worst of times. It was the worst of times. Again.' Representing the Body Politic after Brexit." *Études britanniques contemporaines*, 57, 2019. https://doi.org/10.4000/ebc.7401
Bernard, Catherine (2022). "Vibrant Allegories: Questioning Immunity with Ali Smith's *Seasonal Quartet*". *Études anglaises*, 2022/1, vol. 75, 13-29. https://doi.org/10.3917/etan.751.0013

Bernard, Catherine et ali. (2014). "Recent British Fiction". *Études britanniques contemporaines*, 47/2014. https://doi.org/10.4000/ebc.1992

Bernard, Catherine et ali. (2015). "Recent British Fiction (Part 3)". *Études britanniques contemporaines*, 49/2015. https://doi.org/10.4000/ebc.2753

Biggs, Joanna (2012). "Clytemnestra in Brighton." *London Review of Books*, 34: 6, March 22, 2012.

Black, Naomi (2004). *Virginia Woolf as Feminist*. Ithaca, New York: Cornell University Press.

Boileau, Nicolas Pierre, Hanson, Clare & Tang, Maria (eds.) (2013). "Kay Boyle/Rachel Cusk: (Neo) Modernist Voices." *E-Rea*, 10.2, 2013 https://journals.openedition.org/erea/2966

Boileau, Nicolas Pierre (2013a). "A Novelist in Changing Rooms: Motherhood and Auto/biography." N. Boileau et al. (eds.) (2013) https://journals.openedition.org/erea/3243

Boileau, Nicolas Pierre (2013b). "Not feminine enough? Rachel Cusk's highly-feminised world and unfeminine characters in *Saving Agnes* and *The Country Life*." *Anglistik*, "Focus on the Feminisation of Writing", Barbara Puschmann-Nalenz (ed.), Spring 2013, 39–49.

Boileau, Nicolas Pierre (2014). "Trauma and 'Ordinary Words': Virginia Woolf's Play on Words", in T. Beney et A. Stara (eds.). *The Edges of Trauma*. Cambridge: Cambridge Scholars Publishing, 48-60.

Boileau, Nicolas Pierre (2015). "'In Some Rare and Sacred Dead Time…, there is a Miracle of Silence.' On Not Lifting the Veil in Mc Gregor's and Cusk's Novels." *L'Atelier*, vol.7, No. 2, 2015, http://ojs.u-paris10.fr/index.php/latelier/article/view/428

Boileau, Nicolas Pierre & Estrade, Charlotte, eds. (2021), *Modernist Exceptions*, in *Miranda*, 23: https://doi.org/10.4000/miranda.40824

Boileau, Nicolas Pierre (2022). "Suburbia, or *Para*-urbia: Rachel Cusk's Gendered Readings of Suburban Spaces and the Role of the Writer in *Arlington Park*." M. Bouchet, I. Keller-Privat et al. (eds.) (2022). *Suburbs. New Literary Perspectives*. Rowman and Littlefield.

Boileau, Nicolas Pierre (2023). "*Reading* Hamlet *with Lacan, the Joint of Symptoms, Desire and Time*". J. Tambling (ed.). *The Bloomsbury Handbook of Psychoanalysis and Literature*. London: Bloomsbury Academic.

Bonikowski, Wyatt (2013). *Shell-Shock and the Modernist Imagination, The Death-Drive in post-World War I Fiction*. Burlington: Ashgate.

Bort, Françoise (2002). "Virginia Woolf et Dante: L'enfer de *Mrs Dalloway*". in C. Bernard & Ch. Reynier (eds.) (2002), *Le Pur et l'Impur*, Rennes: Presses Universitaires de Rennes, 91–106.

Bourdieu, Pierre (1986). "L'Illusion biographique". In *Actes de la recherche en sciences sociales*, vol. 62–63, juin 1986, 69–72.

Bowlby, Rachel (2011). "Real Life and its Readers in *Mrs Dalloway*". C. Bernard (ed.), *Woolf as Reader/Woolf as Critic or, The Art of Reading in the Present.* Montpellier: Presses Universitaires de Montpellier, 19–38.

Bradbury, Malcolm & McFarlane, James (eds.) (1976). *Modernism (1890–1930).* London: Penguin Books, reprinted 1991.

Brannigan, John (2005). *Pat Barker.* Manchester: Manchester University Press, "Contemporary British Novelists".

Braun, Alice (2008). *Janet Frame: Le Féminin et la Marge.* Unpublished PhD thesis defended in Paris Nanterre under the supervision of Prof. Claire Bazin.

Brevet, Anne-Laure (2011). "'The shadow of the fifth': Patterns of Exclusion in Doris Lessing's *The Fifth Child*". *La Clé des Langues, Lyon, ENS Lyon, DGESCO (ISSN 2107–7029), December 2011. Last 27/04/2022.* http://cle.ens-lyon.fr/anglais/litterature/litterature-britannique/the-shadow-of-the-fifth-patterns-of-exclusion-in-doris-lessing-s-the-fifth-child

Brintmall, Kent L. (2017). "Psychoanalysis' Tragedy". *Feminist Formations*, vol.29, No. 3.

Brock, Richard (2009). "'No Such Thing as Society': Thatcherism and Derridean Hospitality in *The Fifth Child*." *Doris Lessing Studies*, vol. 28, No. 1, 7–13.

Broughton, Panthea Reid (1987). "'Virginia is Anal': Speculations on Virginia Woolf's Writing 'Roger Fry' and Reading Sigmund Freud". *Journal of Modern Literature*, 14: 1, Spring, 151–157.

Brown, Dennis (2005). "*The Regeneration Trilogy*: Total War, Masculinities, Anthropologies, and the Talking Cure." Monteith et al. (eds.) (2005), 187–202.

Burston, Daniel (2020). *Psychoanalysis, Politics and the Postmodern University.* Basingstoke: Palgrave Macmillan.

Butler Judith (1990). *Gender Trouble, Feminism and the Subversion of Identity.* New York: Routledge.

Butler, Judith (1993). *Bodies that Matter Bodies that Matter.* New York: Routledge, 2011.

Butler, Judith (2005). *Giving an Account of Oneself.* New York: Fordham University Press.

Bynum, W.E. (1994). *Science and the Practice of Medicine in the Nineteenth Century.* Cambridge: Cambridge UP, "Cambridge History of Science Series".

Caminero-Santangelo, Marta (1998). *The Madwoman Can't Speak, Or Why Insanity is Not Subversive.* Ithaca: Cornell University Press.

Canguilhem, Georges (1958). "Qu'est-ce que la psychologie?" in *Revue de Métaphysique et de Morale*, n°1, 12–25.

Canguilhcm, Georges (1966). *Le Normal et le Pathologique.* Paris: Presses Universitaires de France, Quadrige, 2013.

Capé, Anouck (2011). *Les Frontières du délire: écrivains et fous au temps des avant-gardes.* Paris, Honoré Champion.

Casablancas-Cervantes, Anna (2010). "Creating Oneself as a Mother: Dreams, Reality and Identity in Doris Lessing's *The Fifth Child*." *Forum*, Issue 11, Autumn 2010. http://journals.ed.ac.uk/forum/article/view/653/937

Castanet, Hervé (2012). *La Perversion*. Paris: Economica-Anthropos.

Cavalié, Elsa (2015). *Réécrire l'Angleterre: l'anglicité dans la littérature contemporaine*. Montpellier: Presses Universitaires de Montpellier.

Chaney, Sarah (2011). "'A Hideous Torture on Himself': Madness and Self-Mutilation in Victorian Literature". *Journal of Medical Humanities*, 32: 279–289. DOI https://doi.org/10.1007/s10912-011-9152-6

Chesler, Phyllis (1994). *Preface* to Geller Jeffrey L. & Harris Maxine (eds.) (1994). *Women of the Asylum, Voices from behind the Walls, 1840–1945*. New York: Anchor Books.

Childs, Peter (2012). *Contemporary Fiction: British Novelists since 1970*. London: Palgrave Macmillan.

Church, Imogen (2018). "The Picture of Madness – Visual Narratives of Female Mental Illness in Contemporary Children's Literature". *Children's Literature in Education*, 49, 119–139. https://doi.org/10.1007/s10583-016-9286-2

Coates, Kimberly Engdahl (2012). "Phantoms, Fancy (And) Symptoms: Virginia Woolf and the Art of Being Ill". *Woolf Studies Annual*, vol. 18 (2012), 1–28.

Cohn, Dorrit (1978). *Transparent Minds, Narrative Modes for Presenting Consciousness in Fiction*. Princeton: Princeton UP.

Couser, Thomas G. (1997). *Recovering Bodies: Illness, Disability and Life-Writing*. Madison: University of Wisconsin Press.

Cronenberg, David (dir.) (2003). *Spider*, Metropolitan Film Export, with Ralph Fiennes, Miranda Richardson, etc.

Czajka, Isabelle (dir.) (2013), *La Vie domestique*, Agat Film & Cie, France 2 Production, with Emmanuelle Devos, Julie Ferrier, Natasha Regnier and Laurent Poitrenaux.

Danziger, Marie A. (1996). *Text/Countertext, Postmodern Paranoia in Samuel Beckett, Doris Lessing, and Philip Roth*. New York: Peter Lang.

De Bont, Leslie (2021). "'I saw at a glance that your case was exceptional, and that you also were Occult': Comedy, magic and exceptional disabilities in Stella Benson's *Living Alone* (1919)". In N. P. Boileau and Ch. Estrade (eds.). *Modernist Exceptions*, special issue of *Miranda*, 23: 2021. https://doi.org/10.4000/miranda.42498

De Vinne, Christine (2012). "The Uncanny Unnamable in Doris Lessing's *The Fifth Child* and *Ben, in the World*". *Names*, vol. 60, No. 1, March 2012, 15–25.

DeMeester, Karen (2007). "Trauma, Post-Traumatic Stress Disorder, and the Obstacles to Postwar Recovery in *Mrs Dalloway*." Eberly & Henke (eds.) (2007), 77–94.

Denes, Melissa (2003). "A Babel of Voices". *The Guardian*, 19 April, 2003.

Derbyshire, Jonathan (2012). "A Writer with a Splinter of Ice in her Heart". *The New Statesman*, 5 March 2012.

Didi-Hubermann, Georges (1982). *Invention de l'Hystérie*. Paris: Éditions Macula, 2012.

Dobrogoszcz, Tomasz (2021). "Are We In This Together?: The Polarisation of the British Society and the Marginalisation of Otherness in Ali Smith's *Seasonal Quartet.*" *Porównania*, vol. 3 (30), 2021. https://doi.org/10.14746/por.2021.3.9

Downie, Robin (2005). "Madness in Literature: Device and Understanding." C. Saunders and J. McNaughton (eds.), 49–66.

Dumas, Catherine (2008). *The Fifth Child*. Paris: Ellipses.

Dupont, Jocelyn (2006). "Parody and displacement of the Gothic in Patrick McGrath's work." "Rewriting/Reprising". *La Reprise en littérature*, Oct 2006, Lyon, France. hal-02466400

Dupont, Jocelyn (2007). "Récit de l'obsession et obsession du récit chez Patrick McGrath." M. Amfreville and C. Fabre (eds.). *Les Formes de l'obsession, vol. II*. Paris: Michel Houard Éditions, 139–149.

Dupont, Jocelyn (2008). *Intertextualité et autorité dans l'œuvre de Patrick McGrath*, Unpublished PhD thesis.

Dupont, Jocelyn (2009). "'In a Glass Grotesquely': Patrick McGrath's Quaint Old England". *Études britanniques contemporaines*. Montpellier: Presses universitaires de la Méditerranée, 87–98. ⟨10.4000/ebc.3685⟩. ⟨hal-02441379⟩

Dupont, Jocelyn (2010). "Du pastiche idéal à la parodie du pastiche: Patrick McGrath et la fin de l'angoisse de l'influence." J. Dupont & É. Walezak (eds.). *L'Intertextualité dans le roman contemporain de langue anglaise*. Perpignan: Presses Universitaires de Perpignan, 153–169. Available online: https://books.openedition.org/pupvd/32112

Dupont, Jocelyn (2013). "Les psychiatres fous du Dr McGrath." H. Machinal (ed.). *Le savant fou*. Rennes: Presses universitaires de Rennes. Last checked 12/21 http://books.openedition.org/pur/52928

Eaglestone, Robert (ed.) (2018). *Brexit and Literature. Critical and Cultural Response*. London: Routledge.

Easterlin, Nancy (2000). "Psychoanalysis and The Discipline of Love." in *Philosophy and Literature*. vol. 24, No. 2, 261–279.

Eberly, David and Henke, Suzette (2007), *Virginia Woolf and Trauma, Embodied Texts*, New York, Pace University Press.

Edelman, Lee (2003). "Sinthom-osexuality". in P. Matthews & D. McWirter (ed.). *Aesthetic Subjects*. Minneapolis: U of Minnesota P., 230–248.

Ehrenberg, Alain (1998) *La Fatigue d'être soi*. Paris, Odile Jacob.

Éribon, Didier (2005). *Échapper à la psychanalyse*. Paris: Leo Scheer.

Falco, Magali (2007a). *La Poétique néo-gothique de Patrick McGrath*. Paris: Éditions Publibook Université.

Falco, Magali (2007b). *A Collection of Interviews with Patrick McGrath.* Paris: Editions Publibook Université.

Favre, Valérie (2021). "Virginia Woolf et ses 'petites soeurs': Relire *A Room of One's Own* au prisme de sa postérité littéraire, critique et féministe dans l'espace Atlantique anglophone des années soixante à nos jours". Unpublished PhD Thesis, University of Lyon 2, 2021.

Felman Shoshana (1975). "Women and Madness: The Critical Phallacy". *Diacritics,* 5: 4, 2–10.

Felman Shoshana (1978). *Writing and Madness,* Palo Alto: Stanford UP, 2003.

Ferrer, Daniel (1990). *Virginia Woolf and the Madness of Language.* Geoffrey Bennington and Rachel Bowlby (trans.). London: Routledge, 1990.

Foucault, Michel (1963). *Naissance de la Clinique.* Paris: Presses Universitaires de France, "Quadrige grands textes", 2003. For the English version: http://monoskop.org/images/9/92/Foucault_Michel_The_Birth_of_the_Clinic_1976.pdf

Foucault, Michel (1972). *Histoire de la folie à l'âge classique.* Paris: Gallimard, "Tel".

Frances, Allen (2009). "Whither DSM-V?" *British Journal of Psychiatry.* 195:5, 391–392. doi: https://doi.org/10.1192/bjp.bp.109.073932

Freud, Sigmund (1899–1930). *The Interpretation of Dreams.* trans. J.-P. Lefebvre. Paris: Seuil, 'Essais', 2010.

Freud, Sigmund (1912). "Sur la Dynamique du transfert". *La Technique psychana-lytique,* Paris: Presses Universitaires de France, 2013, 57–68.

Freud, Sigmund (1905a). *Jokes and their Relation to the Unconscious.* London: Norton, 1989.

Freud, Sigmund (1905b). *Cinq Psychanalyses.* Paris: Presses Universitaires de France, 2008.

Freud, Sigmund (1919). *L'Inquiétante étrangeté et autres essais.* Paris: Gallimard, 1985.

Freud, Sigmund (1923). "la Disparition du complexe d'Œdipe". *La Vie sexuelle.* Paris: Presses Universitaires de France, trans. Laplanche, 1969.

Freud, Sigmund (1926). *Inhibition, Symptome et Angoisse.* Trans. J. and R. Doron. Paris: Presses Universitaires de France, 1993.

Freud, Sigmund (1931). "On Female Sexuality" trans. "Sur la sexualité féminine", in La Vie sexuelle, Paris: PUF, 1969, 139-155.

Friedan, Betty (1963). *The Feminine Mystique.* London: Penguin, "Modern Classics", 2010.

Froula, Christine (2002). "Mrs. Dalloway's Postwar Elegy: Women, War, and the Art of Mourning." *Modernism/modernity,* Volume 9, Number 1, January 2002, 125–163, https://doi.org/10.1353/mod.2002 [last accessed 21 October 2021]

Frosh, Stephen (1991). "Psychoanalysis, Psychosis, and Postmodernism". *Human Relations,* vol. 44, No 1, 93–104.

Frosh, Stephen (2003). "Psychoanalysis in Britain: The Rituals of Destruction". D. Bradshaw (ed.). *A Concise Companion to Modernism.* Malden: Blackwell Publishing, 116–137.

Gagneret, Diane (2019). *Explorer la frontière: Folie et genre(s) dans la littérature anglophone contemporaine.* Unpublished PhD thesis defended at ENS Lyon, 22.11.2019, under the supervision of Prof. Vanessa Guignery.

Gallagher, Lucy (2011). *The Contemporary Middlebrow Novel.* Unpublished Ph.D. thesis, Newcastle University, 2011.

Gaspard, Jean-Luc (2010). "Nouveaux symptômes et lien social contemporain". L. Jodeau-Belle & L. Ottavi (eds.) (2010). 357–371.

Geller, Jeffrey L. & Harris, Maxine (eds.) (1994). *Women of the Asylum.* New York: Anchor Book.

Germanà, Monica (2017). "Ali Smith: Strangers and Intrusions". J. Acheson. *The Contemporary British Novel Since 2000.* Edinburgh: Edinburgh University Press.

Germanà, Monica & Horton, Emily (eds.) (2013). *Ali Smith: Contemporary Critical Perspectives.* London: Bloomsbury Academic.

Gilbert, Sandra & Gubar, Susan (1984). *The Madwoman in the Attic: The Woman Writer and the Nineteenth Century Literary Imagination.* New Haven: Yale University Press.

Gilman, Sander L. (1982). *Seeing the Insane.* London: Wiley and Son.

Gordon, C., Pryor R. & Watkins, G. (1990). *Sounds from the Bell Jar, Ten psychotic Authors.* London: Macmillan.

Gori, Roland & Del Volgo, Marie-José (2005). *La Santé totalitaire, Essai sur la médicalisation de l'existence.* Paris: Éditions Denoël, "Champs Essais".

Gori, Roland & Del Volgo, Marie-José (2020), *Exilés de l'intime, Vers un Homme neuroéconomique.* Paris: Les Liens qui libèrent.

Graham, Elyse & Lewis, Pericles (2013). "Private Religion, Public Mourning and Mrs Dalloway." *Modern Philology*, vol. 111, n°1, 2013, 88–106.

Gualtieri, Elena (2000). *Virginia Woolf's Essays: Sketching the Past.* London: Macmillan.

Guéguen, Pierre-Gilles (2011). "Lacan américain", *La Cause freudienne*, 2011/3, n°79, 179–182 https://www.cairn.info/revue-la-cause-freudienne-2011-3-page-179.htm# (last checked 09/2020).

Gutleben, Christian (2015). "Serious Play: The Representation of the Thatcher Years in Malcolm Bradbury's *Cuts*, David Lodge's *Nice Work* and Alan Hollinghurst's *The Line of Beauty*." *Études britanniques contemporaines*, 49:2015, doi: https://doi.org/10.4000/ebc.2705

Hannah, Daniel K. (2007). "The Private Life, the Public Stage: Henry James in Recent Fiction." *Journal of Modern Literature*, vol. 30, No. 3, 70–94.

Hawthorn Jeremy (1975). *Virginia Woolf's Mrs Dalloway, A study in Alienation.* London: Sussex University Press, "Text and Context".

Herman, Judith Lewis (1992). *Trauma and Recovery, From Domestic Abuse to Political Terror*. London: Pandora, 2015.

Heynders, Odile (2021). "Dissensus in Ali Smith's *Seasonal Quartet*". *Frame, Journal of Literary Studies*, No. 34.1, May 2021, 35–51.

Hilson, Mica (2012). "'The Odd Man out in the Family?' Queer Throwbacks and Reproductive Futurism." *Doris Lessing Studies*, vol. 30, No. 1, 18–22.

Hitchcock, Peter (2002). "What is Prior? Working-Class Masculinity in Pat Barker's Trilogy." *Genders 35*, http://www.genders.org/g35/g35_hitchcock.html

Hollinghurst, Alan (2004b). "The Middle Fears". in *The Guardian*, Sat. 4 September 2004.

Hopson, Jacqueline (2020). "Malevolent, Mad or Merely Human: Representations of the 'Psy' Professional in English, American and Irish Fiction." PhD defended in September 2020 at the University of Exeter, unpublished: https://search-proquest-com.lama.univ-amu.fr/docview/2497503683?pq-origsite=summon [last checked on 5 May 2020]

Horton, Emily (2012). "'Everything You've Ever Dreamed': Post-9/11 Trauma and Fantasy in Ali Smith's *The Accidental*". *Modern Fiction Studies*. Fall 2012, Vol. 58, No. 3, 637–654.

Hsieh, Meng-Tsung (2010). "Almost Human but Not Quite?: The Impenetrability of Being in Doris Lessing's *Ben, In the World*." *Doris Lessing Studies*, vol. 29, No.1, 14–19.

Hustvedt, Asti (2011). *Medical Muses, Hysteria in Nineteenth-Century Paris*. London: Bloomsbury.

Hutcheon Linda (1988). *A Poetics of Postmodernism, History, Theory, Fiction*. New York: Routledge.

Innes, Catherine L. (2007). *The Cambridge Introduction to Postcolonial Literatures in English*. Cambridge: Cambridge University Press.

Jodeau-Belle, Laëtitia & Ottavi, Laurent (eds.) (2010). *Les Fondamentaux de la psychanalyse lacanienne*. Rennes: Presses Univesitaires de Rennes, 185–197.

Johnson, Allan (2014). *Alan Hollinghurst and the Vitality of Influence*. London: Palgrave Macmillan.

Juranville, Alain (1984). *Lacan et la philosophie*. Paris: Presses Universitaires de France, "Quadrige", 2003.

Kantorowicz, Ernest H (1957). *The King's Two Bodies: a Study in Medieval Political Theology*. Princeton: Princeton University Press, 1981.

Keitel, Evelyne (1989). *Reading Psychosis: Readers, Texts and Psychoanalysis*. London: Blackwell.

Kellaway, Kate (2001). "Mother's ruin." *The Observer*, 9 September 2001.

Kellaway, Kate (2014). Interview of Rachel Cusk, 24 August 2014, last checked May 2022. https://www.theguardian.com/books/2014/aug/24/rachel-cusk-interview-aftermath-outline

Kim, Soo Yeon (2016). "Betrayed by Beauty: Ethics and Aesthetics in Alan Hollinghurst's *The Line of Beauty*". *Texas Studies in Literature and Language*, vol. 58, No.2, summer 2016, 165–188. Doi: https://doi.org/10.7560/TSLL58203

King, Pamela (2018). *L'American Way of Life: Lacan et les débuts de l'ego-psychologie*. Fontenay-le-Comte: Éditions Lussaud.

Knapp, Mona (1984). *Doris Lessing*. New York: Frederick Ungar Publishing Co.

La Sagna, Philippe & Adam, Rodolphe (2020). *Contrer l'universel*. Paris: Éditions Michèle.

Lacan, Jacques (1949). "Le Stade du Miroir comme formateur de la fonction du Je telle qu'elle nous est révélée dans l'expérience psychanalytique". *Écrits I*. Paris: Éditions du Seuil, "Essais Points", 1999, 92–99.

Lacan, Jacques (1966). *Écrits I*. Paris: Éditions du Seuil, "Essais Points", 1999.

Lacan, Jacques (1971). "Lituraterre". *Autres écrits*, 11–20.

Lacan, Jacques (1981). *Le Séminaire*, Livre III, *Les Psychoses* (1955–56). J.-A. Miller (ed.). Paris: Éditions du Seuil.

Lacan, Jaques (2001). *Autres écrits*. Paris: Éditions du seuil, "Champ freudien".

Lacan, Jacques (2013). *Le Séminaire, Livre VI, Le Désir et son interprétation* (1958–1959) J.-A. Miller (ed.). Paris: Éditions de la Martinière.

Lacan, Jacques (2004). *Le Séminaire*, Livre X, *L'Angoisse* (1962–63). J.-A. Miller (ed.). Paris: Éditions du Seuil.

Lacan, Jacques (1973). *Le Séminaire*, Livre XI, *Les Quatre Concepts fondamentaux de la psychanalyse* (1963–64). J.-A. Miller (ed.). Paris: Éditions du Seuil.

Lacan, Jacques (1975). *Le Séminaire, Livre XX, Encore* (1972–73). J.-A. Miller (ed.). Paris: Éditions du Seuil. The English translation by Bruce Fink was published in 1998, "On Feminine Sexuality, the Limits of Love and Knowledge, 1972–1973. New York: Norton, 1999.

Lacan, Jacques (1979). "Lacan pour Vincennes!", *Ornicar?*, 17/18, Spring 1979.

Lacan, Jacques (1991). *Le Séminaire, Livre XVII, Envers de la psychanalyse* (1970). J.-A. Miller (ed.). Paris: Éditions du Seuil.

Lacan, Jacques (2005). *Le Séminaire, Livre XXIII, Le Sinthome* (1975–76). J.-A. Miller (ed.). Paris: Éditions du Seuil.

Lacan, Jacques (2011). *Le Séminaire, Livre XIX, … Ou pire* (1971–72). J.-A. Miller (ed.). Paris: Éditions du Seuil.

Lacan, Jacques (1974). "Les non-dupes-errent", leçon du 19 février, 1974. Unpublished.

Laing, Ronald David (1969). *The Divided Self,* New York, USA: Pantheon.

Lanone, Catherine (1999). "Scattering the Seed of Abraham: The Motif of Sacrifice in Pat Barker's *Regeneration* and *The Ghost Road*." *Literature & Theology* 13: 3, 259–68.

Lanone, Catherine (2007). "Entre accord et écart: l'expérience de lecture selon Virginia Woolf et E. M. Forster". C. Bernard & C. Lanone (eds.), "Woolf lectrice/Woolf critique", *Études britanniques contemporaines*. Montpellier: Presses Universitaires de la Méditerranée, 111–124.

Lapeyre, Michel (2000). *Complexe d'Œdipe et complexe de castration*. Paris: Anthropos.

Latham, Monica (2013). "*Arlington Park:* Variations on Virginia Woolf's *Mrs Dalloway*". Boileau et al. (eds.) (2013) https://journals.openedition.org/erea/3216

Latham, Monica (2016). *A Poetics of Postmodernism and Neomodernism*. New York: Routledge.

Latham, Monica (2021). *Virginia Woolf's Afterlives, The Author as Character in Contemporary Fiction*. London: Routledge.

Latham, Sean (2003). *Am I a Snob? Modernism and the Novel*. Ithaca: Cornell University Press.

Laurent, Éric (2016). *L'Envers de la biopolitique. Une écriture pour la jouissance*. Paris: Editions Navarin, "Le Champ freudien".

Leader, Daria (2014). "Lacan and the Subject", in *Philosophy, Psychiatry and Psychology*, vol.24, No. 4. Dec. 2014, 367–68.

Leavy, Stanley A (2010). "What happened to Psychoanalysis?" *American Imago*, vol. 67, n°1, 73–87.

Lecercle, Jean-Jacques (1996). *La Violence du langage*, Michèle Garlati (trans.). Paris: Presses Universitaires de France.

Lecercle, Jean-Jacques (2004). "Redondance et surclassement: pour une théorie du superflu en littérature". G. Girard (ed.). *Le Superflu chose très nécessaire*. Rennes: Presses Universitaires de Rennes, 17–32.

Lecomte, Héloïse (2020). "The Hapax of Mourning: Ali Smith's *Artful*". *Études britanniques contemporaines*, 58, 2020. https://doi-org.lama.univ-amu.fr/10.4000/ebc.8201

Lee, Hermione (1996). *Virginia Woolf*. New York: Random House, Vintage, 1999.

Lee Hermione (2005). *Virginia Woolf's Nose*. New York: Princeton UP.

Lessing, Doris (2001). "I have nothing in common with Feminists. They never seem to think that one might enjoy men." *The Guardian*, Sept. 9, 2001, https://www.theguardian.com/books/2001/sep/09/fiction.dorislessing

Letissier, Georges (2007), "Queer, Quaint and Camp: Alan Hollinghurst's Own Return to the English Tradition", *Études anglaises*, 2007/2, vol.60, 198–211, 10.3917/etan.602.0198

Letissier, Georges (2019). "L'œuvre romanesque du romancier Alan Hollinghurst: contre-épopée anglaise et généalogie d'une culture alternative". *Itinéraires*, 2019, 2 & 3. 10.4000/itineraires.7020

Ley, James (2020). "Brexit, Pursued by a Bard". *The Sydney Review of Books*. December 4, 2020. https://sydneyreviewofbooks.com/review/smith-autumn-winter-spring-summer/

Lockwood, Patricia (2018). "Why do I have to know what MacDonald's is?" *London Review of Books*, vol. 40, No.9, 10 May 2018, https://www.lrb.co.uk/the-paper/v40/n09/patricia-lockwood/why-do-i-have-to-know-what-mcdonald-s-is

Lodge, David (1992). *The Art of Fiction*, London: Vintage, 2011.

Lucchelli, Juan-Pablo (2009). *Le Transfert de Freud à Lacan*. Rennes: Presses Universitaires de Rennes.

Lucey, Michael (2022). *What Proust Heard and the Ethnography of Talk*. Chicago: The University of Chicago Press.

Luckhurst Roger (2008). *The Trauma Question*. New York: Routledge.

Lyotard, Jean-François (1984). *The Postmodern Condition, A Report on Knowledge*. Minneapolis: University of Minnesota Press.

Maleval, Jean-Claude (1997). *Logique du délire*. Paris: Masson, "Ouvertures Psy", 2000.

Maleval, Jean-Claude (2010). "Comment entendre la voix?". L. Jodeau-Belle & L. Ottavi Laurent (eds.) (2010), 185–197.

Maleval, Jean-Claude (2012). *Étonnantes mystifications, De la psychothérapie autoritaire*. Paris: Éditions Navarin, "Le champ freudien".

Maleval, Jean-Claude (2019). *Repères pour la psychose ordinaire*. Paris: Navarin Éditeurs, 2019.

Marret-Maleval, Sophie (2009). "Le Séminaire XXIII 'Le sinthome'", Introduction à la lecture du Séminaire XXIII, http://www.causefreudienne.net/etudier/le-seminaire-de-lacan/le-seminaire-xxiii-le-sinthome.html, Pdf 5 pages. https://www.causefreudienne.net/le-sinthome/ (last accessed Oct. 19th, 2021)

Marret, Sophie (2010). *L'Inconscient aux sources du mythe moderne: les grands mythes de la littérature fantastique*. Rennes: Presses Universitaires de Rennes.

Marret, Sophie (2017). "Importance et enjeux de la psychose ordinaire". *L'a-graphe*, revue de la section clinique de Rennes 2017–18, Département de psychanalyse de Paris 8, 89–99.

Maslen, Elizabeth (1994). *Doris Lessing: Writers and their Work*. Plymouth, UK: Northcote House.

Masterson, John. "'Don't tell me this isn't relevant all over again in its brand new same old way': Imagination, Agitation, and Raging against the Machine in Ali Smith's *Spring*." Safundi 21.3 (2020): 355–372. https://doi.org/10.1080/17533171.2020.1776961

Mathuray, Mark (ed.) (2017). *Sex and Sensibility in the Novels of Alan Hollinghurst*. London: Palgrave Macmillan.

May, William (2010). *Postwar Literature 1950–1990*, London: York Press.

McAlpin, Heller (2018). "An Epic Conversation Draws to a Close in *Kudos*." https://www.npr.org/2018/06/05/613465563/an-epic-conversation-draws-to-a-close-in-kudos?t=1622381639864 last checked May 2022.

McGrath, Patrick (1989). "A Childhood in Broadmoor Hospital". *Granta*, Dec. 22, 1989. https://granta.com/a-childhood-in-broadmoor-hospital/

McGrath, Patrick (2002), "Problem of Drawing from Psychiatry for a Fiction Writer." *Psychiatric Bulletin*, 26, 140–143.

Messud, Claire (2017). "Fierce, She Got Outside the Moment". *The New York Review of Books*, March, 23rd, 2017: https://www.nybooks.com/articles/2017/03/23/rachel-cusk-transit-fierce-outside-moment/ (checked in May 2022)

Micale, Mark S. (1993). "On the 'Disappearance' of Hysteria: A Study in the Clinical Deconstruction of a Diagnosis". *Isis*, vol.84, n°3, Sept.1993, 496–526.

Micale, Mark S. & Lerner, Patrick (eds.) (2001). *Traumatic Pasts, History, Psychiatry and Trauma in the Modern Age 1870–1930*. Cambridge: Cambridge University Press.

Mijangos, Lynne (2016). "Listening for the Voices of Women: A Close Reading of Virginia Woolf's 'On Being Ill'". *Woolf Miscellany*, 64–65.

Miller, Jacques-Alain (1993). "Clinique ironique". *Revue de la Cause Freudienne*, n°23.

Miller, Jacques-Alain (ed.) (1998). *La psychose ordinaire. La convention d'Antibes*. Paris: Seuil.

Miller, Jacques-Alain (1999). "Les Six Paradigmes de la Jouissance". *La Cause freudienne* No. 43, 7–29.

Miller, Jacques-Alain (2004). "Pièces détachées", *L'Orientation lacanienne*, lesson of 17 November 2004, unpublished.

Miller, Jacques-Alain (2009). "Ordinary Psychosis Revisited" in *Psychoanalytical Notebooks* 19, 139–168: https://static1.squarespace.com/static/5d52d51fc078720001362276/t/6038e36fe6cd371d192a5947/1614340978700/20080707+Miller+Ordinary+psychosis+Psychoanalytic+Notebooks+Vol+19+p139-168+.PDF

Miller, Jacques-Alain (2016). "*Jouissance* is Coupled with Meaning." *The Lacanian Review, Hurly-Burly*, "Sex all Over the Place", 2016, Issue 2, 9–20.

Miller, Jacques-Alain (2018). *L'os d'une cure*. Paris: Navarin éditeur.

Minow-Pinkney Makiko (1987). *Virginia Woolf and the Problem of the Subject*. New Brunswick, Rutgers University Press.

Mitchell, Juliet & Rose, Jacqueline (1985). *Feminine Sexuality, Jacques Lacan and the* école freudienne. London: Norton.

Moi, Toril (1985). *Sexual/Textual Politics*. New York: Routledge, 2002.

Monteith, Sharon, Jolly, Margaretta, Yousaf, Nahem and Ronald, Paul (eds.) (2005). *Critical Perspectives on Pat Barker*. Columbia: University of South Carolina Press.

Moran, Patricia (1996). *Word of Mouth, Body Language in Katherine Mansfield & Virginia Woolf*. Charlottesville: University of Virginia Press.

Moran, Patricia (2007). *Virginia Woolf, Jean Rhys, and the Aesthetics of Trauma*. New York: Palgrave Macmillan.

Mosse, George L. (2000). "Shell-Shock as a Social Disease". *Journal of Contemporary History*, vol.35, n°1, 101–108.

Mulalić, Lejla (2020). "Politics and the Novel in a Post-Brexit World: Ali Smith's *Autumn*". *Journal of Education and Humanities*. Volume 3, No.1, 43–52.

Mullini, Roberta (1989). "'Pardon my folly in writing of folly': Les ouvrages sur la folie de Robert Armin". Max Milner (ed.). *Littérature et Pathologie*. Paris: L'imaginaire du texte, 245–254.

Nathan, T., Blanchet A., et al. (1998). *Psychothérapies*, Paris: Odile Jacob.

Nasio, Juan David (2012). *L'Œdipe*. Paris: Petite Bibliothèque Payot.

Orosz-Réti, Zsófia (2021). "Covidian Metamorphoses: Art and the Poetics of Transformation in Ali Smith's *Seasonal Quartet*". *Acta Universitatis Sapientiae, Philologica*. Vol. 13, No.1, 60–72.

Oyebode, Femi (ed.) (2009). *Misreadings: Literature and Psychiatry*. London: Royal College of Psychiatry Publications.

Paul, Ronald (2005). "In Pastoral Fields: The *Regeneration* Trilogy and Classic First World War Fiction". Monteith et al. (eds.), 147–161.

Pett, Sarah (2019). "Re-Thinking Virginia Woolf's *On Being Ill*". *Literature and Medicine*, volume 37, n°1, Spring 2019, 26–66.

Pollock, Jonathan (2001). *Qu'est-ce que l'humour?* Paris: Klicksieck.

Pommier, Gérard (2004). *Comment les neurosciences démontrent la psychanalyse.* Paris: Flammarion, "Champs Essais".

Poole, Roger (1978). *The Unknown Virginia Woolf.* Cambridge: Cambridge University Press, 1990.

Porter, Roy (2002). *Madness, a Brief History.* Oxford: Oxford University Press.

Prose, Francine (2018). "Real Talk: Rachel Cusk's *Kudos*". *The Sewanee Review*, 126.3, 520–534.

Rabaté, Jean-Michel (ed.) (2003), *The Cambridge Companion to Lacan.* Cambridge: Cambridge University Press.

Rabeyron, T., Evrard, R. et Massicotte, C. (2020). "Psychoanalysts and the Sour Apple: Thought-transference in Historical and Contemporary Psychoanalysis". *Contemporary Psychoanalysis*, 56 (4), 1–41.

Rahimnouri, Zahra & Ghandehariun, Azra (2020). "A Feminist Stylistic Analysis of Doris Lessing's *The Fifth Child* (1988)". *Journal of Language and Literature*, vol. 20, No. 2, 221–230.

Raman, Ratna (2021). *The Fiction of Doris Lessing: Re-envisioning Feminism.* London: Bloomsbury.

Rannou, Isabelle (2013). "'Like journeying through a painting': Travel Writing and the Exploration of Textual Boundaries in Rachel Cusk's *The Last Supper*". *E-rea*, 10.2 | 2013, checked on 27 Dec. 2017. URL: http://journals.openedition.org/erea/3235

Raschke, Debrah (2003). "*The Fifth Child*: From Fairy-Tale to Monstrosity." *Doris Lessing Studies*, Vol. 23, No 1.

Rau, Petra (2018). "*Autumn* After the Referendum". R. Eaglestone (ed.) (2018). 31–43.

Reviron, Floriane (2004). "'Am I a Snob?' de Virginia Woolf: autoportrait d'une femme savante en précieuse ridicule." S. Crinquand (ed.). *Par Humour de soi*, Dijon: Presses Universitaires de Dijon, "Kaléidoscopes", 85–94.

Reynier, Christine (2009). *Virginia Woolf's Ethics of the Short Stories.* New York: Palgrave Macmillan, 2009.

Reynier, Christine (2019). *Virginia Woolf's* Good Housekeeping *Essays.* New York: Routledge.

Reynier, Christine (2021). "Virginia Woolf's Radical Vision of Recycling". In Latham, Monica, Marie, Caroline & Rigeade, Anne-Laure (eds.). *Recycling Virginia Woolf in Contemporary Art and Literature.* Londres: Routledge.

Regard, Frédéric (2002). *La Force du féminin, Sur trois essais de Virginia Woolf.* Paris: La Fabrique Éditions.

Ricœur, Paul (1984). "Entre le temps mortel et le temps monumental: *Mrs Dalloway*". *Temps et récit*, vol. 2, *La Configuration du récit de fiction.* Paris: Éditions du seuil, 1984, 192–212.

Ridout, Alice & Watkins, Susan (eds.) (2009). *Doris Lessing, Border Crossings.* London: Continuum. https://doi.org/10.5040/9781472542403

Rigney, Barbara Hill (1978). *Madness and Sexual Politics in the Feminist Novel, Studies of Brontë, Woolf, Lessing and Atwood.* Madison, USA: the University of Wisconsin Press.

Rivkin, Julie (2005). "Writing the Gay 80s with Henry James: David Leavitt's *A Place I've Never Been* and Alan Hollinghurst's *The Line of Beauty*". *The Henry James* Review, vol. 26, No. 3, 282–292.

Roberts, Adam (2017). "Ogee: The Line of Beauty". In M. Mathuray (ed.), 111–128.

Robbins, Ruth (2009). "'(Not Such) Great Expectations: Unmaking Maternal Ideals in *The Fifth Child* and *We Need to Talk about Kevin*". A. Ridout and S. Watkins (eds.), 92–106.

Ross, Sarah C. E. (2005). "Regeneration, Redemption, Resurrection: Pat Barker and the Problem of Evil." In Acheson & Ross (eds) (2005).

Rothstein, Mervyn (1988). "The Painful Nurturing of Doris Lessing's *Fifth Child*." in *The New York Times*, https://archive.nytimes.com/www.nytimes.com/books/99/01/10/specials/lessing-child.html?_r=1

Rouverol, Alicia J. (2019). "Fragmentary Writing and Globalization in Ali Smith's *Hotel World*". V. Guignery &W. Drag (eds.). *The Poetics of Fragmentation in British and American Contemporary Fiction.* Wilmington: Vernon Press, 67–80.

Rubenstein, Roberta (2009). "Doris Lessing's Fantastic Children". A. Ridout & S. Watkins (eds.), 61–74.

Rundgren, Heta (2016). "Vers une théorie du roman postnormâle: Féminisme, réalisme et conflit sexuel chez Doris Lessing, Märta Tikkanen, Stieg Larsonn et Virginie Despentes". Unpublished PhD thesis Paris 8, France and Helsinki, Finland.

Ryan-Sautour, Michelle (2019). "*Shire* and *How to Be Both* by Ali Smith." *Etudes Britanniques Contemporaines*, 57.

Sadjadi, Bakhtiar (2016). "Investigating Trauma in Narrating World War I: A Psychoanalytical Reading of Pat Barker's *Regeneration*". *Advances in Language and Literary Studies*, Vol. 7, No.6, 10.755/aiac.alls.v.7n.6p.189

Saiful, Islam Muhammad (2013). "Anticipating Apocalypse: Power Structures and the Periphery in Doris Lessing's *The Fifth Child* and *Ben, in the World*". *Romanian Journal of English Studies*, 278–292, doi: https://doi.org/10.2478/rjes-2013-0027

Saudo-Welby, Nathalie (2019). *Le Courage de déplaire. Le roman féministe à la fin de l'ère victorienne*. Paris: Classiques Garnier.

Saunders, Corinne and McNaughton, Jane (eds.) (2005). *Madness and Creativity in Literature and Culture*. London: Palgrave Macmillan.

Scanlan, Margaret (2001). *Plotting Terror, Novelists and Terrorists in Contemporary Fiction*. Charlottesville: The UP of Virginia.

Schlack Beverly Ann (1979). *Continuing Presences: Virginia Woolf's Use of Literary Allusions*. Pennsylvania University Press.

Schlueter, Paul (1973). *The Novels of Doris Lessing*. Carbondale: The Southern Illinois UP.

Seligman, Stephen (2019). "The New Psychoanalysis". *Dissent*, vol.66, No. 1, Winter, 97–103.

Shaw, Kristian (2018), "Brexlit". R. Eaglestone (ed.) (2018). 15–30.

Shorter, Edward (1997). *A History of Psychiatry, From the Era of the Asylum to the Age of Prozac*. New York: John Wiley and Sons, Inc.

Showalter, Elaine (1977). *A Literature of their Own, British Women Novelists from Brontë to Lessing*. London: Virago Press, 1982.

Showalter, Elaine (1985). *The Female Malady, Women, Madness and English Culture, 1830–1980*. London: Virago Press (1985).

Showalter, Elaine (1997). *Hystories, Hysterical Epidemics and Modern Culture*. London: Picador, 2013.

Singsit-Evans, Sharon (2014). "On *Regeneration* (from the *Regeneration* Trilogy) by Pat Barker". *The British Journal of Psychiatry*, 417, doi: https://doi.org/10.1192/bjp.bp.113.139238

Skott-Myhre, Hans (2008). *Who Are We To Become If We Are Not This: Madness, Anti-Psychiatry and literature*. PhD Philosophy, Minnesota.

Smith, Ali (2011). "Once Upon a Life: Ali Smith". *The Guardian*, 29 May 2011, https://www.theguardian.com/lifeandstyle/2011/may/29/once-upon-life-ali-smith

Smith, Ali (2015). "A Gift for John Berger: The Art Critic that contains multitudes". *The New Statesman*, 2 October 2015: https://www.newstatesman.com/culture/2015/10/gift-john-berger

Smith, Ali (2020b). "Before Brexit, Grenfell, Covid-19... Ali Smith on writing four novels in four years". *The Guardian*, August 1ˢᵗ, 2020, https://www.the-guardian.com/books/2020/aug/01/before-brexit-grenfell-covid-19-ali-smith-on-writing-four-novels-in-four-years

Soler, Colette. *L'Aventure littéraire ou la psychose inspirée*. Paris: Champ lacanien, 2001.

Steffens, Karolyn (2014). "Communicating Trauma: Pat Barker's *Regeneration* Trilogy and W.H.R. Rivers's Psychoanalytic Method". *Journal of Modern Literature*, volume 37, No. 3, 36–55.

Stevenson, Sheryl (2005). "The Uncanny Case of Dr. Rivers and Mr. Prior: Dynamics of Transference in *The Eye in the Door*". In Monteith et al. (eds.) (2005), 219–233.

Stone, Jon, et al. (2008). "The 'Disappearance' of Hysteria: Historical Mystery or Illusion?". *Journal of Royal Society of Medicine*, 101, 12–18, DOI: https://doi.org/10.1258/jrsm.2007.070129

Soler Colette (2002). *L'Inconscient à ciel ouvert de la psychose*. Toulouse: Presses Universitaires du Mirail.

Sontag, Susan (1978–1989). *Illness as Metaphor* (1977–78) and *Aids and Its Metaphors* (1988–89). London: Doubleday.

Squier, Susan Merrill (1985). *Virginia Woolf and London, The Sexual Politics of the City*. Chapel Hill: The University of North Carolina Press.

Su, John (2014). "Beauty and the Beastly Prime Minister". *EHL*, vol.81, No3, Fall 2014, 1083–1110.

Suhamy, Henri (1989). "Éloge de la folie ou folie de l'éloge". *Actes des congrès de la Société française Shakespeare*, 7, 9–16.

Szasz, Thomas S. (1961). *The Myth of Mental Illness*. St Albans, UK: Paladin, 1977 [1961].

Szasz, Thomas S. (1970). *Ideology and Insanity: Essays on the Psychiatric Dehumanization of Man*. Syracuse, New York: Syracuse University Press. 1991.

Szasz, Thomas S. (1973). *L'Âge de la folie*. Paris: PUF, 1978 [1973].

Talairach, Laurence (2013). "'Knowledge for its own sake, is the one God I worship': Les Savants fous dans *Heart and Science* de Wilkie Collins". H. Machinal (ed.), *Le Savant fou*, Rennes, Presses Universitaires de Rennes, 127–143: https://books.openedition.org/pur/52903

Tang, Maria (2013). "Bodies at Risk: Ambiguous Subjectivities in *Arlington Park*. A Beauvoirean Perspective". Boileau et al. (eds.), 2013.

Tayler, Christopher (2005). "Imbued... with Exigence". *London Review of Books*, vol. 27, No.18, 22 September 2005, https://www.lrb.co.uk/the-paper/v27/n18/christopher-tayler/imbued-with-exigence

Terzian, Peter (2011). "The Art of Fiction No.214: Interview of Alan Hollinghurst". *The Paris Review*, Issue 1999, Winter 2011.

Thiher, Allen (1999). *Revels in Madness, Insanity in Medicine and Literature*. Ann Arbor: University of Michigan Press, 2004.

Thomas, Sue (1987). "Virginia Woolf's Septimus Smith and Contemporary Perceptions of Shell Shock." *English Language Notes,* vol. 25, No. 2, 49–57.

Tobié, Nathan, Blanchet Alain, Ionescu, Serban, & Zadje, Nathalie (ed.) (1998). *Psychothérapies*. Paris: Odile Jacob.

Tomasi David Lag (2020). *Critical Neuroscience and Philosophy, A Scientific Re-Examination of the Mind-Body Problem*. London: Palgrave Macmillan.

Tollance, Pascale. "Penser l'être-avec: hôtes et parasites dans la fiction d'Ali Smith". *L'Atelier*, 12.2, 2020, 75–91.

Toth, Naomi (2016). *L'Écriture vive, Woolf, Sarraute, une autre phénoménologie de la perception*. Paris: Classiques Garnier, "Perspectives comparatistes, 47".

Trombley, Stephen (1982). *All that Summer She Was Mad, Virginia Woolf: Female Victim of Male Medicine*. New York: Continuum.

Valihora, Karen (2019). "She Got Up and Went Away: Rachel Cusk on Making an Exit". *English Studies in Canada*, 45.1–2 (March/June 2019): 19–35.

Vickroy, Laurie (2004). "A Legacy of Pacifism: Virginia Woolf and Pat Barker". *Women and Language*, vol. 27, No.2, 45–50.

Walezak, Emilie (2021). *Rethinking Contemporary British Women's Writing: Realism, Feminism, Materialism*. London: Bloomsbury.

Wall, Oisin (2018). *The British Anti-Psychiatrists, from institutional Psychiatry to Counter-Culture, 1960–1971*. London: Routledge.

Wally, Johannes. "The Return of Political Fiction? An Analysis of Howard Jacobson's *Pussy* (2017) and Ali Smith's *Autumn* (2016) as First Reactions to the Phenomena 'Donald Trump' and 'Brexit' in Contemporary British Literature", *AAA – Arbeiten aus Anglistik und Amerikanistik*, Issue 43 (2018), online.

Ward, Sean Francis (2016). "Erotohistoriography and War's Waste in Pat Barker's *Regeneration* Trilogy". *Contemporary Literature* 57:3, 320–345.

Westman, Karin E (2005). "Generation Not Regeneration: Screening Out Class, Gender, and Cultural Change in the Film of *Regeneration*". In Monteith et al. (eds.) (2005), 162–172.

Whitehead Anne (2005). "Open to Suggestion, Hypnosis and History in the *Regeneration* Trilogy". Monteith et al. (eds.) (2005), 203–2018.

Whitworth Michael (2005). *Virginia Woolf*. Oxford, Oxford University Press, "Authors in Context".

Wilson, Mary (2013). *The Labors of Modernism Domesticity, Servants, and Authorship in Modernist Fiction*. New York: Ashgate.

Wilson, Elizabeth A. (2004). "Gut Feminism". *A Journal of Feminist Cultural Studies*, 15:3, 66–94.

Wood, Michael (1997). "Mad Love". *The New York Times*, https://archive.nytimes.com/www.nytimes.com/books/97/02/23/reviews/970223.23woodlt.html

Wright, Nicola & Owen, Sara (2001). "Feminist Conceptualizations of Women's Madness: A Review of the Literature", *Journal of Advanced Nursing*, 36(1), 143–150.

Yeager, Myron (2013). "The Topography of Gay Identity: Alan Hollinghurst's 'The Line of Beauty'". *CEA Critic*, November 2013, vol. 75, No. 3, 310–319.

Yebra, José M. (2014). "The Liminoid in Alan Hollinghurst's *The Swimming-Pool Library* and *The Folding Star*". *Revista Canaria de estudios ingleses*, 69, December 2014, 191–203.

Yelin, Louise (1998). "Reading Doris Lessing with Margaret Thatcher: *The Good Terrorist, The Fifth Child*, and England in the 1980s." Yelin, Louise (1998). *From the Margins of Empire, Stead, Lessing and Gordimer*, Cornell University Press, 91–107.

Zakin, Emily (2011). "Psychoanalytic Feminism". *The Stanford Encyclopedia of Philosophy* (Summer 2011 Edition), Edward N. Zalta (ed.), https://plato.stanford.edu/archives/sum2011/entries/feminism-psychoanalysis/

Zhao, Kun (2012). "A Narrative Analysis of Lessing's *The Fifth Child*". *Theory and Practice in Language Studies*, vol. 2, No. 7, July 2012, 1498–1502.

Zizek, Slavoj (1992). *Enjoy your Symptom! Jacques Lacan in Hollywood and Out.* London: Routledge.

Zizek, Slavoj (1999). *Subversions du Sujet, Psychanalyse, Philosophie, Politique.* Rennes: Presses Universitaires de Rennes, "Clinique psychanalytique et psychopathologie".

Index[1]

[1] Note: Page numbers followed by 'n' refer to notes.

© The Author(s), under exclusive license to Springer Nature
Switzerland AG 2023
N. P. Boileau, *Mental Health Symptoms in Literature since Modernism*, Palgrave Studies in Literature, Science and Medicine,
https://doi.org/10.1007/978-3-031-37630-6

SPRINGER NATURE

GPSR Compliance

The European Union's (EU) General Product Safety Regulation (GPSR) is a set of rules that requires consumer products to be safe and our obligations to ensure this.

If you have any concerns about our products, you can contact us on ProductSafety@springernature.com

In case Publisher is established outside the EU, the EU authorized representative is:

Springer Nature Customer Service Center GmbH
Europaplatz 3
69115 Heidelberg, Germany

The manufacturer's authorised representative in the EU is Springer
Nature Customer Service Centre GmbH, Europaplatz 3, 69115 Heidelberg,
Germany. If you have any concerns regarding our products, please
contact ProductSafety@springernature.com

Printed and bound by CPI Group (UK) Ltd, Croydon, CR0 4YY

02/05/2025

01859346-0001